Treating the
Homeless Mentally Ill

Task Force on the Homeless Mentally Ill

The findings, opinions, and conclusions of this report do not necessarily represent the views of the officers, trustees, all members of the task force, or all members of the American Psychiatric Association. The views expressed are those of the authors of the individual chapters. Task force reports are considered a substantive contribution of the ongoing analysis and evaluation of problems, programs, issues, and practices in a given area of concern.

Lawrence Hartmann, M.D.
President, American Psychiatric Association, 1991–1992

Treating the Homeless Mentally Ill

A Report of the Task Force on the Homeless Mentally Ill

Edited by

H. Richard Lamb, M.D.
   Professor of Psychiatry, University of Southern California School of Medicine, Los Angeles

Leona L. Bachrach, Ph.D.
   Research Professor of Psychiatry, Maryland Psychiatric Research Center, University of Maryland School of Medicine, Baltimore

Frederic I. Kass, M.D.
   Professor of Clinical Psychiatry, Columbia University College of Physicians and Surgeons, New York City

American Psychiatric Association
Washington, DC

Note: The authors have worked to ensure that all information in this book concerning drug dosages, schedules, and routes of administration is accurate as of the time of publication and consistent with standards set by the U.S. Food and Drug Administration and the general medical community. As medical research and practice advance, however, therapeutic standards may change. For this reason and because human and mechanical errors sometimes occur, we recommend that readers follow the advice of a physician who is directly involved in their care or the care of a member of their family.

Copyright © 1992 American Psychiatric Association
ALL RIGHTS RESERVED
Manufactured in the United States of America on acid-free paper
First Edition
95 94 93 92   4 3 2 1
American Psychiatric Association
1400 K Street, N.W., Washington, DC 20005

Library of Congress Cataloging-in-Publication Data
American Psychiatric Association. Task Force on the Homeless
    Mentally Ill.
      Treating the homeless mentally ill: a report of the Task Force on
    the Homeless Mentally Ill/H. Richard Lamb, Leona L. Bachrach,
    Frederick I. Kass, editors.—1st ed.
          p.   cm.
      Includes bibliographical references and index.
      ISBN 0-89042-236-2 (alk. paper)
      1. Homeless persons—Mental health services—United States.
    2. Homeless persons—Mental health—United States.   I. Lamb, H.
    Richard, 1929–   .   II. Bachrach, Leona L.   III. Kass, Frederic I.
    IV. Title.
      [DNLM: 1. Community Mental Health Services—United States.
    2. Homeless Persons—psychology—United States.   3. Mental
    Disorders—rehabilitation.   WM 30 A512t]
    RC451.4.H64A44   1992
    362.2′08′6942—dc20
    DNLM/DLC
    for Library of Congress   92–10470
                                                                              CIP

British Library Cataloging in Publication Data
A CIP record is available from the British Library.

Table of Contents

Section II: Treatment and Rehabilitation

Affiliations

Virginia C. Armat is Director of Development and Public Affairs, George Mason University School of Law, Arlington, Virginia. She is co-author with Rael Jean Isaac of *Madness in the Streets: How Psychiatry and the Law Abandoned the Mentally Ill* (Free Press/Macmillan 1990) and lives in Washington, DC.

Leona L. Bachrach, Ph.D., is research professor of psychiatry at the Maryland Psychiatric Research Center of the University of Maryland School of Medicine in Baltimore.

Richard R. Bebout, Ph.D., is associate clinical director for residential services at Community Connections, Inc., in Washington, DC.

Evalina W. Bestman, Ph.D., is research professor in the Department of Psychiatry at the University of Miami School of Medicine in Miami, Florida, and executive director of New Horizons Community Mental Health Center in Miami.

William R. Breakey, M.B., F.R.C.Psych., is associate professor of psychiatry at the Johns Hopkins University School of Medicine in Baltimore, Maryland.

Philip W. Brickner, M.D., is chairman of the Department of Community Medicine at St. Vincent's Hospital and Medical Center of New York in New York City.

Linda Chafetz, R.N., D.N.Sc., is associate professor in the Department of Mental Health, Community, and Administrative Nursing in the School of Nursing at the University of California, San Francisco.

Neal L. Cohen, M.D., is vice-chairman and associate professor in the Department of Psychiatry at Mount Sinai School of Medicine and clinical director at Mount Sinai Hospital in New York City.

Susan Dempsay, B.A., is executive director of Step Up on Second in Los Angeles, California.

Robert E. Drake, M.D., Ph.D., is director of the New Hampshire–Dartmouth Psychiatric Research Center and associate professor of psychiatry at Dartmouth Medical School in Hanover, New Hampshire.

Alan Felix, M.D., is assistant clinical professor of psychiatry at Columbia University College of Physicians and Surgeons in New York City and medical director of the men's shelter psychiatric day programs in the Neuropsychology Service at Presbyterian Hospital in the City of New York.

Pamela J. Fischer, Ph.D., is associate professor of psychiatry at the Johns Hopkins University School of Medicine in Baltimore, Maryland.

Sally Friedlob, L.C.S.W., O.T.R., is clinical coordinator of the University of California, Los Angeles, aftercare clinic.

Stephen M. Goldfinger, M.D., is assistant professor of psychiatry at Harvard Medical School in Boston and associate clinical director of the Massachusetts Mental Health Center.

Maxine Harris, Ph.D., is co-director of Community Connections, Inc., in Washington, DC.

David A. Kahn, M.D., is assistant clinical professor of psychiatry at Columbia University College of Physicians and Surgeons in New York City and associate director of psychiatry in the Neuropsychology Service at Presbyterian Hospital in the City of New York.

Frederic I. Kass, M.D., is professor of clinical psychiatry at Columbia University College of Physicians and Surgeons in New York City.

H. Richard Lamb, M.D., is professor of psychiatry at the University of Southern California School of Medicine in Los Angeles.

Harriet P. Lefley, Ph.D., is a professor in the Department of Psychiatry at the University of Miami School of Medicine in Miami, Florida.

Robert P. Liberman, M.D., is professor of psychiatry at the School of Medicine and director of the UCLA Clinical Research Center for Schizophrenia and Psychiatric Rehabilitation, Los Angeles, California.

Luis R. Marcos, M.D., Sc.D., is senior vice-president of Mental Health and Chemical Dependence Services in the New York City Health and Hospitals Corporation and professor of psychiatry at New York University School of Medicine in New York City.

Kenneth Minkoff, M.D., is chief of psychiatry at Choate Health Systems, Inc., in Woburn, Massachusetts, and a member of the clinical faculty at Harvard Medical School in Boston.

Elane M. Nuehring, Ph.D., M.S.S.W., is a professor in the School of Social Work at Barry University in Miami Shores, Florida.

Roger Peele, M.D., is chairman of the Department of Psychiatry and commission on mental health services at St. Elizabeth's campus in Washington, DC.

Ezra Susser, M.D., M.P.H., is assistant professor at the Nathan Kline Institute for Psychiatric Research at New York University Department of Psychiatry in New York City.

Felicity V. Swayze, M.S.W., is senior clinical supervisor at Community Connections, Inc. in Washington, DC.

John A. Talbott, M.D., is chairman of the Department of Psychiatry at the University of Maryland School of Medicine, Baltimore.

Jerome V. Vaccaro, M.D., is assistant professor of psychiatry at the University of California, Los Angeles, School of Medicine and assistant chief of the Rehabilitation Medicine Service at Brentwood VA Medical Center in Los Angeles.

Elie Valencia, J.D., M.A., is assistant clinical professor of public health in the Department of Psychiatry at Columbia University College of Physicians and Surgeons in New York City and director of services for the homeless in the psychiatry service at Presbyterian Hospital in the City of New York.

Foreword

When *The Homeless Mentally Ill* was published in 1984, it was greeted with great enthusiasm (Lamb 1984). For the first time, the field now had in one place the scientific and experiential information that could inform public policy and, indeed, the policy recommendations contained in the book were significant enough not only to provoke widespread professional discussion but also to warrant serious media and legislative attention.

Since 1984, there has been even more attention paid to the issue—again by psychiatry, the government, and the media. At a national level, the McKinney Act has brought new monies for demonstration programs for the homeless, and the National Institute of Mental Health (NIMH) has initiated new funding for research on the homeless mentally ill. At the state level, most states have attempted to address the problem in their state plans and initiatives. But more important, perhaps largely due to the concentration of the homeless in urban areas, local voluntary organizations and city governmental agencies have increased their attention to this group.

Why, then, when we walk past the missions in Los Angeles or down the Mall in Washington, DC, do we see even more seemingly disturbed and muttering homeless people than before? The answer is for a variety of reasons, explored more fully in this volume, but the bottom line is that we have not implemented the policy recommendations of 1984.

This book, as did its predecessor, provides ample new scientific and experiential data. But it also demonstrates that despite the McKinney Act, NIMH grants, Robert Wood Johnson Foundation 9-Cities demonstration project, and so on, cities and states are still not able to ensure

treatment, care, and rehabilitation of the severely and chronically mentally ill through a comprehensive system of care. Sad to say, we have
advanced quite far in acquisition of knowledge but seemingly have
fallen backward in applying it to solving the problem. Let us hope this
book helps remind society of its obligation to at last take meaningful
action, on a large scale, to address the needs of this long neglected population.

John A. Talbott, M.D.

Reference

Lamb HR: The Homeless Mentally Ill: A Task Force Report of the American Psychiatric Association. Washington, DC, American Psychiatric
Association, 1984

Preface

When we completed the final report of the first American Psychiatric Association's Task Force on the Homeless Mentally Ill in book form (Lamb 1984) and made our recommendations, we believed that we had begun a process that would result in a significant reduction in homelessness among the chronically and severely mentally ill. We believed our recommendations were sound (as we still do) and that their implementation would surely take place. Now 8 years later, we find that very little has been done. There are still editorials in newspapers and on the evening news and statements by persons in public office advocating action, and small steps (relative to the magnitude of the problem) have even been taken here and there to address this issue. Still, the fact of homelessness among the mentally ill is essentially little changed from 1984. That lack of action, more than anything else, spurred us on to write this book. The horror of the chronically and severely mentally ill living on the streets, in constant danger, without the basic necessities of life, let alone treatment, is almost too incredible to contemplate.

Today we know much more about the homeless mentally ill and how to provide services to them, and in this book we have gathered together a group of persons eminently qualified to present this new knowledge and these new techniques. We have again focused on the homeless mentally ill with major mental illnesses (such as schizophrenia, schizoaffective disorder, bipolar disorder, and major depression with psychotic features), for we as mental health professionals have special expertise with this population. Moreover, if we can have an impact in bettering the lives of this long-neglected group, we feel that we will have made a very significant and important contribution.

Input for the summary and recommendations chapter (Chapter 1) was sought from the entire task force, and this input was incorporated. The other chapters represent the views of their authors.

The book is divided into two sections. In the first section, The Context of Treatment, we set the stage for understanding the problems of the homeless mentally ill. This section includes an analytic review of the literature, a discussion of deinstitutionalization, a cross-cultural family perspective, a discussion of why clinicians distance themselves from the homeless mentally ill, and a discussion on training mental health professionals to treat the chronically mentally ill.

In the second section, Treatment and Rehabilitation, we begin with a discussion of clinical work with the homeless mentally ill and go on to address the crucial issues of mobile outreach teams, therapeutic housing, the need-for-treatment standard in involuntary commitment, clinical case management, the needs and treatment of dually diagnosed patients, medical management, day treatment in a shelter, and rehabilitation.

Many persons in addition to the authors of this volume made important contributions to this work. We would like to single out for special commendation Claudia (Corky) Hart of the American Psychiatric Association, who coordinated the task force's efforts and whose exceptional competence helped make this work possible, and Kathy Moriarty Stearman, who helped to give the text its final shape and whose dedication to editorial excellence added much to the quality of this book.

H. Richard Lamb, M.D.
Leona L. Bachrach, Ph.D.
Frederic I. Kass, M.D.

Reference

Lamb HR: The Homeless Mentally Ill: A Task Force Report of the American Psychiatric Association. Washington, DC, American Psychiatric Association, 1984

Chapter 1

Summary and Recommendations

H. Richard Lamb, M.D.
Leona L. Bachrach, Ph.D.
Stephen M. Goldfinger, M.D.
Frederic I. Kass, M.D.

In 1984, the American Psychiatric Association's first Task Force on the Homeless Mentally Ill (Talbott and Lamb 1984) made a series of recommendations for addressing the crisis of homelessness among chronically mentally ill persons (see Appendix). We believe they are as timely and applicable today as they were when they were written. Had they been implemented, they probably would have greatly reduced the prevalence of homelessness among persons with major mental illnesses—persons who are severely and persistently disabled by such disorders as schizophrenia, schizoaffective disorder, bipolar disorder, and major depression.

But these are times of limited resources in terms of housing, social programs, and health care access. Those least able to provide for themselves are, of course, the most vulnerable to any reduction in supports and programs. Chronically mentally ill individuals who suffer from the cognitive and social deficits of their illnesses, left to fend for themselves in the community, are often the most profoundly affected and the most in need of protection and services.

The first task force regarded homelessness as but one symptom of the many problems besetting chronically mentally ill persons throughout the United States, and it called for a comprehensive and integrated system of mental health care that would address the underlying problems that precipitate homelessness among the mentally ill. Such a system of care would include high-quality psychiatric and medical services; an adequate number and range of supervised, supportive housing settings; a well-functioning system of clinically oriented case management; adequate, comprehensive, and accessible crisis intervention capabilities, both in the community and in hospitals; less restrictive laws governing involuntary treatment; ongoing rehabilitative services; and consultation to community agencies and organizations that provide other essential services to homeless populations.

Above all, such a system of care would provide individually prescribed treatments and interventions designed to meet patients where they are, not where the system would like them to be. It would, thus, support assertive outreach to mentally ill individuals living on the streets and in temporary shelters. (These essential system components are dealt with in considerable detail in Section II [Chapters 8 through 16] of this volume.)

Since the first task force report was published in 1984, many efforts have been undertaken to advance our understanding of the homeless mentally ill population (see Chapters 2 and 5). These efforts have been paralleled by a variety of programs designed to provide increased access and improved services to this population (though the numbers served have been relatively small when contrasted with the total population of homeless mentally ill persons in need). Aggressive outreach programs in New York, Washington, DC, and Chicago have combined supportive case management approaches with, when necessary, involuntary hospitalization and treatment (Harris and Bachrach 1990; Marcos et al. 1990; Witheridge, in press). In some communities, large-scale volunteer efforts by mental health professionals of various disciplines have helped supplement underfunded and inadequate state and local services (J.W. Voell, 1991, personal communication). Creative partnerships between providers and recipients of services have resulted in the development of collaborative case management, housing, and day program activities that frequently attract individuals who have avoided more traditional services.

Unfortunately, however, these positive examples aside, efforts on behalf of homeless mentally ill individuals have too often consisted of no more than the provision of temporary shelter residences. And although shelters may at times be necessary as an emergency resource, they address only the symptoms of homelessness among mentally ill individuals and do not really get at the root of the problem. They are only makeshift solutions that do no more than provide people with roofs over their heads from night to night.

Indeed, the very fact that temporary shelters are even offered as solutions for the mentally ill implies an acceptance by society of the notion that mentally ill individuals, whatever their mental status or degree of competence, should be permitted to refuse treatment and live on the streets. It is frequently said that homeless mentally ill individuals live on the streets by choice. That, however, is an allegation that flies in the face of both clinical observation and research data, for the reality is that life on the streets is generally characterized by dysphoria and extreme deprivation. It often leads to victimization by the human predators of the streets and very frequently precipitates the onset of life-threatening medical problems (see Chapter 14). Lipton and his colleagues (1988) have clearly demonstrated that many severely mentally ill homeless individuals will voluntarily accept an offer of safe and supportive housing.

Should chronically mentally ill individuals have a right to "choose" a life on the streets without consideration for their physical health or the extent of their competence to make such a "decision"? We think not. We believe such practices cloak neglect in the banner of freedom and that they are a cruel interpretation of the basic civil rights that are so important to all citizens of the United States. Individuals who are competent to understand the risks and implications of their decisions and who are not a danger to themselves or others cannot, and must not, be deprived of their freedom of choice. However, those individuals whose illness distorts their perceptions and clouds their thinking and puts others and themselves at risk should not be left to make dangerous and irrational decisions (see Chapter 11 for a fuller discussion of these issues).

Perhaps, given funding constraints and competition for resources, complete implementation of the recommendations of the first task force in the near future may be too much to expect. We feel, however, that even partial but more widespread implementation could result in a better life for homeless mentally ill individuals today.

For example, the provision of more clinically oriented case management programs consisting of interventions that have demonstrably positive effects on the lives of homeless mentally ill individuals (see Chapter 12) would represent an important step in the right direction. Assuming adequate housing and treatment resources exist, if effective comprehensive and clinical case management programs could be made an integral part of mental health service systems throughout the United States, we would increase the likelihood that every chronically mentally ill individual could actually be served.

We would also increase the probability that sufficient qualified staff would be available to work intensively with each patient, to take full responsibility for individualized treatment planning, to link patients to needed resources, and to monitor their clinical course. Patients, then, could receive the services they need and would not be lost to the system of care, and the incidence of homelessness could no doubt be reduced. Probably, most of these goals could be accomplished on a voluntary basis. In point of fact, however, although case management is much discussed, too many jurisdictions have done little to implement it.

Can we wait still longer for these improvements to be made? We think not. Indeed, there are strong indications, especially in larger cities, where a high proportion of homeless mentally ill individuals are concentrated, not only that funds are inadequate to implement wide-scale, clinically oriented case management initiatives but also that bureaucracies are often too ponderous and inefficient to allow this to be done (see Chapter 3).

It should be noted as well that many individuals within the homeless mentally ill population tend to resist taking psychotropic medications and, more generally, often appear to resist treatment. They also seem frequently to reject the housing opportunities available to them (Harris and Bachrach 1990; Vernez et al. 1988). These behaviors may, however, result from the fact that we sometimes expect homeless mentally ill individuals to accept unrealistic or inappropriate treatments or placements; or they may result from the fact that the housing and treatment interventions that are offered lack clinical relevance (see Chapter 2). The preferences of the homeless mentally ill persons may also not have been taken into account, and the interventions may be less appealing than they should have been (Susser et al. 1990).

Moreover, many mentally ill individuals, precisely because of their illnesses, may be unable to take advantage of the living situations that are available to them. A recent study (Lamb and Lamb 1990) found that some homeless mentally ill persons who had places to live were too paranoid to live there. In fact, the disabling functional deficits associated with major mental illness also appear to be important contributing factors to homelessness among mentally ill persons (Belcher and Toomey 1988; Herrman 1990). These deficits include disorganized thinking and actions, poor problem-solving skills, and inability to mobilize oneself because of depression (Lamb and Lamb 1990). These are crucial deficits that should lead us as professionals to intervene, preferably with the patient's consent but without it when necessary (Belcher 1988; Bennett et al. 1988). We, of course, want to respect mentally ill persons' freedom of choice. However, during acute exacerbations of illness and periods of incompetence, the imposition of safety and symptom relief may need to prevail over voluntary participation or consent.

In addition to experiencing the symptoms and functional disabilities of their psychotic disorders, many of the homeless mentally ill suffer from a wide range of other impairments. As a group, they are far more likely than their domiciled peers to be debilitated by severe and often life-threatening medical illnesses and to receive little, or inappropriate, medical care (see Chapter 15).

Of particular note in planning and providing adequate services is the high prevalence of serious substance abuse problems within the homeless mentally ill population. Many of these individuals have little if any control over their problems with chemical substances (see Chapter 13) and often have little access to and/or the ability to utilize effective chemical dependency treatment. Moreover, substance abuse among homeless mentally ill individuals tends to exacerbate functional deficits and, like comorbid medical conditions, creates new and difficult challenges in program design and treatment planning.

Recommendations

What, then, should be done? First of all, we strongly endorse the recommendations of the first Task Force, as we did at the time they were drafted, and encourage the launching of wide-scale efforts to implement them.

Further, we believe that the care, treatment, and rehabilitation of chronically mentally ill individuals must be made the highest priority in public mental health and receive the first priority for public funding. This population would, of course, include chronic mentally ill persons who are homeless or at risk for becoming homeless.

Following through on such a priority assignment is utterly dependent upon a continued effort to differentiate those persons within the homeless population who are mentally ill from those who are not (see Chapter 2). Making this distinction does not mean that we have no concern for persons who become homeless for economic or social reasons; it is only a statement of our sense that all subgroups within the homeless population are best served when their varied needs are differentiated.

Too often, unfortunately, taxonomic efforts are rejected on the assumption that acknowledging mental illness among homeless individuals is a form of "victimization" (Alters 1986). We reject this notion and feel, as does Breakey (W.R. Breakey, 1986, personal communication), that a psychiatric diagnosis is not in any sense an indictment; it is merely an attempt to classify and help us know how best to respond to service needs among homeless individuals.

Although the 1984 recommendations generally have lacked widespread application, we can no longer wait for their full implementation. We must take action now to serve the nation's homeless mentally ill population. Thus, although we continue to advocate for comprehensive and coordinated community-based mental health systems to engage homeless mentally ill individuals and help them to accept treatment and suitable living arrangements, we also believe the members of this population must be served immediately.

Nor can we wait for the accumulation of more valid research results and better theoretical constructs before we extend services to these individuals (see Chapter 2). Although we know, for example, that we must find better ways to resolve the problem of residential instability among homeless mentally ill individuals (Harris and Bachrach 1990), we are faced with the need to provide housing now. Clearly, continued investigations into the etiology and prevention of homelessness, the design and operation of more acceptable and effective housing options, and the long-term impact of various treatment alternatives must proceed. We strongly endorse the pursuit of a full complement of research efforts to identify subgroups of the homeless mentally ill population, assess their service needs, study alternative clinical interventions, and evaluate the outcomes of our efforts. We cannot, however, sit idly by waiting for the results of these research endeavors. We must plan and provide services even as a better knowledge base is being developed.

Further, we believe that a range of treatment interventions encompassing both community and hospital alternatives is necessary. Many individuals able to live in the community may, at times of crisis, require more intensive support and structure. Community workers serving the homeless mentally ill must receive training in the recognition and assessment of both functional strengths and dangerous degrees of disability. Those who serve the homeless mentally ill must neither glorify autonomy nor dismiss individual rights. The individual in need must be given access to appropriate care. This care may involve voluntary acceptance of a specific intervention. However, there are those individuals so incapacitated by their psychiatric disorders that they have serious deficits in insight, judgment, and awareness regarding their physical surroundings, needs, and potential personal dangers.

Accordingly, we conclude that until our knowledge is more complete, and until our resources have expanded sufficiently, hospitalization must be an available option within the system of care. For some individuals, inpatient stays will be brief, until a crisis is resolved; for others, more extended hospital care will be required. However, we believe that outreach teams that include psychiatrically trained personnel must be permitted to bring to the hospital those individuals who are incompetent to make decisions about treatment, who present a danger to themselves or others, or who are gravely disabled. No persons meeting these criteria should be left living on the streets. Hospital admission should be voluntary whenever that is possible; but, if need be, it must be involuntary.

Do people have a right to live on the streets? It is our strong belief that this question should be phrased differently—Does society have a right to deny treatment to the members of this population (see Chapter 11)? We believe the answer to the second question is *No,* because homeless mentally ill individuals have a more fundamental right to treatment even if the treatment must at times be involuntary (Lamb and Mills 1986). The care of chronically mentally ill individuals should be based on an understanding, derived from our clinical experience, that these persons frequently ask for the opposite of what they want and need. It is not unusual for these patients to test for limits, nor is it unusual for them to respond with relief and a lessening, or even remission, of symptoms when the limits have been set. And it is not uncommon for these patients to inform us after the fact that setting limits on them has served them well.

Thus, for example, we favor the initiation of advance directives for psychiatric treatment, a model being put forward by various persons, including persons who have been mentally ill, professionals, and family members (Appelbaum 1991). Many individuals recognize that when they are most severely symptomatic, they often reject interventions that they acknowledge as invaluable once they are restabilized. Therefore, while stable and competent, they sign a "will" authorizing the use of "involuntary" interventions in the event of a future decompensation. This strategy, combining dignity and choice with necessary protection and treatment, may provide a novel and practical solution for many patient care dilemmas.

We believe that for those homeless mentally ill persons who must be hospitalized, inpatient stays preferably should be relatively brief, but their exact length should be based on the individuals' clinical needs. Appropriate living arrangements in the community, with on-site treatment capabilities, must be made available to discharged individuals. Further, we believe that residential and treatment standards for homeless mentally ill individuals should measure up fully to the standards of care needed for severely disabled individuals and that they should be capable of being monitored.

However, we cannot in good conscience support leaving homeless mentally ill individuals to remain on the streets while we wait for such standards to be developed and for the requisite resources to be marshalled. In the short run, we shall probably be compelled to settle for facilities and services that are acceptable, if less than ideal. Cost must also, unfortunately, be a consideration in the development of services, and we must do everything possible to mobilize support for increased and adequate mental health funding. But, whatever the outcome of our efforts, in the end we must be prepared to work within the limits of what society is willing to spend, even as we advocate for additional resources.

We believe that the provision of housing opportunities, the provision of psychotropic medications, and the provision of structure, in varying amounts, are each important and interrelated matters in serving the members of the homeless mentally ill population and that it is essential to acknowledge the varied needs of its members with this in mind. For instance, most chronically and severely mentally ill individuals are better served by placement in supervised housing: mainstream housing in which people live alone in their own apartments and manage by themselves may be simply beyond the capabilities of most of these persons (see Chapter 10). As we continue to develop and collect data on alternative residential models, we will, we hope, move even further in our efforts to maximize independence while maximizing mentally ill persons' safety and stability.

We also believe that it hardly needs to be stated that psychotropic medications, including neuroleptics, antidepressants, and lithium, are critical in treating homeless mentally ill individuals. Given the frequency with which noncompliance with medications is associated with symptom exacerbation and decompensation, every effort should be made to establish therapeutic partnerships with patients and maximize their understanding of the nature and importance of their medications. Of course, there will be times when involuntary medication, as part of a larger crisis intervention or an involuntary hospitalization, may be required. Moreover, given the high prevalence of comorbid substance abuse and psychiatric problems in this population, a range of treatment settings must be made available to meet the special needs of such individuals (see Chapter 13).

Finally, structure (Lamb 1980) is a critical concept in the care of homeless mentally ill persons. Like those of domiciled chronically mentally ill individuals, the needs of homeless mentally ill persons for structure fall on a continuum; some need only modest amounts, some need moderate amounts, and some require highly structured kinds of environments. Homeless mentally ill individuals often require supervised living situations in which their medications are monitored and in which they may be given as much freedom as they can handle but not more. For some, a full schedule of useful and meaningful activities is an important way to provide structure; for others, however, a locked setting for a limited, or even an extended, time, may be a necessary form of structure. At the present time, many patients are probably being placed inappropriately in unstructured community settings (see Chapter 3).

Whether or not a particular patient needs a moderate or a high degree of structure should not be seen as an ideological issue but, rather, as a clinical decision based on a pragmatic assessment of that patient's needs. Does the patient have sufficient internal controls to organize himself or herself to cope with life's demands? To what degree do we need to add external structure to compensate for a lack of internal controls?

That segment of the homeless mentally ill population that needs the degree of structure that only hospitals can afford should receive the highest quality of inpatient care, and our hospitals must be upgraded toward that end. Once again, however, there will be times when we cannot wait for the ideal to be offered. We believe that, if funds are not available, it is more humane to place individuals in hospitals whose charts and even staffing standards fall somewhat short of high accreditation standards than it is to leave these neglected human beings living on the streets.

Similarly, although we believe that all competent chronically mentally ill individuals are, if they wish, entitled to live in a safe and high quality community facility, it is clear that the resources to provide such opportunities do not currently exist. We recognize that although they are far less desirable, interim living arrangements that are less than ideal will continue to provide the only domiciles for many of these individuals. Although clearly a compromise, such residences, if they provide regular, assigned beds, safety, decent physical surroundings, and caring professional staff, are far preferable living situations to the streets or to most "temporary" shelters.

Finally, it is our belief that the time for endless (and often fruitless) discussion is long past. There has been more than enough wringing of hands. The time for action on behalf of homeless mentally ill persons is long overdue, and the directions we must take are clear. We must be bold and strong of will. We must be prepared to mount a large-scale operation that will give relief to all persons who are homeless and mentally ill. The fate of these persons, who have such profound service needs and who are at great risk for harm, cannot be left in the hands of the fainthearted.

References

Alters A: Roots of homelessness debated at conference. Boston Globe, 28 March 1986, p 16

Appelbaum PS: Advance directives for psychiatric treatment. Hosp Community Psychiatry 42:983–984, 1991

Belcher JR: Defining the service needs of homeless mentally ill persons. Hosp Community Psychiatry 39:1203–1205, 1988

Belcher JR, Toomey BG: Relationship between the deinstitutionalization model, psychiatric disability, and homelessness. Health Soc Work 13:145–153, 1988

Bennett MI, Gudeman JE, Jenkins L, et al: The value of hospital-based treatment for the homeless mentally ill. Am J Psychiatry 145:1273–1276, 1988

Harris M, Bachrach LL: Perspectives on homeless mentally ill women. Hosp Community Psychiatry 41:253–254, 1990

Herrman H: A survey of homeless mentally ill people in Melbourne, Australia. Hosp Community Psychiatry 41:1291–1292, 1990

Lamb HR: Structure: the neglected ingredient of community treatment. Arch Gen Psychiatry 37:1224–1228, 1980

Lamb HR, Lamb DM: Factors contributing to homelessness among the chronically and severely mentally ill. Hosp Community Psychiatry 41:301–304, 1990

Lamb HR, Mills MJ: Needed changes in law and procedure for the chronically mentally ill. Hosp Community Psychiatry 37:475–480, 1986

Lipton FR, Nutt S, Sabatini A: Housing the homeless mentally ill: a longitudinal study of a treatment approach. Hosp Community Psychiatry 39:40–45, 1988

Marcos LR, Cohen NL, Nardacci D, et al: Psychiatry takes to the streets: the New York City initiative for the homeless mentally ill. Am J Psychiatry 147:1557–1561, 1990

Susser E, Goldfinger SM, White A: Some clinical approaches to work with the homeless mentally ill. Community Ment Health J 26:468–480, 1990

Talbott JA, Lamb HR: Summary and recommendations, in The Homeless Mentally Ill: A Task Force Report of the American Psychiatric Association. Edited by Lamb HR. Washington, DC, American Psychiatric Association, 1984

Vernez G, Burnam MA, McGlynn EA, et al: Review of California's Program for the Homeless Mentally Disabled. Santa Monica, CA, RAND Corp, 1988

Witheridge TF: The active ingredients of assertive outreach. New Dir Ment Health Serv (in press)

Section I:

The Context of Treatment

Chapter 2

What We Know About Homelessness Among Mentally Ill Persons: An Analytical Review and Commentary

Leona L. Bachrach, Ph.D.

How much of the homeless population suffers from chronic mental illness? Has deinstitutionalization precipitated an increase in homelessness among mentally ill persons? What kinds of programs—what specific services—should homeless mentally ill individuals be offered? During the past decade, as a participant in nearly 100 seminars and workshops on service development for homeless mentally ill persons throughout the United States, I have found that these three questions in one form or another consistently dominate discussion. In this chapter I shall analyze and comment on the current literature on the homeless mentally ill population by using these questions as points of departure.

Taken together, the three questions cover considerable ground. The first, which is essentially epidemiological in nature, seeks to establish some broad statistical parameters. Although asked in a variety of ways, it frequently takes the following form: "What percentage of the homeless population is mentally ill?" This analysis will not answer the question definitively and will explain why it is unable to do so. Indeed, the limitations that preclude a valid answer to this question are so critical to the conduct of replicable research that a major portion of the analysis will be devoted to discussing them.

The second question—"What is the relationship between deinstitutionalization and the apparent growth of the homeless mentally ill pop-

This chapter is based on the first Philip R. A. May Memorial Lecture, delivered at the University of California, Los Angeles, Neuropsychiatric Institute and Hospital, October 1, 1990.

ulation?"—lies in the area of policy assessment and is of critical concern to scholars, clinicians, and policymakers alike. Once again this analysis will provide no definitive statistics. It will, however, examine why the question as stated is subject to considerable misinterpretation and might best be reconceptualized.

Nor will this analysis provide a conclusive answer to the third question, one that lies in the area of program planning and service development: "Where and how should homeless mentally ill individuals be served?" However, several issues that surround programming for the population will be examined, and some emerging concepts of care will be discussed.

Like that in the first task force report (Bachrach 1984a), this analysis will pay special attention to the body of research literature. It draws on popular writings in addition to professional sources, since the former sometimes offer important perspectives on the population (Bachrach 1990b). Selected "fugitive" literature that has come to my attention— documents and reports not readily found through standard bibliographic searches—will also be covered.

The Question of Prevalence

Precisely what percentage of the homeless population is mentally ill? This is without doubt the single question that I hear most often as I travel throughout the United States. It is as if people need a numerical fix on the members of this population in order to deal with the problems affecting them. However, there is little in the literature to aid these individuals in their quest, for the question is deceptively difficult to answer. Five factors were reported in the first task force's report as confounding the question: absence of a standardized definition of homelessness; difficulties in establishing the presence of mental illness among homeless individuals; overlap of the homeless mentally ill population with other subgroups of mentally ill individuals; diversity within the population; and temporal and spatial variations in the population's distribution (Bachrach 1984a). These problems, which continue to interfere with defining, counting, and classifying people who are homeless and mentally ill, have had a marked impact on research and policy development.

Defining Homelessness

Since the earliest expressions of professional concern about the homeless mentally ill population, the body of knowledge has been hampered by the absence of a standard definition of homelessness (Bachrach

1984b; Barrow et al. 1989; Milburn and Watts 1986; Rossi et al. 1987; Susser et al. 1990a). More than a matter of semantics, this difficulty reflects a basic inability, or perhaps at times an unwillingness, by writers and researchers to take a broad view of their subject. Indeed, not only is the field marked by the absence of a standard definition; but, with few exceptions, most writings on the homeless mentally ill population do not even bother to define homelessness for their own purposes.

Yet the meaning of this term is anything but self-evident, and an examination of the literature reveals little consensus. Experts sometimes argue over whether a cardboard box, a reed hut, or an automobile might reasonably be construed as a home, particularly under benign climatic conditions like those that prevail in southwestern portions of the country. Similar debates take place over whether a simple lack of shelter is by itself sufficient to render an individual homeless. These circumstances have led certain advocacy groups in Great Britain to introduce the concept of "houselessness" in contradistinction to homelessness (Bailey 1977). While houselessness implies the simple absence of physical residence such as might occur when one's house burns down, homelessness is a term that is reserved for conditions of more generalized deprivation.

To add to the confusion, having a home does not constitute a variable with binary values: housed or not housed. Thus, Roth and Bean (1986) have developed a three-part typology based on utilization patterns in shelters; and Rossi and his colleagues (1987) have distinguished people who are "literally" homeless from those who are precariously housed and at risk for becoming homeless.

That many homeless individuals are often "invisible" to researchers (Hope and Young 1986; Pitt 1989; Ropers 1988) further complicates defining and counting the population. Most current definitions appear to agree, either implicitly or explicitly, that in order for homelessness to be present, the absence of physical residence must occur under conditions of social isolation or disaffiliation. Thus, homeless people are generally viewed as individuals who lack the resources and the community ties that they need in order to divest themselves of their houselessness. The absence of housing is one part of the equation; the lack of resources and community ties—that is, the lack of social margin—is the other part.

A proper definition of homelessness should also, ideally, contain a temporal dimension that provides some notion of how long the disaffiliation and lack of housing must endure in order for a person to be regarded as homeless. Is one day long enough? If not, what is an appropriate cutoff point? Most current research definitions are cross-sectional: they seek to establish whether an individual is undomiciled at the moment that he or she is screened for inclusion in a particular study.

However, this practice may be misleading, for research in Arizona has demonstrated that the number of homeless individuals may be increased substantially with only a slight longitudinal refinement in qualifying criteria (Santiago et al. 1988).

Thus, while 22% of individuals with psychiatric emergency admissions to the Kino Community Hospital in Tucson were homeless according to a cross-sectional definition, half again as many (33%) could be so defined when they were asked whether they had lived on the streets, in a shelter, or in an automobile at some time during the 3 months prior to admission.

Assessing Mental Illness in the Homeless Population

In addition to problems associated with the definition of homelessness per se, there are difficulties in confirming the presence of psychopathology among persons who are homeless. Under the best of circumstances defining chronic mental illness is a complicated endeavor (Bachrach 1988a); under conditions of homelessness the difficulty increases (Barrow et al. 1989).

To put the matter simply, it may be difficult to establish the presence of psychopathology in an individual who is suffering extreme physical deprivation. Baxter and Hopper (1982, p. 402) have written that if at least some homeless individuals who are regarded as mentally ill could receive "several nights of sleep, an adequate diet, and warm social contact, some of their symptoms might subside." In addition, because homeless people are often shy, withdrawn, and frightened, it may take months just to approach some of them, let alone question them. Many abuse alcohol and other substances, and they are likely to have a subculture that encompasses entirely different values, norms, and expectations from those familiar to most mental health workers and researchers—all circumstances that make differential diagnosis difficult (Barrow et al. 1989; Drake et al. 1989; Linn et al. 1990).

When difficulties surrounding the definition of homelessness are combined with those that impede psychiatric diagnosis, it becomes easy to play "number games" with homeless mentally ill people (Bachrach 1985). Speculation and rhetoric appear to replace efforts to derive reliable estimates, and political concerns override considerations of objectivity—a situation illustrated by the failure of the federal government to suggest credible numbers.

In 1983, the Alcohol, Drug Abuse, and Mental Health Administration estimated that there were approximately 2 million homeless people in the United States and that about half suffered from alcohol, drug abuse, or mental health problems (Department of Health and Human

Services 1983). However, in the following year, the U.S. Department of Housing and Urban Development (1984) effectively rejected that estimate by releasing another of only 250,000 to 350,000 homeless people in the country. Both estimates were methodologically flawed (General Accounting Office 1988), and the latter, particularly, was widely criticized for seeking out homeless individuals in only a few nonrepresentative communities, aggregating rather than extrapolating from those counts, and virtually ignoring street people and others who were difficult to locate (Rich 1986; U.S. Congress 1984). Not surprisingly, a number of critics felt that the estimate had been released for political reasons: if homeless people do not exist in large numbers, one need not think about how to serve them (Prewitt 1987).

The federal government has not issued a definitive estimate since the 1984 figure.

Overlap With Other Populations

A third problem related to defining and counting homeless mentally ill people is the overlap between this population and other subgroups of mentally ill persons—what some statisticians call "between-group variation." The characteristics of homeless mentally ill people as a population are not easily distinguished from those of certain other groups discussed in the literature—for example, "urban nomads" (Appleby et al. 1982), "revolving door patients" (Geller 1982), "chronic crisis patients" (Bassuk and Gerson 1980), and "young adult chronic patients" (Pepper et al. 1981). Studies at San Francisco General Hospital have identified some patients who actually fit all of these descriptions (Chafetz and Goldfinger 1984; Goldfinger et al. 1984).

The homeless mentally ill population is also, incidentally, sometimes difficult to distinguish from certain population groups in jails and other correctional facilities (Belcher 1988). Lamb and Grant (1982, 1983), for example, have reported that 36% of male and 42% of female inmates in Los Angeles County jail facilities who were referred for psychiatric evaluation had been living as transients on the streets, on the beach, or in shelters at the time of their arrests.

Diversity Within the Population

A fourth problem in defining and counting the homeless mentally ill population resides in the extreme diversity of its membership (Wright 1989), or "within-group variation." Much of the current literature agrees that like homeless people in general (and also chronically mentally ill people in general), homeless mentally ill individuals are not uniform diagnostically, demographically, in terms of their residential or treatment histories, nor certainly in terms of their treatment needs. This situation makes it difficult to extract characteristics common to the entire population.

Thus, an evaluation of five programs for homeless mentally ill individuals, all in New York City, has revealed that each serves a distinctive subgroup of the population (Barrow et al. 1989). Indeed, as noted in the first task force report (Bachrach 1984a), homeless mentally ill people do not even constitute a uniform group in appearance. Project HELP, an outreach program that has been given a mandate to serve the most severely psychiatrically disabled people that workers can locate on the streets of New York City, offers this description of its target population:

> Primary visual indicators include an extremely dirty and disheveled appearance; torn, dirty, or layered clothing; clothing inappropriate to the weather (layers of heavy coats and woolen hats in midsummer and no coats in midwinter); and a collection of belongings in bags, boxes, or shopping carts. Primary behavioral indicators include walking in traffic, urinating or defecating in public, lying on a crowded sidewalk, and remaining mute and withdrawn. (Cohen et al. 1984, p. 922)

Although this familiar description reinforces a common stereotype of people widely considered to be prototypically homeless and mentally ill, it may be contrasted with a description by Reich and Siegel (1978) of another subgroup of mentally ill street people in New York City:

> Most of these men are intelligent and have better than the usual education found on the Bowery. They present a fairly intact appearance even when undergoing severe inner disturbance and thus can avoid unwanted hospitalization even when their situation destabilizes and there is a threat of erupting violence. (pp. 195–196)

Many reports readily acknowledge the diversity of the homeless mentally ill population. However, few speak so eloquently as Pia McKay (1987), a schizophrenic homeless woman who lives in Washington, DC:

> In my view the big mistake people make in trying to help the homeless is that they expect, or hope, that one single solution will solve the problems of all of us. . . . In fact, the solution for one of us can spell disaster for another. Low-cost housing, for example, is a wonderful idea for many of us. Yet that "solution" would be no more than a sentimental gesture for women who throw rolls of toilet paper down the toilet or, forgetting to take their tranquilizers, tear off refrigerator doors.

Variations in Time and Space

Last, but certainly not least, it is difficult to define and count the homeless mentally ill population because its membership exhibits considerable geographical and temporal variation (Bachrach 1987). Although these individuals are often associated with inner-city residence, they are also found in small cities, suburban and rural areas, and remote districts (Bachrach 1986; Institute of Medicine 1988; Jones 1986; Patton 1987; Roth and Bean 1986). Variations in the duration of homelessness add to the confusion: homelessness may be quite temporary, or it may be a more or less permanent circumstance. Several research reports have distinguished between "permanent" street people and individuals who are episodically homeless (Appleby and Desai 1987; Arce et al. 1983; Drake et al. 1989; Roth and Bean 1986; Sosin et al. 1988).

In addition, the population varies in its practices of diurnal or seasonal movement within defined geographic areas. Some people live more or less constantly in one place, sometimes as small as a few city blocks. Others, however, while remaining essentially in a single neighborhood, are more difficult to locate, because they branch out as shelters and other services become available to them, or as their specific needs for subsistence and health care shift. Some shelters contribute to this kind of movement by imposing a time limit on the number of nights an individual is permitted to remain in residence (Kates 1985). One variant of such local migration is illustrated in the case of the so-called subway homeless in New York City (Pitt 1989): persons who regularly board subway trains at the World Trade Center in lower Manhattan and ride to the end of the line in Queens. The journey, lasting 1 hour and 50 minutes, represents for many their only opportunity to get some sleep and avoid the cold (Verhovek 1988).

A third kind of mobility affecting the homeless mentally ill population concerns migration over wide geographic areas. Although many individuals appear to remain in the same general geographic area (Benda and Dattalo 1988; Rosnow et al. 1986), some move extensively among regions of the United States. The Tucson Homeless Mentally Ill Study has shown that homeless men referred for psychiatric screening in a public general hospital emergency room have, on the average, lived in the Tucson area for only 5 months. The same study has shown that the average for women is less than 1 month (Bachrach et al. 1988). There are also reports from the Montana State Hospital, located in rural Warm Springs, that mentally ill individuals from all parts of the country arrive there voluntarily and may be admitted for brief stays. They get a night or two of sleep and some food before being sent on their way (Bachrach 1988c).

Mobility over wide geographic areas is now reported for homeless mentally ill individuals in the District of Columbia and a number of different states, including Arizona, California, Colorado, Hawaii, Virginia, Washington, and Wisconsin (Bachrach 1989, Blaska 1984; Brown et al. 1983; Chambers 1986; Chmiel et al. 1979; Citizens Coalition for Shelter 1983; Cleveland 1990; Kimura et al. 1975; Seattle-King County Human Resources Coalition 1984; Streltzer 1979; van Winkle 1980). Even Alaska is not immune (Bachrach 1986).

These gross migration patterns are sometimes reinforced—and in some cases perhaps even precipitated—by certain informal practices. For example, there are reports of homeless mentally ill individuals who are recruited into temporary migrant labor streams, transported over considerable distances to work sites, and then, after the temporary agricultural work is finished, released to wander in the areas to which they have been taken (Henry 1983; Herman 1979). Similarly, there is documentation for a practice ironically referred to as Greyhound therapy (Cordes 1984; van Winkle 1980)—providing homeless mentally ill people with one-way bus tickets out of town, ostensibly because they belong in some other catchment area and are not entitled to local services.

Together, these three sources of mobility appreciably increase difficulties in defining and counting the homeless population—a situation that has distinct political overtones. This is especially true in the case of gross geographical mobility, which inevitably is tied up with expectations by service providers concerning which individuals "belong" at which service sites. Some providers who wish to expand their service bases for humanitarian or financial reasons may understate mobility in the population. Others, however, may exaggerate it as a way to reduce their service rolls, and they are assisted in this effort by the practice of catchmenting.

Thus, it is hardly surprising that the research literature contains reports that minimize the effects of geographical movement. A St. Louis study found that although 56% of homeless individuals using emergency shelters had lived outside the city during the previous year, 22% had lived in only one other city and 9% in only two other cities (Morse et al. 1985). The investigators concluded, on the basis of these data, that "the vast majority of the homeless should be considered permanent residents of St. Louis." Similarly, researchers in Ohio concluded that since 64% of the homeless population had either been born in the counties where they currently resided or had lived there for longer than 1 year, the state's homeless population should not be regarded as "highly transient" (Roth and Bean 1986). And a Baltimore study concluded that since 60% of sheltered homeless persons had lived in that city for 10 years or longer, the population was essentially "native," not "transient" (Fischer et al. 1986).

One may infer from such statements that mobility is of negligible importance. However, such an interpretation may be flawed, for there is reason to question whether raw percentages are appropriate indicators of either clinical need or system impact. Geographically mobile individuals who constitute a numerical minority may also be disproportionately representative of those in the population who are the most severely disabled. Who is to say whether 36%, 40%, or 44% constitutes a significant portion of that population?

The potential danger of reducing service delivery problems to numerical rankings is illustrated in a service utilization study of persons with schizophrenia. Although only 1% of the American population suffers from schizophrenia at any given time, 40% of all long-term care days and 25% of all hospital beds are utilized by individuals with this diagnosis (Talbott et al. 1986).

Circumscribing the Universe

The limitations inherent in defining and counting the homeless mentally ill population lead to the conclusion that we are dealing with a situation resembling a large and complex jigsaw puzzle (Bachrach 1984b). Every so often, one or another study offers a valid description of a piece of the puzzle, and occasionally two or three pieces seem to interlock. But the bottom line is that we cannot really complete the puzzle because we are unable to lay down a perimeter. Nor shall we be able to do so until we have agreed on the puzzle's outline by adopting a more or less standardized definition of the population. Such a definition would require both a complex conceptual and statistical model (Burnam and Koegel 1988) and an ability to reduce the population's parameters to simple language.

If anything, this predicament has become more acute since it was first noted in the earlier task force report (Bachrach 1984a). With a substantial increase in literature have come increasingly varied conceptualizations of the homeless mentally ill population—a situation that makes it ever more difficult to compare findings across studies (Burt and Cohen 1989). Because the population is so diverse, and because we really do not even know how to characterize it, we must guard against unwarranted descriptions that oversimplify its dimensions or minimize its service needs.

For example, some of the existing research reveals substantial differences between homeless mentally ill men and women in terms of their demography, treatment histories, and service needs (Bachrach 1987,

1990a; Bachrach et al. 1988; Crystal 1984; Santiago et al. 1988). There is also reason to suppose that homeless mentally ill people living in shelters differ from those living on the streets or those who show up in general hospital emergency rooms (Gelberg and Linn 1989; Koegel et al. 1986). The Tucson Homeless Mentally Ill Study has shown, for example, that men are more heavily represented than women in a street population of homeless mentally ill individuals but that women outnumber men in a sheltered population (Bachrach et al. 1990).

Thus, when people seek a numerical estimate of the prevalence of mental illness within the homeless population, they are often asking a question that is, at the present time, virtually impossible to answer. Current estimates from communities throughout the United States generally run from about one-third to one-half of the total homeless population (General Accounting Office 1985). But it is immediately clear to those who have observed the problem in different parts of the country that there are places where 90% or more of the homeless population are mentally ill, just as there are other places, particularly facilities or neighborhoods that regulate their gatekeeping effectively, where probably no more than 5% are mentally ill. And if we add to this the fact that the "new poor" within the homeless population are apparently increasing very rapidly in many places (Hope and Young 1986), the question of what percentage of all homeless people are mentally ill may well turn out to be the "unquestion" of the 1990s.

Accordingly, the answer to the first question—What percentage of the homeless population is chronically mentally ill?—must be, "It depends." The percentage depends utterly on how one defines the population and on what portion of the population one is viewing.

Indeed, this question may not always be the question that people wish to ask after all, for it is frequently confused with a second question that reverses the numerator and denominator. Thus, although the major portion of current literature is concerned with establishing the prevalence of mental illness within a homeless population, another smaller portion focuses on the prevalence of homelessness within a population of mentally ill individuals (Belcher and First 1987–1988; Drake et al. 1989; Mowbray et al. 1987). Although the difference between them is too often overlooked (Bachrach 1984b), these are entirely different epidemiological questions with distinctive implications for service planning.

Is it any easier to answer the prevalence question when the numerator and denominator are reversed, and the alternative question is posed? It appears not. Morrison (1989) has classified a group of patients in San Francisco according to definitions of homelessness culled from the research literature and found that, depending on the definition employed, homelessness rates range from 22% to 57% of mentally ill individuals—a finding that has caused the investigator to conclude that "'homelessness' is by no means a unitary concept; definition is key" (p. 953).

The Question of Deinstitutionalization

Do we fare better with the policy question, "What is the relationship between deinstitutionalization and homelessness among mentally ill persons?" than with the epidemiological question? Apparently not, for once again the response is limited by semantic and conceptual concerns. And once again the best answer appears to be the equivocal and unsatisfactory, "It depends." Just as the terms "homelessness" and "chronic mental illness" lack standardized definitions, so is "deinstitutionalization" open to various interpretations; and it is well to recognize at least three theoretically distinct aspects of deinstitutionalization in any analysis of its effects.

First, deinstitutionalization is a *fact*, an objective series of events manifested in a massive shift in the locus of care for chronic mental patients. Unpublished estimates from the National Institute of Mental Health reveal that there are currently some 103,000 patients in the nation's state mental hospitals on any given day—a dramatic reduction from the 559,000 reported in 1955. Even more striking is the drop in resident-patient rates. In 1955, 339 of every 100,000 people living in the United States resided as patients in state mental hospitals. Today, the nation's base population has increased to about 250 million (from 165 million in 1955), and only 41 of every 100,000 people reside in state mental hospitals on any given day.

However, deinstitutionalization is also a *philosophy* with roots in post–World War II America, when a variety of civil rights protests were gaining widespread support. Early in its history, deinstitutionalization reflected the optimism of an era dominated by a strong belief that the world could be made a better place through positive social action. Chronic mental patients were seen as victims of inhumane conditions inside state mental hospitals, and there was a conviction that community-based care would offer them a more therapeutic and humane alternative. These ideas were, of course, reinforced by our expanding ability to contain patients' most obvious symptoms through pharmacological advances, for patients were beginning to *seem* less sick than they had been in the past.

This idealism was coupled with another philosophical stream that was preoccupied with reducing the costs of care for mentally ill persons. As a result, deinstitutionalization philosophy quickly came to represent a coalition of ideologies: a marriage of such unexpected bedfellows as fiscal reformers and social reformers. Indeed, the ability of these ordinarily antagonistic factions to agree on the goal of changing the primary locus of care was essential to the widespread acceptance of deinstitutionalization as a concept and to the many rapid efforts mounted to implement that concept.

Third, deinstitutionalization is a *process*, in that it reflects extensive and profound social change: a movement away from one orientation in patient care to another that is radically different. It thus implies an ongoing series of accommodations and shifting boundaries among service delivery agencies that, not surprisingly, has generated severe disequilibrium in the system of care. The very process of change has, in fact, created its own momentum, so that deinstitutionalization now involves all elements of the mental health service system and all the individuals who receive care in, or are rejected by, that system.

As a process, deinstitutionalization constantly shapes the patient careers of chronically mentally ill people. Before its advent, most such individuals sooner or later ended up in state mental hospitals, where they tended to stay for a very long time, often for life. Today, precisely as the result of deinstitutionalization, most admissions to state mental hospitals last a few days or weeks, not a few months or years, much less a lifetime. Increasing numbers of chronically mentally ill individuals are never admitted to state mental hospitals at all (Pepper et al. 1981).

Nevertheless, despite its complexity, deinstitutionalization is often defined narrowly in the literature and is equated solely with state hospital depopulation, an interpretation that gives rise to some curious and basically erroneous conclusions. An appropriate understanding of the concept should allow for the variety of gatekeeping practices, sometimes euphemistically referred to as admission diversion, that keep many mentally ill people from ever using state mental hospitals in the first place. It should also subsume the prevailing climate of civil rights, which, while having had positive effects in protecting the citizenship of some people who are mentally ill, has at the same time discouraged others from seeking help in the mental health service system.

When the definition of deinstitutionalization is broad enough to cover state hospital depopulation, diverted admissions, and unserved individuals, that policy may be viewed as having a pronounced, if not readily quantified, influence on homelessness among chronically mentally ill individuals (Bennett et al. 1988; Institute of Medicine 1988; Marcos et al. 1990; Rossi 1989; Torrey 1988). Many persons, disabled by their psychiatric illnesses and unable to access suitable housing on their own, experience a unique form of eviction in being excluded from state mental hospitals that historically have performed many functions in their behalf, including that of providing a stable residential environment.

Thus, the answer to the question of how deinstitutionalization has affected homelessness among chronically mentally ill individuals depends utterly on our willingness to view the effects of that policy in a global and comprehensive manner, instead of focusing only on easily counted discharged state hospital patients.

The Question of Services

The discussion of the effects of deinstitutionalization leads logically to the third question guiding this analysis and commentary: "Where and how should we serve homeless mentally ill people?" And, once again, the best answer to this question appears to be the equivocal, "It depends."

Given the fact that the homeless mentally ill population is so varied, posing general questions about what is best for the population as a whole seems almost absurd. Planning must obviously respond to the needs of specific individuals within the population, not to an undifferentiated mass.

Even beyond this, however, there is an issue of goals. Before we can answer the question of how to serve homeless mentally ill individuals, we must have some idea of what goals we hold for them, for communities vary in this matter extensively. If a community seeks to clear the streets of these persons, the question of how to plan services is easily answered: it need only expand the capability of its state mental hospitals by whatever means possible, a decidedly humane solution compared to others that have sometimes been pursued (Bachrach 1990b). On the other hand, if a community seeks to offer individualized treatments that have some relevance to the specific pathologies and disabilities of homeless mentally ill people, the question of what to do becomes more complex. Individualizing care means stretching resources and changing priorities, factors that complicate service planning and resource allocation.

The third question must thus be addressed with these caveats in mind, for there are no simple answers in service planning. Although we know something about how to help some homeless mentally ill people some of the time, we are still in the process of learning how to conceptualize the dimensions and the requirements of the population. Very often, planning relevant services puzzles us, bewilders us, and frustrates us, for homeless mentally ill persons frequently appear to ignore our offerings and reject us.

Nevertheless, several contributions to the literature about treatment of homeless mentally ill people are noteworthy.

First, although such a principle is difficult to establish empirically, strong overtones found in both professional and popular writings suggest that services are best offered within a supportive climate that regards homeless mentally ill individuals as legitimate users of the service system. The importance of an acceptant milieu in which these individuals are perceived as sick and deserving, not as lazy and worthless, is tacitly assumed to be basic to the provision of effective services.

A second area of general consensus concerns the need to apply proven program planning principles in developing services for individuals who are both homeless and mentally ill. These principles, discussed in the first task force report (Bachrach 1984a) and widely reiterated since (Goldfinger 1990), include such basic concerns as having a flexible and multifaceted service system, providing individualized but culturally relevant treatments, and having service delivery agencies that work together and talk to one another. In other words, these concepts relate to providing individualized treatments, comprehensive care, and continuity of care, although, as we shall see, they tend to have unique connotations for homeless mentally ill individuals who generally have nothing and need everything (Lamb 1990; Lipton et al. 1988).

Third, the literature frequently underscores the need for service providers to be prepared to approach homeless mentally ill individuals in nontraditional ways (Goldfinger 1990; Susser et al. 1990b). A recent volume by Cohen (1990), *Psychiatry Takes to the Streets*, focuses on the need to alter traditional concepts of time and space in reaching today's chronic mental patients and summarizes a variety of outreach approaches that appear to work with different segments of the population. It also documents the need for new and imaginative treatment interventions that respond to homeless mentally ill people wherever they are, both psychologically and physically, not where we might expect or want them to be. The metaphor in the title of Cohen's book is most apposite.

In this connection the literature also notes that homeless mentally ill individuals vary in their readiness for certain kinds of service interventions. Thus, for example, although rehabilitation or skills training is an excellent ultimate goal for us to hold on their behalf, we must also recognize that some in the population cannot immediately respond to such interventions, and that, for those who are not ready for skills training, a full array of prevocational and nonvocational rehabilitative interventions must be offered.

Fourth, the literature reveals that some of the life circumstances experienced by homeless mentally ill persons act like intervening variables in altering their service needs. The very absence of appropriate protection from the elements, the frequent abuse of chemical substances, the exposure to violence and danger, and the tendency toward geographical instability affect homeless mentally ill individuals in such a basic and overwhelming manner that traditional service planning concepts must, as noted above, be altered to suit their needs. Some writers, for example, speak of "shelterization" (Gounis and Susser 1990), which Grunberg and Eagle (1990) define as a "process of acculturation endemic to shelter living . . . characterized by a decrease in interpersonal responsiveness, a neglect of personal hygiene, increasing passivity, and an increasing dependency on others" (pp. 22–23). Just as institutionalization in the past created extraordinary life circumstances that had to be ameliorated, so does shelterization create its own set of unique service needs. The same may be said of living on the streets (Martin 1990).

Thus, the first task force report (Bachrach 1984a) noted that the services required by this population are remarkable both for their extensiveness and for the fact that many are outside the scope of traditional offerings. Homeless mentally ill individuals frequently need services that planners rarely consider (Ball and Havassy 1984), such as easy access to toilets, mailboxes where Supplemental Security Income checks may be collected, delousing facilities, and even private spaces where they may escape from constant noise or threats of violence. Ready access to telephones may be critical—a situation illustrated by the story, not apocryphal, of a homeless mentally ill individual who, in trying to call a homeless hotline, reached an answering machine asking him to leave a telephone number. And, of course, not to be overlooked is the fact that the need for medical and surgical care in this population is so staggering that it falls well outside the bounds of what a traditional mental health service agency might offer (Gelberg and Linn 1989; Gelberg et al. 1990).

Agencies are generally hard-pressed to ensure these kinds of services, for they are usually not prepared to respond to patients' basic health, subsistence, and sanitary needs. Yet, psychotherapeutic and rehabilitative interventions will probably have little positive effect until those needs have been met (Cohen et al. 1984).

Finally, the literature strongly suggests that effective service planning requires both clinical and cultural sensitivity to the realities of life among people who are both homeless and mentally ill (Cohen 1989; Goldfinger 1990; Graves 1985; Shaner 1989; Susser et al. 1990b). The need for sensitivity is commonly discussed in the literature and has been noted by Stephen M. Goldfinger of Boston, who often speaks in workshops about how we, in all good faith, may give a homeless mentally ill individual an appointment to come to the clinic at noon in ignorance of the fact that the individual may have no way of knowing when noon is. Worse yet, by giving the person such an appointment, we may be forcing him or her to make a choice between the clinic and getting noontime lunch at a soup kitchen.

The Role of Residential Planning

The sense of the foregoing discussion may be summarized in the statement that homeless mentally ill persons need what other chronically mentally ill individuals need. The fact that they are homeless, far from mitigating service needs, tends to render them more acute. Nonetheless, a substantial portion of the literature overlooks this fact and focuses on residential care as the single element that is central to effective service provision. Indeed, residential planning is sometimes raised to a status of such primacy that the population's other requirements are virtually ignored (Culhane 1990; Hartman 1986).

Such a disproportionate focus on residential planning reflects an oversimplified view of reality, one that is conceptually flawed and perhaps dangerous. Obviously, the provision of appropriate and relevant housing must be a primary concern for homeless mentally ill individuals (Lipton et al. 1988), but it does not stand alone.

Lamb and Lamb (1990) have persuasively outlined the importance of coming "face to face with [the] clinical reality" of homeless mentally ill people and about what we need to do "to provide them with support, protection, treatment, and rehabilitation" (p. 305). In this catalog of needs, housing is one of several requirements, and it always has to be balanced against the others.

Indeed, housing may be only minimally correlated with the success of other services, a point that is supported by findings from an in-depth study of 25 homeless mentally ill women in Washington, DC (Harris and Bachrach 1990). Two years after the women had been enrolled in a special clinical case management program, 19 were still in treatment, even though they had changed residences frequently. Having spent a total of 406 months in the program, the women had moved 138 times, or 5.5 times per woman. The median tenure for their residential stays was 3.8 months. The critical finding from this research in the present context is that it is possible to engage at least some homeless mentally ill persons in community-based care, even to a point that improvements in their symptomatology and levels of functioning may be measured, but that does not mean that they will necessarily "stay put" in the residences that are offered to them. They may still move in and out of housing with great frequency, and they often even return to the streets for a short while, all without losing contact with the treatment agency.

Thus, it appears that two variables in interaction—what I have referred to elsewhere as rootlessness and restlessness (Bachrach 1989)—affect the service needs of at least some homeless mentally ill persons. What is more, the two variables may be largely independent of one another, so that some of the rootlessness can be reduced without apparent alteration of the restlessness.

Residential planning, in short, must be seen as a very complicated endeavor, a fact that is belied by research and policy that focus primarily on rootlessness—an absence of affiliation and a place in the community—but that largely overlook restlessness: the fact that, even under benign clinical conditions, some individuals seem to need *not* to remain in one residence, at least in the beginning of treatment. And it is essential for us to know more about both the sociology and the clinical antecedents of restlessness if we are to plan services properly.

Some portion of restlessness may relate to sociologically entrenched patterns of coping (Stokols and Shumaker 1982). Many of the women in the District of Columbia study, for example, recalled childhoods in which a standard familial response to crisis was to pick up and move to a new location. Such an explanation is not, incidentally, inconsistent with a finding by Susser and his colleagues (1987) that the experience of residential mobility in childhood is positively correlated with adult homelessness.

It is likely, however, that sociological factors commonly interact with clinical factors to exacerbate restlessness among some homeless mentally ill persons. Corin (1990) has provided a thoughtful description of the need that some chronically mentally ill individuals exhibit to relate to others "without having to be personally committed in personal interactions" (p. 176). They often desire to be close to others, even as they need to keep their distance. Residential instability may be one means for responding to such a need.

Lamb's (1982) poignant description of persons he has called "new drifters" underscores this point. Typically, these chronically mentally ill persons

wander from community to community seeking a geographic solution to their problems; hoping to leave their problems behind, they find that they have simply brought their difficulties to a new location. . . . [Some] drift in the community from one living situation to another, and some, though they remain in one place, can best be described as drifting through life. (p. 467)

Lamb has explained the movement of these individuals as coming from both a "desire to outrun their problems, their symptoms, and their failures," and great difficulty in achieving closeness and intimacy (p. 467).

At times, the disproportionate importance assigned to residential planning is translated in the literature into a quest for permanent housing for people who are homeless and mentally ill (Kanter 1989). This is, however, a questionable practice, for as Barrow and her associates (1989) have concluded, "Obtaining housing, though a necessary part of achieving residential stability, is only part of the process. . . . [For those] whose patterns of homelessness tend to be episodic, movement into housing [may be] part of a cycle rather than representing an end to homelessness" (p. 158).

This point is brought into focus when we view the analogous situations of homelessness and joblessness among mentally ill persons. Joblessness and homelessness are closely related events in that most mentally ill people who are homeless are also jobless. Yet few clinicians are likely to prescribe employment as a total solution for the circumstances of jobless mentally ill individuals. Work might be proposed as part of a broader rehabilitative effort, but it would almost certainly not be viewed as a totally independent variable in changing the life circumstances of a jobless mentally ill person.

Carrying this analogy further, we may note that when work is promoted as part of a broader treatment plan, it is probably desirable that the plan not call for a single permanent job. This is so for several reasons. First, we readily recognize that, like many things in American life, the permanence of jobs is not certain. Jobs come and go, depending on the economy, the composition of the labor force, and changes in a community's demography. Second, something about holding a person to a single permanent job flies in the face of what might be termed the American dream. Occupational mobility—moving up in the world—is deeply ingrained in our culture, and this means basically that jobs are generally best viewed as sometime things. Third, and most important, we recognize that mentally ill people frequently experience job-related stresses that interfere with their ability to persevere. Consequently, we are disposed to give these individuals a certain amount of space and freedom with respect to employment, a principle that is prominent in such well-known supported employment programs as Fountain House (Propst 1987).

It seems reasonable to conclude that similar concerns should inform residential planning for homeless mentally ill individuals. Like not having a job, not having a home is definitely a circumstance to be reversed. But housing must be provided cautiously and flexibly. It certainly must be individualized and made part of a more organized treatment plan. And it may be most effective if expectations of permanence are not superimposed upon it.

Conclusions

I began this analysis and commentary by posing three broad, frequently asked questions about the homeless mentally ill population. Although the existing corpus of literature is extensive and contains some impressive contributions, it still fails to provide the kinds of information that would permit these questions to be answered in any definitive manner. Does the failure come from some lack in the literature? Or does it result because the questions, as stated, are irrelevant ones? It appears that both factors contribute to the situation: the literature does indeed have some serious gaps, but the questions are also conceptually naive.

Nonetheless, attempting to answer these questions is a useful exercise, for it suggests some important avenues of inquiry. Among other things, it demonstrates the futility of focusing on numerical questions when the conceptual framework within which they might be interpreted is weak or nonexistent. Alonso and Starr (1987) have argued quite appropriately that statistics describing sociological concerns must be interpreted cautiously because they "reflect propositions and theories about the nature of society . . . and they are sensitive to methodological decisions made by complex organizations with limited resources" (p. 1). Starr (1987), in fact, has written a chapter named "The Sociology of Official Statistics" in a book with an equally provocative title, *The Politics of Numbers* (Alonso and Starr 1987).

In concluding this analysis and commentary, it is well to ask what we have learned about this population since publication of the first task force report. What do we know today that we did not know then? Although the number of both professional and popular reports has increased dramatically, it appears that this question must be answered with some equivocation. On the one hand, our base of knowledge has expanded considerably. A number of research projects have reported on the characteristics, epidemiology, and unique service needs of homeless mentally ill people; and we have begun to amass quite an array of facts and figures. However, conceptually we remain at the kicking-off point and still have a long way to go.

Should we be discouraged? Emphatically not. We must realize that understanding the composition and the needs of the homeless mentally ill population is necessarily a slow and gradual process and the fact that we are moving forward in accumulating some important information about these vulnerable individuals is encouraging. Perhaps the most dramatic summary statement that can be made in concluding this chapter is that, despite gaps in our knowledge, this analytical review could not have been written a decade ago, for the literature needed to support it was not available then.

Where do we go from here? There are a number of important considerations that must guide the next generation of studies of homeless mentally ill individuals.

First, it is apparent that we must make an effort to clarify our concepts and define our terms with greater precision. Loose definitions and fuzzy concepts have paved the way for misunderstandings and word games (Bachrach 1985) that may do great harm to members of this population. Shared consensual definitions are essential not only for standardizing research but also for facilitating consensus and compromise in service planning, for planners cannot communicate unless they understand each other.

On the level of policy, there is a critical need for federal direction in these matters. It is not enough for the government in Washington to adopt a laissez-faire attitude that favors the states' prerogatives in responding to the problems of homeless mentally ill individuals. The federal government must take a firm stand, first, in promoting a shared definition of the population and, beyond that, in proposing guidelines for comprehensive program development. Although individual local programs must be specialized so that they are relevant to the specific concerns of the portion of the homeless mentally ill population they are attempting to reach, such problems as establishing a locus of responsibility for geographically mobile individuals and ensuring their access to entitlements are national in scope and must be approached accordingly. It is much too easy under present circumstances for a community or state to refuse care to and exclude or extrude a person who is an outsider. All too often that person is an outsider everywhere.

Finally, it is important that we attempt to reduce the political influences that adversely affect the conduct of research on homeless mentally ill individuals. Too often, the problems of this population are seen not as clinical concerns but as political fodder (Bachrach 1988b; Marcos and Cohen 1986). For example, homeless mentally ill individuals are sometimes said to be undomiciled by choice, even though a variety of studies contradict such a conclusion (Herrman 1990; Lamb and Lamb 1990; Wright 1989). The words of one chronically mentally ill woman place "choice" among homeless mentally ill persons in perspective.

> Someone who has been on the streets and is homeless and jobless and who has a disability, who doesn't have a car or food or a friend, and

doesn't know what to do about the situation, is in pain. Most people would probably agree that if given a choice, they would trade that level of emotional pain for some good old-fashioned physical hurt anytime. But there is no choice. If you talk to people who have been there, they will tell you they were alone and afraid. So afraid that help doesn't look like help, but like more torture. (Anonymous 1988)

Above all, identifying homeless persons as mentally ill must not be viewed, as some writers have (Hyde 1985; Snow et al. 1986), as a "labeling" issue. To diagnose an individual is neither an encroachment upon his or her civil rights nor an indictment of his or her behavior. It is merely an aid to appropriate and humane service planning. For persons whose primary reason for being homeless is an economic one, providing a "boost up," employment, and access to appropriate housing may be the most important and timely answer. On the other hand, for those whose homelessness is related to mental illness, service planning must be more comprehensive and more oriented toward clinical realities.

For successful service planning, it is essential to consider the full array of disabilities typically endured by homeless mentally ill persons. Like other chronically mentally ill individuals, they experience at least three types of disability, as described by Wing and Morris (1981). The primary disabilities, those directly related to and symptomatic of the illness, are often best treated through judicious pharmacological intervention. The secondary disabilities, those that derive from individuals' personal responses to the experience of illness, are often best reversed through individualized and sensitive counseling, psychotherapy, and rehabilitative skills training. And the tertiary disabilities, those externally imposed "disablements" that result from stigma and lack of societal opportunity, require focused efforts to change service systems and to make them more responsive to the needs of the most disabled individuals they must serve. Changes at all three levels must be pursued simultaneously if the members of this population are to be served in any comprehensive manner.

This analysis reveals that we have taken some important first steps in understanding the needs of homeless mentally ill persons. It is now time to move forward conceptually, so that we may begin to improve the lives of these individuals. They are, in the most basic sense, victims. They are victims of their illnesses, which are serious, debilitating, and often painful conditions. They are victims of a society that stigmatizes them and frequently denies their humanity. And, until planning efforts can respond to them as individuals whose needs for clinical and supportive services are complex and unique, they will also be victims of service systems that, deliberately or knowingly, fail to respond to them.

References

Alonso W, Starr P: Introduction, in The Politics of Numbers. Edited by Alonso W, Starr P. New York, Russell Sage Foundation, 1987, pp 1–6

Anonymous: Someone who has been there. Newsletter of New Beginnings, Elgin, OK, Summer 1988

Appleby L, Desai PN: Residential instability: a perspective on system imbalance. Am J Orthopsychiatry 57:515–524, 1987

Appleby L, Slagg N, Desai PN: The urban nomad: a psychiatric problem?, in Current Psychiatric Therapies, Vol 21. Edited by Masserman JH. New York, Grune & Stratton, 1982, pp 253–262

Arce AA, Tadlock M, Vergare MH, et al: A psychiatric profile of street people admitted to an emergency shelter. Hosp Community Psychiatry 34:812–817, 1983

Bachrach LL: The homeless mentally ill and mental health services: an analytical review of the literature, in The Homeless Mentally Ill: A Task Force Report of the American Psychiatric Association. Edited by Lamb HR. Washington, DC, American Psychiatric Association, 1984a, pp 11–53

Bachrach LL: Interpreting research on the homeless mentally ill: some caveats. Hosp Community Psychiatry 35:914–917, 1984b

Bachrach LL: Slogans and Euphemisms: The Functions of Semantics and Mental Health and Mental Retardation Care. Austin, TX, Hogg Foundation, 1985

Bachrach LL: Service delivery in Juneau. Hosp Community Psychiatry 37:669–670, 1986

Bachrach LL: Geographic mobility among the homeless mentally ill. Hosp Community Psychiatry 38:27–28, 1987

Bachrach LL: Defining chronic mental illness: a concept paper. Hosp Community Psychiatry 39:383–388, 1988a

Bachrach LL: Programs and politics: toward new coalitions. Hosp Community Psychiatry 39:927–928, 1988b

Bachrach LL: Transient patients in a western state hospital. Hosp Community Psychiatry 39:123–124, 1988c

Bachrach LL: An In-Depth Analysis of Services for Homeless Mentally Ill Women: The Community Connections Homeless Women's Project Study. Quarterly Evaluation Report 2. Washington, DC, Community Connections, 1989

Bachrach LL: Homeless mentally ill women: a special population, in Women's Progress. Edited by Spurlock J, Robinowitz CB. New York, Plenum, 1990a, pp 189–201

Bachrach LL: The media and homeless mentally ill persons. Hosp Community Psychiatry 41:963–964, 1990b

Bachrach LL, Santiago JM, Berren MP, et al: The homeless mentally ill in Tucson: implications of early findings. Am J Psychiatry 145:112–113, 1988

Bachrach LL, Santiago JM, Berren MP: Homeless mentally ill patients in the community: results of a general hospital emergency room study. Community Ment Health J 26:415–423, 1990

Bailey R: The Homeless and Empty Houses. Middlesex, England, Penguin, 1977

Ball FLJ, Havassy BE: A survey of the problems and needs of homeless consumers of acute psychiatric services. Hosp Community Psychiatry 35:917–921, 1984

Barrow SM, Hellman F, Lovell AM, et al: Effectiveness of Programs for the Mentally Ill Homeless. New York, New York State Psychiatric Institute, 1989

Bassuk EL, Gerson S: Chronic crisis patients: a discrete clinical group. Am J Psychiatry 137:1513–1517, 1980

Baxter E, Hopper K: The new mendicancy: homeless in New York City. Am J Orthopsychiatry 52:393–408, 1982

Belcher JR: Are jails replacing the mental health system for the homeless mentally ill? Community Ment Health J 24:185–195, 1988

Belcher JR, First RJ: The homeless mentally ill: barriers to effective service delivery. Journal of Applied Social Sciences 12:62–78, 1987–1988

Benda BB, Dattalo P: Homelessness: consequence of a crisis or a long-term process? Hosp Community Psychiatry 39:884–886, 1988

Bennett MI, Gudeman JE, Jenkins L, et al: The value of hospital-based treatment for the homeless mentally ill. Am J Psychiatry 145:1273–1276, 1988

Blaska D: Street life makes city "place to be." Madison (WI) Capital Times, June 27, 1984, pp 1, 7

Brown C, MacFarlane S, Paredes R, et al: The Homeless of Phoenix: Who Are They? And What Should Be Done? Phoenix, AZ, Phoenix South Community Mental Health Center, 1983

Burnam MA, Koegel P: Methodology for obtaining a representative sample of homeless persons: the Los Angeles Skid Row Study. Evaluation Review 12:117–152, 1988

Burt MR, Cohen BE: America's Homeless: Numbers, Characteristics, and Programs that Serve Them. Urban Institute Report 89-3. Washington, DC, Urban Institute, 1989

Chafetz L, Goldfinger SM: Residential instability in a psychiatric emergency setting. Psychiatr Q 56:20–34, 1984

Chambers M: Tolerant policy on homeless divides Santa Monica. New York Times, March 23, 1986, p 28

Chmiel AJ, Akhtar S, Morris J: The long-distance psychiatric patient in the emergency room. Int J Soc Psychiatry 25:38–46, 1979

Citizens Coalition for Shelter: Interviews with 786 Homeless People on the Streets of Denver. Aurora, CO, Citizens Coalition for Shelter, 1983

Cleveland MM: Letter to New York Times, March 14, 1990, p A28

Cohen M: Social work practice with homeless mentally ill people: engaging the client. Social Work 505–509, 1989

Cohen NL (ed): Psychiatry Takes to the Streets: Outreach and Crisis Intervention for the Mentally Ill. New York, Guilford, 1990

Cohen NL, Putnam JF, Sullivan AM: The mentally ill homeless: isolation and adaptation. Hosp Community Psychiatry 35:922–924, 1984

Cordes C: The plight of the homeless mentally ill. APA Monitor, February 1984, pp 1, 13

Corin EE: Facts and meaning in psychiatry: an anthropological approach to the lifeworld of schizophrenics. Cult Med Psychiatry 14:153–188, 1990

Crystal S: Homeless men and homeless women: the gender gap. Urban and Social Change Review 17:2–6, 1984

Culhane DP: Letter to New York Times, March 14, 1990, p A28

Department of Health and Human Services: Alcohol, Drug Abuse, and Mental Health Problems of the Homeless. Rockville, MD, Alcohol, Drug Abuse and Mental Health Administration, 1983

Department of Housing and Urban Development: A Report to the Secretary on the Homeless and Emergency Shelters. Washington, DC, U.S. Department of Housing and Urban Development, 1984

Drake RE, Wallach MA, Hoffman JS: Housing instability and homelessness among aftercare patients of an urban state hospital. Hosp Community Psychiatry 40:46–51, 1989

Fischer PJ, Shapiro S, Breakey WR, et al: Mental health and social characteristics of the homeless: a survey of mission users. Am J Public Health 76:519–524, 1986

Gelberg L, Linn LS: Assessing the physical health of homeless adults. JAMA 262:1973–1979, 1989

Gelberg L, Linn LS, Usatine RP, et al: Health, homelessness, and poverty: a study of clinic users. Arch Intern Med 150:2325–2330, 1990

Geller MP: The "revolving door": a trap or a lifestyle? Hosp Community Psychiatry 33:388–389, 1982

General Accounting Office: Homeless Mentally Ill: Problems and Options in Estimating Numbers and Trends. Washington, DC, U.S. General Accounting Office, 1988

General Accounting Office: Homelessness: A Complex Problem and the Federal Response. Washington, DC, U.S. General Accounting Office, 1985

Goldfinger SM: Homelessness and schizophrenia: a psychosocial approach, in Handbook of Schizophrenia, Vol 4: Psychosocial Treatment of Schizophrenia. Edited by Herz MI, Keith SJ, Docherty JP. New York, Elsevier North-Holland, 1990

Goldfinger SM, Hopkin JT, Surber RW: Treatment resisters or system resisters? Toward a better service system for acute care recidivists. New Dir Ment Health Serv 21:17–27, 1984

Gounis K, Susser E: Shelterization and its implications for mental health services, in Psychiatry Takes to the Streets: Outreach and Crisis Intervention for the Mentally Ill. Edited by Cohen NL. New York, Guilford, 1990, pp 231–255

Graves M: Working with homeless women: a transcultural experience. Spectrum (Newsletter of the American Psychiatric Association/National Institute of Mental Health Fellows), November 1985, pp 3–6

Grunberg J, Eagle PF: Shelterization: how the homeless adapt to shelter living. Hosp Community Psychiatry 41:521–525, 1990

Harris M, Bachrach LL: Perspectives on homeless mentally ill women. Hosp Community Psychiatry 41:253–254, 1990

Hartman C: The housing part of the homelessness problem. New Dir Ment Health Serv 30:71–85, 1986

Henry N: The long, hot wait for pickin' work. Washington Post, October 9, 1983, pp A1, A16

Herman R: Some freed mental patients make it, some do not. New York Times, November 19, 1979, pp B1, B4

Herrman H: A survey of homeless mentally ill people in Melbourne, Australia. Hosp Community Psychiatry 41:1291–1292, 1990

Hope M, Young J: The Faces of Homelessness. Lexington, MA, DC Heath, 1986

Hyde P: A state mental health director's perspective. Psychosocial Rehabilitation Journal 8:21–25, 1985

Institute of Medicine: Homelessness, Health, and Human Needs. Washington, DC, National Academy Press, 1988

Jones BE (ed): Treating the Homeless: Urban Psychiatry's Challenge. Washington, DC, American Psychiatric Press, 1986

Kanter AS: Homeless but not helpless: legal issues in the care of homeless people with mental illness. Journal of Social Issues 45:91–104, 1989

Kates B: The Murder of a Shopping Bag Lady. San Diego, CA, Harcourt Brace Jovanovich, 1985

Kimura SP, Mikolashek PL, Kirk SA: Madness in paradise: psychiatric crises among newcomers in Honolulu. Hawaii Med J 34:275–278, 1975

Koegel P, Farr RK, Burnam MA: Heterogeneity in an inner-city homeless population: a comparison between individuals surveyed in traditional Skid Row locations and in voucher hotel rooms. Psychosocial Rehabilitation Journal 10:31–45, 1986

Lamb HR: Young adult chronic patients: the new drifters. Hosp Community Psychiatry 33:465–468, 1982

Lamb HR: Will we save the homeless mentally ill? Am J Psychiatry 147:649–651, 1990

Lamb HR, Grant RW: The mentally ill in an urban county jail. Arch Gen Psychiatry 39:17–22, 1982

Lamb HR, Grant RW: Mentally ill women in a county jail. Arch Gen Psychiatry 40:362–368, 1983

Lamb HR, Lamb DM: Factors contributing to homelessness among the chronically and severely mentally ill. Hosp Community Psychiatry 41:301–305, 1990

Linn LS, Gelberg L, Leake B: Substance abuse and mental health status of homeless and domiciled low-income users of a medical clinic. Hosp Community Psychiatry 41:306–310, 1990

Lipton FR, Nutt S, Sabatini A: Housing the homeless mentally ill: a longitudinal study of a treatment approach. Hosp Community Psychiatry 39:40–45, 1988

Marcos LR, Cohen NL: Taking the suspected mentally ill off the streets to public general hospitals. N Engl J Med 315:1158–1161, 1986

Marcos LR, Cohen NL, Nardacci D, et al: Psychiatry takes to the streets: the New York City initiative for the homeless mentally ill. Am J Psychiatry 147:1557–1561, 1990

Martin MA: The homeless mentally ill and community-based care: changing a mind set. Community Ment Health J 26:435–447, 1990

McKay P: We bag ladies aren't all alike. Washington Post, December 27, 1987, pp C1, C2

Milburn NG, Watts RJ: Methodological issues in research on the homeless and the homeless mentally ill. International Journal of Mental Health 14:42–60, 1986

Morrison J: Correlations between definitions of the homeless mentally ill population. Hosp Community Psychiatry 40:952–954, 1989

Morse G, Shields NM, Hanneke CR, et al: Homeless People in St. Louis: A Mental Health Program Evaluation, Field Study, and Follow-up Investigation. Jefferson City, MO, Missouri Department of Mental Health, 1985

Mowbray CT, Johnson VS, Solarz A: Homelessness in a state hospital population. Hosp Community Psychiatry 38:880–882, 1987

Patton LT: The Rural Homeless. Washington, DC, Health Resources and Services Administration, 1987

Pepper B, Kirshner M, Ryglewicz H: The young adult chronic patient: overview of a population. Hosp Community Psychiatry 32:463–469, 1981

Pitt DE: New strategy for homeless in subways. New York Times, July 22, 1989, pp 27, 28

Prewitt K: Public statistics and democratic politics, in The Politics of Numbers. Edited by Alonso W, Starr P. New York, Russell Sage Foundation, 1987, pp 261–274

Propst RN: A normal life for the mentally ill, in Homelessness: Critical Issues for Policy and Practice. Boston, MA, Boston Foundation, 1987, pp 39–42

Reich R, Siegel L: The emergence of the Bowery as a psychiatric dumping ground. Psychiatr Q 50:191–201, 1978

Rich S: HUD homeless data still questioned. Washington Post, June 8, 1986, p A13

Ropers RH: The Invisible Homeless: A New Urban Ecology. New York, Human Sciences Press, 1988

Rosnow MJ, Shaw T, Concord CS: Listening to the homeless: a study of homeless mentally ill persons in Milwaukee. Psychosocial Rehabilitation Journal 9:64–77, 1986

Rossi PH: Down and Out in America: The Origins of Homelessness. Chicago, IL, University of Chicago Press, 1989

Rossi PH, Wright JD, Fisher GA, et al: The urban homeless: estimating composition and size. Science 235:1336–1341, 1987

Roth D, Bean J: New perspectives on homelessness: findings from a statewide epidemiological study. Hosp Community Psychiatry 37:712–719, 1986

Santiago JM, Bachrach LL, Berren MR, et al: Defining the homeless mentally ill: a methodological note. Hosp Community Psychiatry 39:1100–1102, 1988

Seattle-King County Human Resources Coalition: The Seattle-King County Emergency Shelter Study. Seattle, WA, Seattle-King County Human Resources Coalition, 1984

Shaner A: Asylums, asphalt, and ethics. Hosp Community Psychiatry 40:785–786, 1989

Snow DA, Baker SG, Anderson L, et al: The myth of pervasive mental illness among the homeless. Social Problems 33:407–423, 1986

Sosin MR, Colson P, Grossman S: Homelessness in Chicago: Poverty and Pathology, Social Institutions and Social Change. Chicago, IL, Chicago Community Trust, 1988

Starr P: The sociology of official statistics, in The Politics of Numbers. Edited by Alonso W, Starr P. New York, Russell Sage Foundation, 1987, pp 7–57

Stokols D, Shumaker SA: The psychological context of residential mobility and well-being. Journal of Social Issues 38:149–171, 1982

Streltzer J: Psychiatric emergencies in travelers to Hawaii. Compr Psychiatry 20:463–468, 1979

Susser E, Struening EL, Conover S: Childhood experiences of homeless men. Am J Psychiatry 144:1599–1601, 1987

Susser E, Conover S, Struening EL: Mental illness in the homeless: problems of epidemiologic method in surveys of the 1980s. Community Ment Health J 26:391–414, 1990a

Susser E, Goldfinger SM, White A: Some clinical approaches to the homeless mentally ill. Community Ment Health J 26:463–480, 1990b

Talbott JA, Goldman HH, Kaup B: The economic costs of schizophrenia. Paper presented at the annual meeting of the American Psychiatric Association, Washington, DC, May 1986

Torrey EF: Nowhere to Go: The Tragic Odyssey of the Homeless Mentally Ill. New York, Harper & Row, 1988

U.S. Congress: HUD Report on Homelessness. Washington, DC, U.S. Government Printing Office, 1984

van Winkle WA: Bedlam by the bay. New West, December 1980, p 1

Verhovek SH: For shelter, homeless take the E train. New York Times, November 21, 1988, pp A1, B8

Wing JK, Morris B: Clinical basis of rehabilitation, in Handbook of Psychiatric Rehabilitation Practice. Edited by Wing JK, Morris B. Oxford, England, Oxford University Press, 1981

Wright JD: Address Unknown: The Homeless in America. New York, Aldine de Gruyter, 1989

Chapter 3

Deinstitutionalization in the Nineties

H. Richard Lamb, M.D.

Probably nothing more graphically illustrates the problems of deinstitutionalization than the shameful and incredible phenomenon of the homeless mentally ill. The conditions under which they live are symptomatic of the lack of a comprehensive system of care for the long-term mentally ill in general. Though the homeless mentally ill have become an everyday part of today's society, they are nameless; the great majority are not on the caseload of any mental health professional or mental health agency. Hardly anyone is out looking for them, for they are not officially missing. By and large the system does not know who they are or where they came from.

We can see firsthand society's reluctance to do anything definitive for them; for instance, stopgap measures such as shelters may be provided, but the underlying problem of a lack of a comprehensive system of care is not addressed (Talbott and Lamb 1984). We can see our own ambivalence about taking the difficult stands that need to be taken—for instance, advocating changes in the laws for involuntary treatment and the ways these laws are administered.

When we get to know homeless mentally ill persons as individuals, we often find that they are not able to meet the criteria for the programs that most appeal to us as professionals. For the citizenry in general, the homeless mentally ill represent everything that has gone wrong with deinstitutionalization, and their circumstances have persuaded many that deinstitutionalization was a mistake (Lamb 1988).

Readers interested in the history of deinstitutionalization are referred to the report of the first American Psychiatric Association task force on homelessness (Lamb 1984).

Many things have gone *right* with deinstitutionalization. For instance, the chronically mentally ill enjoy much more liberty, in the majority of cases appropriately so, than when they were institutionalized. Further, we have learned what is necessary to meet their needs in the community, and we have begun to understand the plight of families and how to enlist their help in the treatment process. Yet major problems remain. The purpose of this chapter is twofold: to examine the problems of deinstitutionalization—with regard to not only the homeless mentally ill but also the long-term mentally ill generally—and to draw upon our experience, especially our clinical experience, in working with them to develop strategies for solving these problems.

The New Long-Term Patients

Before deinstitutionalization, those patients, who are now called the new long-term patients or the young adult chronic patients, were institutionalized indefinitely and often for life. Sometimes they improved in the hospital and were discharged, but at their next decompensation were rehospitalized, this time never to return to the community. Thus, after their initial failures to cope with the vicissitudes of life and of living in the community, they were no longer exposed to these stresses: they were given permanent asylum from the demands of the world. Now hospital stays tend to be brief. In this sense, most of the new long-term patients are products of deinstitutionalization (Lamb 1982a). It is this new generation of chronically mentally ill persons that constitutes the greatest challenge to deinstitutionalization, that poses the most difficult clinical problems in community treatment, and that has swelled the ranks of the homeless mentally ill.

What is life like for these new long-term patients in the community? One study of long-term severely disabled psychiatric patients (in a board-and-care home in Los Angeles) showed that significantly more patients under age 30 than those over age 30 had set goals to change something in their lives (Lamb 1979). In the same study, a strong relationship was found between age and history of hospitalization; three-fourths of those under age 30 had been hospitalized during the preceding year, compared with only one-fifth of those over age 30. What do these findings mean? Perhaps they reflect a process of coming to terms with limited capabilities after a more hopeful but also more stormy earlier course. As these patients become older, they may experience repeated failures in dealing with life's demands and in achieving their earlier goals. They have had more time to lower or set aside their goals and to accept a life without goals and a low level of functioning that does not exceed their capabilities.

Young people who are just beginning to deal with life's demands and to make their way into the world are struggling to achieve a measure of independence, to choose and succeed at a vocation, to establish satisfying interpersonal relationships and attain some degree of intimacy, and to acquire some sense of identity. Because mentally ill persons lack ego strength, the ability to withstand stress, and the ability to tolerate intimacy and form meaningful interpersonal relationships, their efforts to reach their goals often fail. The result may be a still more determined, even frantic, effort characterized by a greatly increased level of anxiety that begins to border on desperation.

For a person predisposed to retreat into psychosis, repeated failures lead to a stormy course with acute psychotic breaks and hospitalizations and/or periods of living on the streets. The situation becomes compounded when such persons are in an environment in which unrealistic expectations emanate not just from themselves but also from family and mental health professionals. Denial of illness and the rebelliousness of youth may also contribute to repeated decompensations, hospitalizations, and homelessness.

Some chronically dysfunctional and mentally disordered individuals gradually, over a period of years, succeed in their strivings for independence, a vocation, intimacy, and a sense of identity. Deinstitutionalization, for them, has become a triumph. Many others, however, eventually give up the struggle and find face-saving rationalizations for their limited degree of functioning and accomplishments. For instance, a middle-aged woman may console herself that she would have raised her children if someone had not lied to the judge who ordered them to be taken away from her; or someone in his middle years might report being retired on Social Security when in fact he receives Supplemental Security Income (from the Social Security Administration) because of a disabling psychiatric disorder.

Similar rationalizations are heard from chronically dysfunctional persons who have come to feel they must passively submit to overwhelming forces that control their destinies and impede their progress. Often an individual may adopt a constricted, passive attitude toward life without offering any rationalizations. An example would be the patient who seems to look no further than his next cigarette.

All too often there is a tendency to forget that long-term, severely mentally ill patients are affected by the stresses and concerns of each phase of the life cycle, and that they have the same existential concerns as do we all. Life in the community exposes chronically disabled patients to the same standards of success or failure by which their non-mentally ill peers are judged.

Concerns about getting older but having little to show for their lives are felt not only by those in the involutional period but also by those who are approaching age 30 and even by those still in their mid-twenties (Lamb 1982a). Chronically disabled patients in both the younger and the older age groups feel disheartened and depressed, just as we would be, about not having goals, about not being able to reach goals, and about experiencing repeated failures instead. For patients in their thirties, the contrast between their own lives and those of their non-mentally ill peers, who are in the process of "settling down," marrying or establishing a permanent relationship, and launching a career, may be particularly painful.

On the other hand, long-term studies of individuals with schizophrenia, with mean lengths of follow-up ranging from 22.4 to 36.9 years, have demonstrated considerable degrees of improvement over time (Bleuler 1968; Ciompi 1980; Harding et al. 1987; Huber et al. 1980; Tsuang et al. 1979). These findings are not surprising, for they are consistent with everyday clinical experience that schizophrenia in the middle and later years of a patient's life tends to be more benign and far less stormy than in the earlier years. Goals have been lowered and expectations lessened. Many persons with limited abilities to cope and deal with stress gradually as they reach their fifties and sixties become able to function in both vocational and domestic roles, meeting lowered expectations of others and themselves.

With time, the fires of youth burn lower. Because of their greater maturity, older patients with schizophrenia may present a far different picture than they did when they were younger, less experienced, and striving to meet higher aspirations.

Ideology Versus Clinical Reality

A major problem in the implementation of deinstitutionalization has been preconceived ideology. Reality intrudes at every step in our clinical work with the chronically mentally ill, and cherished theories and ideologies, if rigidly held, take a pounding. If we fail to heed reality, proceeding instead as if these patients need what we want them to have, the resulting exacerbations of psychosis, dysphoria, and perhaps homelessness forcibly remind us that we were wrong.

Thus, we may want our patients to be independent, to be free, and to function at higher levels. If, instead, they need to be dependent and controlled and are able to be only marginally functional, their illness tells us that in no uncertain terms. Practicality is the watchword; without it we are of little value to our chronically and severely ill patients.

Unfortunately, many in this field cling to ideologies, regardless of the clinical realities and the consequences to the patients. Vocational rehabilitation can serve as an example. Everyone wants chronically and severely mentally ill persons to experience the heightened self-esteem and gratification that a life of working at a job, of feeling needed, and of being productive provide. Our own needs and ideology, however, must give way to the clinical reality that most of these persons cannot handle the stress of non-sheltered, competitive employment and that for the minority who can, entry-level, low-stress jobs should most often be the goal. Otherwise, we simply give the patient another experience of failure and further lower his or her self-esteem. We will see that ideology is often a major problem when we come to the discussion of hospital versus community, independence versus dependency, and involuntary treatment.

Hospital or Community

Has deinstitutionalization gone too far in attempting to treat long-term mentally ill persons in the community? We now have more than 3 decades of experience to guide us. Probably only a relatively small minority of long-term mentally ill persons require a highly structured, locked, 24-hour setting for adequate intermediate or long-term management (Dorwart 1988). It may well be, however, that the proportion of homeless mentally ill who need such care may be higher (Marcos et al. 1990). There is an increasing belief that we have a professional obligation to provide such care to those who need it (Group for the Advancement of Psychiatry 1982), either in a hospital or in an alternative setting such as California's locked, skilled-nursing facilities with special programs for psychiatric patients (Lamb 1980).

Where to treat should not be an ideological issue; it is a decision best based on the clinical needs of each person. Unfortunately, deinstitutionalization efforts have, in practice, too often confused locus of care and quality of care (Bachrach 1978; Minkoff 1987). Where mentally ill persons are treated has been seen as more important than how they are treated. Care in the community has often been assumed almost by definition to be better than hospital care. In actuality, poor care can be found in both hospital and community settings.

The other issue that requires attention is appropriateness of care. The long-term mentally ill are not a homogeneous population; what is appropriate for some is not appropriate for others. For instance, some members of the population are characterized by such problems as assaultive behavior; severe, overt major psychopathology; lack of internal controls; reluctance to take psychotropic medications; inability to adjust to open settings; problems with drugs and alcohol; and self-destructive behavior. When these persons have been treated in open community settings, they have required an inordinate amount of time and effort from mental health professionals, various social agencies, and the criminal justice system. Many have been lost to the mental health system and are on the streets or in jail.

Moreover, both mentally ill persons and mental health professionals have often considered these results as evidence of failures by both groups. As a consequence, many long-term mentally ill persons have become alienated from a system that has not met their needs, and some mental health professionals have become disenchanted with their treatment.

Unfortunately the heat of the debate over whether to provide intermediate and long-term hospitalization for such patients has tended to obscure the benefits of community treatment for the great majority of the long-term mentally ill who do not require such highly structured, 24-hour care.

Since the great majority of long-term mentally ill persons are able to live in the community, we must ask ourselves if we have truly established this group as the population with the highest priority in public mental health. If so, does this priority include commitments of our resources and our funding, as well as our concern? We have learned a great deal about the needs of the long-term mentally ill in the community. Thus, we know that this population needs a comprehensive and integrated system of care (Bachrach 1986); such a system would include an adequate number and range of supervised, supportive housing settings; adequate, comprehensive, and accessible crisis intervention, both in the community and in hospitals; and ongoing treatment and rehabilitative services, all provided assertively through outreach when necessary.

We know the importance of a system of case management (see Chapter 12) in which every long-term mentally ill person is on the case load of a mental health agency that will take full responsibility for providing individualized treatment planning that links patients to needed resources and monitors them so that they not only receive the services they need but also are not lost to the system. Have we done enough to put our knowledge into practice? For most parts of this nation, the answer, clearly, is no (Talbott 1985).

Therapeutic But Realistic Optimism

Nothing is more important than therapeutic optimism if we are to work successfully with the long-term mentally ill. But equally important is a need for a realistic appraisal of these persons' capacities. On the basis of such an appraisal we can mount vigorous treatment and rehabilitation efforts for those with the potential for high levels of functioning and strive for other goals, such as improving quality of life, for patients with less potential.

An important issue related to goal setting is that the kinds of criteria that theorists, researchers, policy makers, and clinicians use to assess social integration have a distinct bias in favor of the values held by these professionals and by middle-class society generally (Shadish and Bootzin 1981). Thus, holding a job, increasing one's socialization and relationships with other people, and living independently may not be goals that are shared by a large proportion of the long-term mentally ill, especially as they grow older.

Likewise, what makes the patient happy may be unrelated to these goals. Patients may want (or need) to avoid the stress of competitive employment, or even sheltered employment, and of living independently. They may experience more anxiety than gratification from the threat of intimacy that accompanies increased involvement with other people. Furthermore, many relatives may be primarily concerned that their family member simply be provided decent custodial care (Thomas 1980).

Moreover, if we use expectations applicable to the higher-functioning patients as our only model, we will neglect the large population who function at a lower level and cannot respond to these expectations. And, in fact, in many jurisdictions this population has been neglected. We can only speculate about why. One possible reason is the failure by some mental health professionals to recognize that there are many different kinds of long-term patients, who vary greatly in their capacity for rehabilitation and for change (Lamb 1982b).

Long-term mentally ill persons differ in their ability to cope with stress without decompensating and developing psychotic symptoms. They differ, too, in the kinds of stress and pressure they can handle; for instance, some who are amenable to social rehabilitation cannot tolerate the stresses of vocational rehabilitation, and vice versa. What may appear, at first glance, to be a homogeneous group turns out to be a group that ranges from persons who can tolerate almost no stress at all to those who can, with some assistance, cope with most of life's demands.

Such a view is supported by the very marked variations of course and outcome in both the shorter-term follow-up studies of schizophrenia (Hawk et al. 1975; World Health Organization 1979) and the longer-term studies discussed earlier. For some long-term patients, competitive employment, independent living, and a high level of social functioning are realistic goals; for others, just maintaining their present level of functioning should be considered a success (Solomon et al. 1980).

A patient's degree of dependency, and how professionals react to it, may well be another important factor. Gratifying dependency needs and nurturing are crucial activities of the helping professions. And we learn to do this in such a way that patients do not experience a loss of self-esteem from knowing that they need our help and support (Lamb 1986). Not only may this process be draining to professionals, it may be sorely disappointing when the growth that is expected does not come, even though the potential for the growth we seek may not be there. As a result, we may give less attention, resources, and effort to lower-functioning patients.

Moreover, most of us, as products of our culture and our society, tend to highly value independence and morally disapprove of persons who have "given in" to their dependency needs, who have adopted a passive, inactive lifestyle, and who have accepted public support instead of working (Lamb 1982b). Perhaps this moral disapproval helps to explain why programs whose goals are rehabilitating patients to high levels of functioning, or "mainstreaming" them, attract the most attention and the most funding. Such programs are very much needed for those chronically mentally ill persons capable of higher functioning.

If, however, professionals attempt to raise patients' low levels of functioning without making a realistic appraisal of the capabilities of each individual to cope with the pressures of life, the result may be an acute exacerbation of psychosis. Probably no problems are harder to overcome in the treatment of the long-term mentally ill than the reluctance of professionals to come to terms with the fact that some persons are unable or unwilling (or both) to give up a life of dependency.

Nothing is more difficult for many long-term mentally ill persons to attain and sustain than independence (Harris and Bergman 1987). The issue of supervised versus unsupervised housing provides an example (see Chapter 10). Professionals want to see their patients living in their own apartments and managing on their own, perhaps with some outpatient support. But the experience of deinstitutionalization has been that most long-term severely mentally ill persons living in unsupervised settings in the community find the ordinary stresses of managing on their own more than they can handle. After a while they tend to not take their medications, to neglect their nutrition, and to let their lives unravel and become disorganized. Eventually they find their way back to the hospital or the streets (Lamb 1984).

Mentally ill persons highly value independence, but they very often underestimate their dependency needs. Professionals need to be realistic about their patients' potential for independence, even if the patients are not.

A lack of appreciation by some professionals of the rewards of treating patients who function less well and of forming an enduring relationship over many years with both patient and family also may contribute to the focus on higher-functioning patients. Even when the patient's potential for higher functioning is limited, we can derive an immense amount of satisfaction from helping to transform a chaotic, dysphoric lifestyle into a stable one that affords at least some opportunity for pleasure and contentment for both the mentally ill person and the family.

Asylum and Sanctuary in the Community

The fact that the chronically mentally ill have been deinstitutionalized does not mean that they no longer need social support, protection, and relief (either periodic or continuous) from the pressures of life. In short, they need asylum and sanctuary *in the community* (Lamb and Peele 1984). Unfortunately, because the old state hospitals were called asylums, the word asylum took on a bad, almost sinister connotation. Only in recent years has the word again become a respectable part of our language that denotes the function of providing asylum rather than simply asylum as a place.

The concept of asylum and sanctuary becomes important because although some chronically mentally ill patients eventually attain high levels of social and vocational functioning, many others cannot meet simple demands of community living, even with long-term rehabilitative help. Many consciously limit their exposure to external stimuli and pressure, not from laziness but from a well-founded fear of failure. Professionals must realize that whatever degree of rehabilitation is possible for each patient, whether at a high or a low level of functioning, it cannot occur unless support and protection—whether from family, treatment program, therapist, or board and care home—are provided at the same time. If we do not take into account the need for asylum and sanctuary among those living in the community, it may not be possible for many patients to live in the community at all.

Involuntary Treatment

Involuntary treatment presents us with an extremely difficult dilemma. Our beliefs in civil liberties come into conflict with our concern for the welfare of our patients. This dilemma can be resolved if we believe that the mentally ill have a right to involuntary treatment (Lamb and Mills 1986; Rachlin 1975) when, because of severe mental illness, they present a serious threat to their own welfare or that of others and at the same time are not mentally competent to make a rational decision about accepting treatment.

Reaching out to patients and working to encourage them to accept help on a voluntary basis is certainly an important first step. But if that fails and the patient is at serious risk, helping professionals need to see that ethically they cannot simply stop there. As discussed in Chapter 11, there is a need for changes in the laws that will facilitate involuntary treatment for such persons or for changes in the way the laws for involuntary treatment are administered. These changes would result in patients' prompt return to acute inpatient treatment when it was clinically indicated and use of ongoing measures, such as conservatorship, commitment to outpatient treatment, and appointment of a payee for the patient's Supplemental Security Income check, when they were indicated.

What is needed is a treatment philosophy that recognizes that such external controls are a positive, even crucial, therapeutic approach for those in the long-term mentally ill population who lack the internal controls to deal with their impulses and to organize themselves to cope with life's demands. Such external controls may interrupt the self-destructive, chaotic life of a patient who is on the streets and in and out of jails and hospitals.

For instance, in some parts of California, conservatorship has become an important therapeutic modality for such persons. It is particularly useful when conservators are psychiatric social workers or persons with similar backgrounds and skills who use their court-granted authority to become a crucial source of stability and support for chronically mentally ill persons. Conservatorship, thus, can enable persons who might otherwise be long-term residents of hospitals to live in the community and achieve a considerable measure of autonomy and satisfaction in their lives.

If we do not take a firm stand on these issues, we risk being viewed by society, not to mention by the long-term mentally ill themselves, as uncaring and even inhumane. The plight of the homeless mentally ill dramatically illustrates the seriousness of this obligation.

Strategies for Making Deinstitutionalization Work

What do we need to do to get deinstitutionalization back on course? The following strategies should be considered.

- Recognize the problems that the new long-term patients face when they try to cope with the demands of living in the community.

- Let what we learn from our clinical experience with our patients determine our ideology rather than letting preconceived ideology determine what we do with our patients.
- Acknowledge that while deinstitutionalization was a positive and correct step, for some severely mentally ill persons it has gone too far. Only some long-term mentally ill now in the community need intermediate or long-term, highly structured, 24-hour residential care, but for those who do, we should provide it. When we do not, the resulting problems and debate obscure the benefits of community treatment for the great majority who do not require highly structured, continuous care.
- Truly make the long-term mentally ill our priority in public mental health in terms of both resources and funding. In making this commitment, we should join with our natural allies, the families.
- Establish a comprehensive and coordinated system of care for the long-term mentally ill.
- Refuse to settle for stopgap solutions—for instance, maintaining a system of shelters for the homeless mentally ill, instead of dealing with the underlying problem of the lack of a comprehensive system of care for the long-term mentally ill generally.
- Possess the therapeutic optimism needed to treat the long-term mentally ill, but temper this optimism with realistic, individualized goals.
- Emphasize that the long-term mentally ill are a highly heterogeneous population.
- Be aware that the values and goals of psychiatrically disabled persons may be different from those projected onto them by well-meaning professionals.
- Continue to mount a vigorous rehabilitation effort aimed at achieving higher levels of functioning, both social and vocational, for those long-term mentally ill persons who can benefit from it. At the same time, we should give high priority to those among the long-term mentally ill who function at lower levels and not focus only on persons with higher functioning.
- Realize the gratification that can be derived from helping to change the chaotic and painful life of a patient who is on the streets and in and out of jails and hospitals into a stable life that offers the possibility of at least some contentment, even if we cannot rehabilitate that patient to a high level of functioning.
- Come to grips with the bureaucracy, politics, and inefficiency of our largest cities, where the greatest number of long-term mentally ill persons live. It is there that the politics are the most complex, the pressure from special interest groups on local politicians

the most effective, the bureaucracies the largest and most cumbersome, and the battles for power and turf the fiercest (Elpers 1986; Keill 1985; Marcos 1988). There, too, the administrative costs of providing care tend to be high (often as much as 50% of the budget), leaving an insufficient amount for actual services to patients. If not corrected, these factors inevitably lead to inadequate care of the long-term mentally ill. A solution to these problems may require removing responsibility for the long-term mentally ill from the cities in favor of another administrative solution, for instance, turning the responsibility over to the states.

- Participate as mental health professionals in actively advocating involuntary treatment, both emergency and ongoing, for persons for whom it is clinically indicated.

Conclusion

We have now had more than 3 decades of experience with deinstitutionalization. Most of what we know about community treatment of the long-term mentally ill we have learned the hard way—through experience. We need to be guided by that hard-won knowledge, look at each long-term mentally ill person as an individual with unique strengths, weaknesses, and needs, and do what our experience and clinical judgment tell us is necessary to maximize the benefits of deinstitutionalization for each individual.

References

Bachrach LL: A conceptual approach to deinstitutionalization. Hosp Community Psychiatry 29:573–578, 1978

Bachrach LL: The challenge of service planning for chronic mental patients. Community Ment Health J 22:170–174, 1986

Bleuler M: A 23-year longitudinal study of 208 schizophrenics and impressions in regard to the nature of schizophrenia, in The Transmission of Schizophrenia. Edited by Rosenthal D, Ketty SS. Oxford, England, Pergamon, 1968, pp 3–12

Ciompi L: Catamnestic long-term study on the course of life and aging of schizophrenics. Schizophr Bull 6:606–618, 1980

Dorwart RA: A ten-year follow-up study of the effects of deinstitutionalization. Hosp Community Psychiatry 39:287–291, 1988

Elpers JR: Dividing the mental health dollar: the ethics of managing scarce resources. Hosp Community Psychiatry 37:671–672, 1986

Group for the Advancement of Psychiatry: The Positive Aspects of Long-Term Hospitalization in the Public Sector for Chronic Psychiatric Patients (GAP Report No 110). New York, Mental Health Materials Center, 1982

Harding CM, Brooks GW, Ashikaga T, et al: The Vermont longitudinal study of persons with severe mental illness, II: long-term outcome of subjects who retrospectively met DSM-III criteria for schizophrenia. Am J Psychiatry 144:727–735, 1987

Harris M, Bergman HC: Differential treatment planning for young adult chronic patients. Hosp Community Psychiatry 8:638–643, 1987

Hawk AB, Carpenter WT, Strauss JS: Diagnostic criteria and 5-year outcome in schizophrenia: a report from the International Pilot Study of Schizophrenia. Arch Gen Psychiatry 32:343–347, 1975

Huber G, Gross G, Schuttler R, et al: Longitudinal studies of schizophrenic patients. Schizophr Bull 6:592–605, 1980

Keill SL: Politics and public psychiatric programs. Hosp Community Psychiatry 36:1143, 1985

Lamb HR: The new asylums in the community. Arch General Psychiatry 36:129–134, 1979

Lamb HR: Structure: the neglected ingredient of community treatment. Hosp Community Psychiatry 37:1224–1228, 1980

Lamb HR: Young adult chronic patients: the new drifters. Hosp Community Psychiatry 33:465–468, 1982a

Lamb HR: Treating the Long-Term Mentally Ill. San Francisco, CA, Jossey-Bass, 1982b

Lamb HR (ed): The Homeless Mentally Ill: A Task Force Report of the American Psychiatric Association. Washington, DC, American Psychiatric Association, 1984

Lamb HR: Some reflections on treating schizophrenics. Arch Gen Psychiatry 43:1007–1011, 1986

Lamb HR: Deinstitutionalization at the crossroads. Hosp Community Psychiatry 39:941–945, 1988

Lamb HR, Mills MJ: Needed changes in law and procedure for the chronically mentally ill. Hosp Community Psychiatry 37:475–480, 1986

Lamb HR, Peele R: The need for continuing asylum and sanctuary. Hosp Community Psychiatry 35:798–802, 1984

Marcos LR: Dysfunctions in public psychiatric bureaucracies. Am J Psychiatry 145:331–334, 1988

Marcos LR, Cohen NL, Nardacci D, et al: Psychiatry takes to the streets: the New York City Initiative for the homeless mentally ill. Am J Psychiatry 147:1557–1561, 1990

Minkoff K: Beyond deinstitutionalization: a new ideology for the postinstitutional era. Hosp Community Psychiatry 38:945–950, 1987

Rachlin S: One right too many. Bull Am Acad Psychiatry Law 3:99–102, 1975

Shadish WR Jr, Bootzin RR: Nursing homes and chronic mental patients. Schizophr Bull 7:488–498, 1981

Solomon EB, Baird B, Everstine L, et al: Assessing the community care of chronic psychotic patients. Hosp Community Psychiatry 31:113–116, 1980

Talbott JA: The fate of the public psychiatric system. Hosp Community Psychiatry 36:46–50, 1985

Talbott JA, Lamb HR: Summary and recommendations, in The Homeless Mentally Ill: A Task Force Report of the American Psychiatric Association. Edited by Lamb HR. Washington, DC, American Psychiatric Association, 1984

Thomas S: A survey of the relative importance of community care facility characteristics to different consumer groups. Paper presented at the meeting of the Midwestern Psychological Association, St. Louis, MO, 1980

Tsuang M, Woolson R, Fleming J: Long-term outcome of major psychoses, I: schizophrenia and affective disorders compared with psychiatrically symptom-free surgical conditions. Arch Gen Psychiatry 36:1295–1301, 1979

World Health Organization: Schizophrenia: An International Follow-Up Study. New York, Wiley, 1979

Chapter 4

Homelessness and Mental Illness: A Transcultural Family Perspective

Harriet P. Lefley, Ph.D.
Elane M. Nuehring, Ph.D., M.S.S.W.
Evalina W. Bestman, Ph.D.

Families of mentally ill persons have obvious reasons to be concerned about homelessness. The cognitive deficits and impaired judgment that may cause a loved one to end up on the streets will also render that person exceptionally vulnerable to assault, exploitation, and life-threatening self-neglect.

As Hatfield and colleagues (1984) note, "To come to the point where one's vulnerable mentally ill relative is forced to survive as best [he or she] can in the hostile climate of an urban street is the culmination of a family's worst fear" (p. 279). These fears are compounded by guilt and self-recrimination if the family feels responsible for not having prevented the deterioration that led to this state, or even worse, for having extruded a disruptive mentally ill loved one from the family home.

What conditions contribute to the separation of a dependent, dysfunctional person from a helping network? Homelessness, like mental illness itself, is a multifaceted phenomenon. The locality, time of year, and length of time in which one has lived without shelter; current community attitudes; availability of supportive resources; and the individual's physical and psychological capability for finding and utilizing opportunities for survival are all important factors in determining how one tolerates and overcomes homelessness.

In this process, cultural variables are extremely relevant. They may affect the genesis, phenomenology, duration, and periodicity of the homeless condition, as well as the potential for change. Among persons

The authors are indebted to Mrs. Eleanor Gale of Hanson, Massachusetts, co-chairperson of the NAMI Network on Homeless and Missing Mentally Ill Persons, for information on the network.

with psychiatric disorders, cultural values and practices may determine who becomes homeless and under what conditions, who succumbs and who survives, and who may become reunited with a caring network.

In this chapter, accordingly, we deal with the relationship of families and their homeless mentally ill relatives in terms of two interrelated perspectives. In the first section, we begin with generic issues that appear to apply transculturally to almost all family situations. Because little empirical research on this subject exists, our observations are derived primarily from writings and experiences of members of the National Alliance for the Mentally Ill (NAMI), reports in family support groups, and experiences and opinions of primary consumers, many of whom have been homeless. Later, we tap into ethnographic data and some empirical research that may teach us about how homelessness of mentally ill persons is experienced in a cross-cultural context.

Common Issues Among Families of Homeless Mentally Ill Persons

The homelessness of a mentally ill person may be the result of many deficiencies and operational breakdowns. These shortcomings may be found in the individual, the familial and social network, the mental health and criminal justice systems, or societal policies whose parameters extend from housing availability to legal definitions of dangerousness to self. These definitions determine the degree to which society, including family members, can interfere with the self-destructive behavior typically associated with selective homelessness of mentally ill persons. Similarly, legal constraints affect the extent to which family members can track a disappearing mentally ill relative through the labyrinth of the service delivery system, not only in their own localities but in other cities and states.

Efforts to Locate Mentally Ill Relatives

A family may have a good idea of the city to which a relative has gravitated, or even the names of the hospitals to which he or she may have been taken. In many cases, however, hospitals refuse to share information with the family over the phone and sometimes even in person. Policies of confidentiality, designed to protect the anonymity of patients, have long plagued anxious families trying to locate a missing relative through the crisis emergency rooms and inpatient facilities of strange cities. And all too often, staff members have ensured the continued homelessness of mentally ill patients by neglecting or refusing to ask the patients for permission to talk with their families or by failing even to convey to them their family's concern before they are discharged.

The anguish of a family searching for a homeless mentally ill loved one is reflected well by a letter received by NAMI's central office. The following excerpt was published in an open letter to NAMI membership in October 1990 from president Tom Posey, who noted that NAMI receives hundreds of letters like this one every week.

> I don't know where else to turn. My son has been missing for 2 months and the police won't help me. I see all these homeless people on the streets and wonder how many, like my child, are mentally ill. My son once called the homeless "invisible people." Now he is one of them. Will anyone help him? As a father I thought I would always be able to protect and provide for my children. But instead, we are now living a nightmare. When will it end. . . .

Fortunately, NAMI operates a national Network on Homeless and Missing Mentally Ill that helps locate missing psychiatrically disabled persons and reunite them with their families. National coordinators are often able to enlist local Alliance for the Mentally ill (AMI) members and to obtain the cooperation and services of sympathetic police. Mentally ill persons listed on the national police computer are identified as endangered adults rather than as missing persons to facilitate the search and ensure appropriate handling. In the coordinator's experience, persons who have never run off before will stay away for a week or two, but will come back to their families. But the search for those who have been away longer becomes far more rigorous.

The homeless network has developed a sophisticated methodology for finding missing mentally ill persons. A coordinator contacts the Social Security Administration (SSA) to determine whether there has been any current action, although SSA will not divulge a recipient's address. The network also advertises on television and enlists the aid of the missing persons department of the police in that locality. Some police departments will take pictures of a mentally ill street person who matches a circulated description and send it to the network for identification by the family. The coordinators constantly take calls from different parts of the country and cultivate contacts at shelters, Travelers' Aid, the Salvation Army, local agencies, and state hospitals. In some states, AMI members have even trained the police in how to locate and deal with homeless mentally ill persons.

The coordinators have also developed a handbook for families of missing mentally ill persons. The book outlines a procedure for searching for a person who has disappeared and the appropriate steps for evaluating the person once found. Families are advised to contact professionals to find out how to treat a relative who has been missing.

The network also offers nationwide services to practitioners who are trying to identity homeless mentally ill persons to determine where they were previously treated and, if possible, to link them up with relatives. The following vignettes indicate how the network uses the basic identifiers of date of birth and Social Security numbers to locate missing mentally ill persons.

> NAMI received a call from a social worker in South Dakota who had found a mentally ill young man on the street. It had taken a month to learn the man's whole name and Social Security number. Because the digits indicate the state and parts of the state in which the Social Security number was first issued, the network was able to trace the number to Minneapolis. The local AMI contacted several Minneapolis psychiatric facilities where the young man may have been a patient. They were able to obtain a last known address and located the parents who were then reunited with their son.
>
> A 17-year-old schizophrenic girl had run away from her community residence in New England. She stayed with a girlfriend for a few days and then disappeared. The network subsequently received a call from an AMI member in a midwestern city, saying she had located a mentally ill street person she couldn't identify. Because the AMI member knew the girl's Social Security number, age, and birthday, the network, as in most cases, was able to match the date of birth and Social Security number with the missing young woman.

When Mentally Ill Relatives Reject Help

Most families feel a commitment to kin and will go to considerable sacrifice to provide resources for a homeless member. Some families face rejection in this endeavor, however, because their relatives will indicate they do not want to be found. There are a number of reasons why mentally ill homeless people refuse help, particularly if they have been without medication for a considerable period of time. The first is the presence of acute psychosis that precludes judgment and recognition of a life-threatening condition (Lamb and Lamb 1990).

In this situation, a psychotic person will cling to the familiar; inertia is probably less threatening than change. The patient apparently is too confused and frightened to accept help and is likely to deteriorate rapidly. Legal remedies are probably inevitable.

A somewhat more functional group of homeless mentally ill people who are able to communicate their wishes overtly reject control by others. In many cases, runaway mentally ill adults have still not resolved the conflicts of independence and dependency characteristic of adolescence and are still acting out their rebellion against parental authority. In other cases, mentally ill persons who for too long have felt dominated by the decisions and regimens of psychiatric institutions may reject help out of a desire for self-affirmation. The values of street people and domiciled people inevitably differ with respect to necessities of life. It is often hard for people who are not homeless to understand that many homeless patients, even those who have not become desensitized to the deprivations of street life, prefer their autonomy to basic creature comforts of life.

However, such individuals frequently confuse true autonomy with a desire to be left alone and to be allowed to give up. Their rejection of help from others often masks a fear of the demands of structured programs and a rejection of ordinary role responsibilities of day-to-day life. Reunification with family members will inevitably mean yielding to some measure of communal rules and regulations—whether in the shelter or in a relative's home.

Mentally ill individuals may reject help because any suggestion of control by others reminds them of one of the most fearful aspects of the psychotic condition, the loss of the known self. For persons with multiple hospitalization experiences, this feeling of loss is compounded by loss of control of one's own history. In our mainstream culture, which values individualism to the highest degree, these fears can be exacerbated by the paternalism of others. The message that others know what is best—that they have the right to take over all decision making from the patient—can speed decompensation in some individuals even faster than physical neglect. As we shall see, decision making by others is far less likely to be perceived as a threat in more traditional ethnic groups in which family paternalism is a cultural norm.

Finally, help is sometimes rejected because of antagonism toward family members. The anger may stem from the family's participation in previous involuntary commitments. Hostility may also be the result of prior conflicts, recollections of real or imaginary abuse, resentment because the family members cannot or will not have the patient live with them, or the patient's envy of the relatives' more fortunate life conditions and status. Homeless patients may feel tainted and inferior because of their psychiatric history and current destitution and then project these feelings onto the family. They may try to alienate those who profess to love them and test the limits of their love with angry rejection.

It may take a great deal of gentle urging and patience to persuade a homeless mentally ill person to accept proffered aid. In most cases, the

effort is best made by service providers because family members sometimes lack the skill, patience, and emotional distance to conduct this
campaign. Family members frequently have endured a history of toler-
ating disruptive behaviors, spending enormous amounts of time and
money in negotiating the mental health system, and sacrificing a good
deal of their own plans and those of other family members in dealing
with the patient's illness. Many have suffered verbal and sometimes
physical abuse from patients. If the system does not offer decent housing and good case management, family members may find themselves
in the position of cajoling a person who has caused numerous hardships into a life situation that may renew hardships for themselves.

Whatever the reason that mentally ill relatives reject help, the
families' options are limited. They can hope to convince the homeless
relative to seek or accept help; try to provide their own case management; offer housing and resolution of the relative's dependency needs,
which may upset their own lives and be maladaptive for other family
members; or seek involuntary commitment for the relative. The latter
course often generates a self-defeating loop. Families must seek ex
parte orders to hospitalize the patient against his or her will and face
repeated scenarios of partial stabilization and discharge that may return the patient to the streets.

Families play a delicate role when they try to balance their own desires for their relatives' safety with a patient's desire to control his or
her own fate. This is particularly difficult when the family members
feel they have a consensual, reality-based view of what is right and
necessary in life, based on commonly held social values and believe the
patient's view would be perceived as unrealistic or even delusional by
most sensible people. Yet the family's urge to protect the patient cannot
be restricted to the physical dangers of homelessness. It is essential that
both families and service providers try to protect the patient from af-
fronts to his or her dignity as a human being. It is doubly important to
evidence respect for the avowed wishes of individuals whose illness
embodies threats to the integrity and control of the self.

Iatrogenic Homelessness

Sometimes, the mental health provider system tends to facilitate rather
than prevent homelessness of its most psychotic patients. These cases
involve 1) failure to erect barriers against housing eviction and loss of
therapeutic contact, 2) rejection of communication with families, and
3) provision of counter-therapeutic advice to caregivers.

The community-based mental health system is effective in preventing homelessness only to the extent that it provides comprehensive

services, including housing, with an emphasis on follow-up and continuity of care. Mental health professionals have been extremely inconsistent in their attitudes toward housing adult patients with their families, who frequently consist of aging parents incapable of fulfilling a permanent caregiver's role (Lefley 1987). Providers have often used families as a first and last resort for postdischarge housing while at the same time advocating against family tenure.

When alternative housing is arranged, however, the providers rarely insist on a no-reject, no-eject policy that ensures that persons with psychotic disorders, regardless of difficult behavior, will be referred and maintained within the system. In too many community-based services, the patient is placed in a board-and-care home, single-room-occupancy unit, or other housing operated by landlords who will evict their tenants for disruptive behavior. While landlords may legitimately refuse to tolerate abusive or bizarre behavior and property destruction, it is not legitimate for the mental health system to allow an evicted mentally ill patient to return to the streets.

Before the days of case management, that was all too common. Lacking continuity of care, patients placed in community residences frequently stopped taking medications, decompensated, and erupted in psychotic behavior that led to their loss of residence. The system's failure to provide ongoing contact and oversight often led directly to the homelessness of its sickest patients. Even today, when most states have developed case management systems, the staff-patient ratio is often so unrealistic that case managers cannot find suitable housing for all of the people in their case loads. In many situations, also, transitional housing has been phased out to provide added case management, so that oversight is provided but without adequate resources to compensate for the loss of these residential units.

Other iatrogenic factors that contribute to homelessness are the noncommunicative distance and even hostility maintained toward families by many professionals. This approach is in sharp contrast to practices in other parts of the world, where families are often welcomed and treated as partners in service delivery (Lefley 1985). In our culture, these behaviors are an outgrowth of older etiological paradigms that considered the family culpable for the patient's illness or eschewed communication with the patient's family because of possible contamination of transference and the therapeutic alliance.

Many families have been kept in such profound ignorance regarding the nature of their relatives' illnesses that they have no basis on which to make judgments or develop role expectations consistent with the patients' actual capabilities. Thus, parents, thinking that their son or daughter is cured after a hospital stay, may insist that he or she perform in roles that are perfectly appropriate but that a mentally ill person is incapable of fulfilling.

This expectation can generate a preventable cycle of psychotic reaction, family disruption, and rehospitalization. The ordeal of the psychotic episode is so devastating (Group for the Advancement of Psychiatry 1986; Lefley 1987) that after several such cycles, the family may be wary of taking the patient back. To date, despite the demonstrated success of family psychoeducation (Hogarty et al. 1986), few hospitals or community mental health centers offer family education as a service to their patients.

Mental health professionals' failure to communicate with families has typically been rationalized by the mandate for confidentiality (Bernheim 1990). Although the initial aims were for practitioners to avoid revealing the patient's disclosures and for clinical facilities to protect patients' anonymity, confidentiality has subsequently become a means of withholding from the family information that may be essential for the patient's survival (Zipple et al. 1990). While confidentiality is important for protecting the patient's rights, the avowed purpose of avoiding identification of mental hospital patients has also prevented families from locating their missing relatives. In arbitrarily denying information to families, rather than allowing patients to make the decision for revelation and contact, mental health providers fail to use two important therapeutic tools: to empower patients to control their own confidentiality and to facilitate the patient's renewed bonding with a needed support system.

At the other end of the spectrum are professionals who offer families counterproductive advice. Too often this advice is also based on tenuous etiological models. Some professionals advise extruding the patient from the home on the assumption that families reinforce psychotic behavior by fostering dependency. Both psychodynamic and systems theories contend that allowing the patient to live with the family is countertherapeutic. The rationale is that the family acts to impede separation and individuation, often because the family system needs the patient's symptoms to avoid confronting other problems that threaten it.

The premise of such theories seems to be that once free of the family, the patient will no longer need to act out his or her symptomatology and, moreover, will become motivated to seek independent solutions for survival. When the patient is seriously mentally ill, this expectation is astonishingly naive and may even be life-threatening.

A case history described by Hatfield and associates (1984) is an excellent example of how psychodynamic attributions of dependency and concomitant "tough love" cures may create a path to homelessness for difficult psychotic patients. This rather typical case involves a psychotic 25-year-old man with a pattern of stopping medications and re-volving-door crisis admissions. When his desperate mother sought guidance from a psychiatrist, she was advised to evict her son from their apartment and refuse his periodic importuning to return home. After her son spent weeks of homeless wandering and was subjected to severe assaults, infection, and sickness, the mother realized, "[This was] a crazy solution to a difficult problem. Today, 10 years later, Mrs. J. is haunted by the terrible experience of seeing her son on the street . . . feels terribly guilty, and has lost trust in a mental health profession that could offer no better solution to her son's problems" (p. 288).

Unfortunately, there are many similar cases in which advice by mental health professionals to extrude a mentally ill relative has led to dire consequences of homelessness, incarceration, and exposure to severe brutalities that could only make the illness worse.

Cross-Cultural Aspects of Homelessness

The anthropological and cross-cultural psychiatric literature suggests that family structure and belief systems may play an important part in patterns of homelessness. Culture determines whether family structure is likely to be nuclear or extended; whether normal adult development decrees separation of unmarried adult children from their parents' home; whether a disabled family member is likely to live with or apart from blood relations; and whether the family is likely to expel or retain a nonproductive and perhaps disruptive member.

The availability and accessibility of an auxiliary helping network is often culturally patterned. Residential proximity of kin, beliefs regarding familial obligations, and tolerance of deviant behavior are all likely to be involved in patterns of homelessness.

Cultural factors may also determine whether a homeless person lives with relatives intermittently or whether he or she (typically he) is homeless on a continuous basis. These factors will also determine whether homeless members follow patterns of migration through an extended kinship network. The culture may offer a homeless person the possibility of staying with one relative or another for a few days, weeks, or even longer or, alternatively, tapping known sources of community help for food and money.

Family structure is extremely important because it determines whether caregivers can tolerate the strains of living with a seriously mentally ill individual. Forty years ago, noted medical sociologists Parsons and Fox (1952) predicted that the nuclear family of the Western world would be incapable of taking care of persons with chronic illnesses. They suggested that because typically only one or two adults were available to take caregiving roles, there would be little margin for "shock absorption" and considerable danger of emotional overload because of the demands of illness. Common elements of family burden have since been confirmed across a range of long-term developmental, physical, and psychiatric conditions (Lefley 1987). The extent of family burden in mental illness, of course, is an ongoing issue (Noh and Turner 1987).

Concomitantly, a cross-cultural literature has emerged, linking family structure, family burden, and prognosis in schizophrenia. This literature suggests that high expressed emotion in patients' families (a tendency toward hostile criticism and emotional overinvolvement) is relatively rare both in developing countries (Wig et al. 1987) and in traditional ethnic groups in the United States (Jenkins et al. 1986). Leff (1988) has linked the dual phenomena of low expressed emotion and better prognosis for schizophrenia in developing countries (Sartorius et al. 1986) to the extended or joint family structure of these cultures.

The assumption behind Leff's conclusion is that the availability of multiple caregivers diffuses burden and defuses conflict in contrast to the overcharged atmosphere of the nuclear family of the West. Other commentators have linked a more benign course of illness with a cultural worldview that embodies tolerance of aberrant behavior, acceptance of fate, and belief in supernatural causality (Jenkins et al. 1986; Lefley 1990; Lin and Kleinman 1988).

In the United States, ethnic minority cultures typically have been more communally or group oriented and less focused on individual needs, in contrast to mainstream middle-class culture. Lin and Kleinman (1988) have suggested that sociocentric cultures tend to be characterized by long-term social relationships, extended helping networks, and little social isolation. Ethnic minority status has also coexisted with lower socioeconomic status and in many cases larger family size compared with the small nuclear family. Under these conditions, crowded housing has been a normative reality, and sharing a residence is consistent with a value system that shares resources within the group.

In extended African American families, for example, the worldview is that everyone has a right to be housed, but not necessarily a right to separate housing. Families are expected to share a roof with relatives who do not have one. In group-oriented cultures, proprietary values may be very different from those of the homeowner, whose home symbolizes achievement and status rather than simply a place of shelter.

We may hypothesize that in traditional subcultures with group-oriented values, mentally ill persons are more likely to be incorporated in a familial or quasifamilial setting, either permanently or intermittently, and are less likely to be voluntarily homeless. However, substance-induced violence and other highly disruptive behaviors are unlikely to be tolerated in any cultural setting; and since these behaviors pit individual against group needs, they may be particularly upsetting in a sociocentric context (Tessler et al. 1990).

Data on Homelessness and Families

The empirical literature on families of mentally ill adults, on homelessness, on homeless mentally ill persons, and on homeless families is expanding rapidly. However, no research of which we are aware addresses in any depth families whose mentally ill relatives are also homeless, either from the perspective of the family or of the homeless individual. Furthermore, most studies of homelessness present only limited insight into family dimensions as one aspect of the social support systems of homeless persons.

A large-scale investigation of homelessness in South Florida, however, has provided some interesting findings about families and mentally ill homeless. In addition, we have begun an investigation of family relations of homeless mentally ill clients of the New Horizons Community Mental Health Center in Miami. Some of the findings are summarized below.

South Florida Homelessness Study

A comprehensive study of homelessness in South Florida was conducted in 1988–1989 by a collaborative team of seven highly experienced social scientists from four universities (Fike et al. 1990). The research involved six interrelated substudies that focused on the metropolitan areas of Palm Beach County, Fort Lauderdale, and Miami. Three of the substudies—those by Andrew Cherry, George Warheit, and J. Bryan Page and associates—are of particular interest here, although none focused in depth on variables relating to families of homeless persons. Based on his four stages of enumeration in shelters, agencies, and street sites in three South Florida counties, Cherry (1990) estimated the total of homeless individuals ranged from 6,472 in November 1988 to 7,284 in August 1989. Metropolitan Miami-Dade County accounted for over half of the homeless population. Most homeless persons in Miami-Dade County, as in New York City, are African American (56%), 14% are Hispanic, and the balance are non-Hispanic whites.

Cherry's structured interviews with a sample of 448 homeless people highlighted a finding consistent with our expectations: 37% of African American and 7% of white respondents had family in the local area; another 21% of African American and 10% of white respondents had family somewhere in the state. A total of 82% of African American and 71% of white respondents had been in contact with their families in the past year, and 79% and 64% of the two groups, respectively, had visited with their families in the past year. These data suggest that the general population of homeless adults, of both racial groups, are more likely than severely mentally ill homeless people to remain in touch with family.

George Warheit, a well-known psychiatric epidemiologist, conducted extensive structured interviews with 107 men and 103 women in Miami homeless shelters focusing on mental illness and substance abuse. He asked hundreds of questions, including all items on the Diagnostic Interview Schedule. He prepared a detailed analysis with controls for race and gender. Warheit found a 58% prevalence rate of severe mental illness among homeless adult men and women in Miami, which was much higher than the average rate (25%) reported in other studies of homeless in other urban areas of the United States. Summarizing the findings, Fike and colleagues (1990) wrote:

> About 15% seem to be schizophrenic and about 43% seem to suffer from severe depression. The depression appears to be more than circumstantial. It would be longstanding, present in better times as well as worse times, and debilitating. *Current efforts of the mental health system have been inadequate to bring these people into the system and to rehabilitate them.* (p. 14, original emphasis)

In Warheit's sample, 67% indicated they used drugs. African American males were the most likely to report having used drugs (82%). Only 36% of Warheit's sample, however, met criteria for having had a diagnosis of drug abuse at any time in their lives. The group with the highest rate of drug abuse diagnoses, affecting approximately two-thirds, was white American men. White males also had the highest rates of alcohol abuse or dependence (71%), and 37% met criteria for having ever had a DSM-III-R diagnosis (American Psychiatric Association 1987). If serious mental illness and substance abuse are combined, recognizing that there is some obvious overlap, it becomes clear that Warheit's shelter sample reflects a high rate of impairment.

Family linkages were apparently tenuous in a good half of the cases. Warheit (1990) noted:

> About two-thirds of the sample said they had close relatives to help them as needed. . . . Our estimation is that no more than one-half the sample rarely, if ever, sought assistance from close relatives or family members.

... Only about half the sample believed they could get assistance from their families, even if their problems were serious ones. A small proportion expected to return to living with family, with about a fifth of women of both races and black men, and 5% of white men, expressing this anticipation. (p. 41)

The third South Florida homelessness substudy of interest is an ethnography conducted by anthropologist J. Bryan Page and his associates. After mapping the areas in which homeless people lived and sampling the sites where groups greater than five persons congregated, the researchers stated:

There is a fundamental difference based on ethnicity, among the homeless. Among Hispanics and Haitians, it is a general cultural principle that the only way one can become completely homeless is losing one's family. If there is family around, one can live with them in almost all cases. African American and Anglo-American homeless individuals often will have family but will be estranged from them. Probably these are central facts explaining the low proportions of Hispanics and Haitians among the homeless. *This cultural difference should be noted in transitional programs, with family contact relevant in all cases and the reuniting of families especially prominent as a goal in Hispanic and Haitian cases.* (Fike et al. 1990, p. 12, original emphasis)

The New Horizons Project for Homeless Mentally Ill Persons

We have begun to investigate family relations of homeless mentally ill clients of the New Horizons Community Mental Health Center in Miami. It is possible to make some preliminary observations now based on an inspection of clients' case records. Because both the cross-cultural literature and the South Florida study suggest there are cultural differences in the genesis and characteristics of homelessness, we have been interested in studying the role of ethnic background in experiences of homelessness in this sample.

New Horizons is a comprehensive community mental health center that has served an inner-city, multiethnic catchment area for more than 16 years. Affiliated with the University of Miami department of psychiatry, New Horizons for many years employed a model of culturally sensitive treatment in which seven ethnic community teams provided services to the major groups in the catchment area: African American, Bahamian, Cuban, Haitian, Puerto Rican, and white and African American elderly (Lefley and Bestman 1984). The academic-practitioner staff subsequently developed a national cross-cultural training institute for mental health professionals (Lefley and Pedersen 1986).

The center has unique capabilities for working with multicultural groups, and its current homeless program serves a rich ethnic mix of clients. Initiated by the National Institute of Mental Health Community Support Program (CSP) and McKinney funds, the program offers housing, day treatment, vocational rehabilitation, and an array of outpatient and case management services to homeless persons with a diagnosed mental illness.

We sought to identify material in case records that would expand our understanding of families, culture, and homelessness among mentally ill adults. A random sample of 20% of active cases was examined. Consistent with the findings of the South Florida Homelessness Studies, New Horizons' homeless clients are predominantly African American. Hence, a repeat random sample of remaining non-Hispanic white and Hispanic clients was drawn to even the numbers for comparison. Cases were eliminated if the individual did not exhibit severe mental illness based on a DSM-III-R diagnosis of a major mental disorder or had not had three or more psychiatric inpatient episodes.

This process yielded a total group of 59 homeless and severely mentally ill adults. The racial breakdown was 36% African Americans, 32% Hispanics (primarily Cubans but also Puerto Ricans and other Central and South Americans), 22% non-Hispanic whites, and 10% Haitians. Forty-nine subjects, or 83%, were male; the mean age was 37 ± 10 years. Thirty-five subjects had been diagnosed as schizophrenic; 7 had major mood disorders; and 13 had dual diagnoses of mental illness and substance abuse or addiction. Over 80% had had multiple admissions to psychiatric inpatient programs; seven had had only one recorded hospitalization, and four had never been inpatients. Forty-two percent came from relatively large families of three or more siblings. This was more likely to be true for the African Americans (53%) and Haitians (60%) than for the Hispanics (38%) and white Americans (20%).

Case records often indicated that the client was unwilling to discuss his or her family or provided vague, noncommittal information for the psychosocial history. In any event, rich, qualitative family data were unfortunately not forthcoming from the records. However, one variable was always carefully documented on both the agency's incoming referral form and its financial and demographic face sheet: the name and address of a contact person named by the client and that person's relationship to the client.

Consistent with our assumptions about minority families, race or ethnicity was associated with a person's contact of record ($\chi^2 = 27$, $df = 15$, $P = .03$). The records of the 13 non-Hispanic white clients were the most likely not to contain the name of a contact person (46%). The 21 African Americans were more likely than any other group to name their mothers (38%). If mother, sister, father, brother, and adult child are combined into one nuclear family category, the six Haitian clients were almost sure to name some nuclear family member (80%). A member of the nuclear family was named by 62% of African Americans, 41% of Hispanics, and 24% of white Americans.

Only six clients, but no white Americans, named an extended family member (aunt, uncle, cousin, or grandparent). Eleven listed an unrelated friend or ex-spouse; most of these were non-Hispanic whites and Cuban refugees with no family members living stateside.

In a pilot effort to test a protocol for further data collection, the authors also conducted structured interviews in focus groups with 18 members of the homeless project, 15 men and 3 women. Included were eight African American and six Hispanic men and women and four non-Hispanic white men. Preliminary findings indicated that at least half of each group were in contact with local or distant family, and that 75% of the African Americans, 66% of the Hispanics, and 25% of the white men had lived with a family member within the last 5 years.

Minorities were less likely to have been separated from their families for long periods of time and were also less likely to blame family members for their homeless condition. However, family deterioration, with substance abuse components, was cited prominently as the reason for homelessness by African Americans. It will be of great interest to see if these patterns persist when the interviewing process is expanded to include a larger number of homeless mentally ill persons and their families.

Conclusions

Data from a variety of sources are beginning to indicate cultural differences in families' adaptation to the mental illness of a loved one. A recent study by Tessler and his associates (1990) reported that African American and white families differ significantly about the aspects of a family members' mental illness that are experienced as most burdensome. For African American families, disruptive behavior is most difficult; for white families, the patient's failure to fulfill role responsibilities in the home causes the most disturbance. It is of interest that most African Americans in our New Horizons focus groups were separated from their families because of substance-induced disruptive behaviors.

Homelessness, the separation of people from their support networks, suggests that the homeless person either lacks or is estranged from the family. In the latter case, a mentally ill person may be too sick or too angry to seek out kin. Anger comes about when the mentally ill person blames the family for perceived wrongs, ranging from their fail-

ure to prevent involuntary commitment to their inability to fulfill unrealistic and often grandiose expectations. A young man will not go
home because he fantasizes that his sister stole the royalty checks for
the hit songs that he wrote, although neither songs nor checks were
ever a reality. Another believes the family is withholding a massive in-
heritance. Still another is furious because nobody bailed him out of jail,
although the family had no way of knowing where or when he was
incarcerated.

A local success story came about when siblings, who had long tried
to get their psychotic sister off the street, enlisted a local newspaper
reporter to do a story about a schizophrenic bag lady. Cleaned up and
medicated, the former bag lady now lives in an apartment affiliated
with a psychosocial rehabilitation center and works full-time in competitive employment.

Some family members go to great lengths to retrieve a mentally ill
relative from homelessness. Social exchange theory would predict that
these efforts might be particularly urgent if the mentally ill member
had made a contribution to the family in the past. A story in *The New
York Times Magazine* of African American families in Chicago housing
projects described how a formerly hard-working member of a family
decompensated, spent some time in a mental hospital, and later became homeless. In this family, George, the patient, had been "the
steady, dutiful son, the only one willing to throw himself wholeheart-
edly into a strong-back trade. . . . Over the years, he had baby-sat,
brought over food when the family ran out of food, and otherwise
acted as a stabilizing force." But various stressors in his life "pushed
him over the edge into emotional instability" (Lemann 1991, p. 36).
After psychiatric hospitalization, George somehow ended up homeless
on the West Coast. His was a very large, economically stressed family
with many dysfunctional members. But one of George's brothers left
Chicago to look for him, found him on the streets of Los Angeles, and
brought him home for Thanksgiving.

Homelessness continues to be a tragedy for society, the mentally ill,
and their families. We have discussed the relationship of families and
the homeless from a cross-cultural perspective because there seem to
be some lessons to be learned from the way other cultural groups treat
their mentally ill citizens and how they view their families. For example, Jenkins and her associates (1986) clearly showed that Mexican
Americans living in Los Angeles tended to be tolerant and accepting of
a schizophrenic family member and to be highly noncritical compared
with Anglo-American families.

An analysis holding social class constant found that 57% of Mexican
American families were characterized by low levels of expressed emo-

tion compared with 17% of their Anglo-American counterparts (*P* = .003) (Jenkins and Karno 1990). As Page has noted (Fike et al. 1990), there are very few Hispanic and Haitian homeless persons, mentally ill or otherwise, in an area of the country that has large numbers of these ethnic groups. Our New Horizons data on homeless mentally ill persons indicated that white patients were significantly less likely than members of African American and Hispanic groups to name a relative on whom they could rely.

We have attempted in this chapter to present some hypotheses on a subject that is almost totally missing from the research literature—the families of homeless mentally ill persons. Although much of this chapter has focused on the family's experience, culled from the NAMI network and similar sources, our empirical data have been limited to tangential information from an existing research base on homeless mentally ill persons. So far, no systematic attempt to research the family perspective has been undertaken. It is time for the cursory attention paid thus far to family issues in studies of homeless persons to be enriched by more complex and detailed investigations.

To this end, we have tried to make a case for exploring kinship networks and relationships in cross-cultural perspective. The ethnographic literature suggests that homelessness of mentally ill individuals is less likely to occur in cultures in which families expect to take care of their disabled relatives, in which relatives tend to tolerate rather than criticize bizarre behavior, and in which large kinship networks offer alternative helping resources to alleviate burden.

In these cultures, paternalistic attitudes by family members are more likely to be culturally normative and, thus, less likely to be resented by patients as threats to their integrity as separate human beings. Cultures that value interdependence rather than individualism are more likely to accept dependency and less likely to transmit disparaging messages to their disabled members (Lefley 1985, 1990).

Yet even traditional cultures face reduced housing resources and diminishing helping networks, and nuclear families are rapidly replacing the joint families of old. In the modern world, these cultural norms of family caregiving will not continue indefinitely. It seems evident that social and legal solutions must be found to provide permanent community housing for the mentally ill in order to prevent their being catapulted into homelessness and to alleviate family responsibilities both now and in the future.

References

American Psychiatric Association: Diagnostic and Statistical Manual of Mental Disorders, 3rd Edition, Revised. Washington, DC, American Psychiatric Association, 1987

Bernheim KF: Principles of professional and family collaboration. Hosp Community Psychiatry 41:1353–1355, 1990

Cherry AL Jr: The South Florida Homelessness Studies, Vol 1: The Magnitude and Nature of Homelessness in South Florida. Unpublished report. Miami, FL, Barry University, 1990

Fike DF, Cherry AL, Dluhy MJ, et al: The South Florida Homelessness Studies of 1989: A Summary of Key Findings. Unpublished report. Miami, FL, Barry University, 1990

Group for the Advancement of Psychiatry: A Family Affair: Helping Families Cope With Mental Illness: A Guide for the Professions (GAP Report No 119). New York, Brunner/Mazel, 1986

Hatfield AB, Farrell E, Starr S: The family's perspective on the homeless, in The Homeless Mentally Ill: A Task Force Report of the American Psychiatric Association. Edited by Lamb HR. Washington, DC, American Psychiatric Press, 1984, pp 279–300

Hogarty GE, Anderson CM, Reiss DJ, et al: Family psychoeducation, social skills training, and maintenance chemotherapy in the aftercare treatment of schizophrenia. Arch Gen Psychiatry 43:633–642, 1986

Jenkins JH, Karno M: Inside the black box called "expressed emotion": a theoretical analysis of the construct in psychiatric research. Unpublished paper. Cleveland, OH, Case Western Reserve University, 1990

Jenkins JH, Karno M, de la Selva A, et al: Expressed emotion in cross-cultural context: familial responses to schizophrenic illness among Mexican Americans, in Treatment of Schizophrenia: Family Assessment and Intervention. Edited by Goldstein MJ, Hand, I, Halweg K. Berlin, Springer-Verlag, 1986, pp 35–49

Lamb HR, Lamb D: Factors contributing to homelessness among the chronically and severely mentally ill. Hosp Community Psychiatry 41:301–305, 1990

Leff J: Psychiatry Around the Globe: A Transcultural View, 2nd Edition. London, Gaskell, 1988

Lefley HP: Families of the mentally ill in cross-cultural perspective. Psychosocial Rehabilitation Journal 8:57–75, 1985

Lefley HP: Aging parents as caregivers of mentally ill adult children: an emerging social problem. Hosp Community Psychiatry 38:1063–1070, 1987

Lefley HP: Culture and chronic mental illness. Hosp Community Psychiatry 41:277–286, 1990

Lefley HP, Bestman EW: Community mental health and minorities: a multiethnic approach, in The Pluralistic Society: A Community Mental Health Perspective. Edited by Sue S, Moore T. New York, Human Sciences Press, 1984, pp 116–148

Lefley HP, Pedersen PB (eds): Cross-Cultural Training for Mental Health Professionals. Springfield, IL, Charles C Thomas, 1986

Lemann N: Four generations in the projects. New York Times Magazine, January 13, 1991, pp 16–21, 36–38, 49

Lin K-M, Kleinman AM: Psychopathology and clinical course of schizophrenia: a cross-cultural perspective. Schizophr Bull 14:555–567, 1988

Noh S, Turner RJ: Living with psychiatric patients: implications for the mental health of family members. Soc Sci Med 25:263–271, 1987

Parsons T, Fox RC: Illness, therapy, and the modern urban American family. Journal of Social Issues 8:31–44, 1952

Sartorius N, Jablensky A, Korten A, et al: Early manifestations and first contact incidence of schizophrenia in different cultures. Psychol Med 16:909–928, 1986

Tessler RC, Fisher GA, Gamache GM: Dilemmas of kinship: mental illness and the modern American family. Unpublished paper. Amherst, MA, University of Massachusetts Social & Demographic Research Institute, 1990

Warheit GM: The South Florida Homelessness Studies, Vol 3: Mental Health and Psychosocial Well-Being Among Shelter Residents in South Florida. Unpublished report. Miami, FL, Barry University, 1990

Wig NN, Menon K, Bedi H, et al: Distribution of expressed emotion components among relatives of schizophrenic patients in Aarhus and Chandigarh. Br J Psychiatry 151:160–165, 1987

Zipple AM, Langle S, Spaniol L, et al: Client confidentiality and the family's need to know: strategies for resolving the conflict. Community Ment Health J 26:533–545, 1990

Chapter 5

Mental Health Problems Among Homeless Persons: A Review of Epidemiological Research From 1980 to 1990

Pamela J. Fischer, Ph.D.
Robert E. Drake, M.D., Ph.D.
William R. Breakey, M.B., F.R.C.Psych.

In this chapter we provide an overview of representative epidemiological research conducted during the 1980s concerning the homeless mentally ill population. Our discussion emphasizes findings from studies of homeless populations in which people with mental illness are compared with those without mental illness and, where empirical data are available, with those in household surveys.

The daunting methodologic problems in studying homeless mentally ill populations are discussed by Bachrach in this volume (Chapter 2) and by Fischer (1991) and others (Lovell et al., in press; Morrissey and Dennis 1986; Robertson 1986) elsewhere. Because methods used for sampling, diagnosis, and other assessments vary from study to study, great caution must be exercised in generalizing from a particular study. Nevertheless, a series of carefully designed epidemiological studies in recent years has led to certain general conclusions regarding the prevalence of mental disorders in homeless people and the characteristics of homeless mentally ill individuals.

Prevalence

Much of the research between 1980 and 1990 addressed the prevalence of mental disorders among particular homeless populations. Most

The chapter was adapted from a review prepared for and funded by the National Institute on Alcohol Abuse and Alcoholism and the National Institute of Mental Health (Fischer PJ: Alcohol, Drug Abuse and Mental Health Problems Among Homeless Persons: A Review of the Literature, 1980–1990. Rockville, MD, U.S. Department of Health and Human Services, 1991).

studies focused on single people living in shelters. Some examined young mothers. Few included men and women in such a way that their clinical characteristics could be compared, and few attempted to sample systematically from populations on the streets. Because of the heterogeneity of research designs and samples, results varied greatly. The prevalence of mental health problems ranged from 2% to 90%, alcohol problems from 4% to 86%, and other drug problems from 1% to 70%—ranges that, obviously, are too wide to be useful in projecting needs for services (Fischer 1991). As shown in Table 5–1, prevalence estimates were affected by assessment methods and sampling sites.

Using epidemiologic techniques to reduce these ranges, Fischer (1991) estimated that about one-third of homeless adults have mental health problems (about one-quarter of men and nearly half of women), whereas rates for family samples (nearly two-fifths) are intermediate between single men and women. Median rates reported for children (43%) and youth (52%) are among the highest reported. Alcohol problems are observed in about half of homeless men—more than twice the rate reported among homeless women. Between 10% and 20% of homeless men and women have drug problems, but homeless adolescents

Table 5–1.   Recent estimates of prevalence of alcohol, drug, and mental health problems among homeless populations, by method of assessment and sampling site

Study variable	Alcohol		Drug		Mental health	
	No. of studies	Prevalence (%)	No. of studies	Prevalence (%)	No. of studies	Prevalence (%)
Assessment method						
Psychiatric examination	6	8.0–68.0	6	1.0–23.1	6	12.3–48.6
Standardized scale	16	16.1–66.8	9	8.0–48.0	24	19.0–89.3
Prior/current treatment	8	13.0–45.3	4	6.0–14.0	30	10.6–59.0
Records review	25	6.9–80.0	19	1.7–70.0	16	10.6–52.8
Self-report	29	4.0–86.0	25	2.0–61.2	2	18.8–54.0
Provider assessment	3	12.4–44.7	3	2.3–38.0	11	2.0–68.6
Total	87	4.0–86.0	66	1.0–70.0	89	2.0–89.3
Sampling site						
Clinic/hospital	13	12.6–76.0	10	1.9–70.0	9	12.3–52.8
Shelter	51	7.0–86.0	37	1.0–61.2	49	12.0–89.3
SRO	4	4.0–41.7	2	12.5–31.0	1	54.2

may have twice the rate of drug problems as older homeless people. Around one-fifth of homeless people have both a mental health and a substance use disorder (including both drugs and alcohol). Tessler (1990) reviewed a smaller set of studies that used standardized instruments and arrived at similar estimates.

Several studies, shown in Table 5–2, contrasted homeless samples with community populations, usually from the Epidemiologic Catchment Area (ECA) household survey (Regier et al. 1984). In general, the rate and distribution of specific disorders differed substantially in homeless populations compared with the household population of the ECA study. Anxiety disorders, major affective disorders, and substance use disorders were more common than the major mental illnesses in the

Table 5–2.   Prevalence of selected DSM-III disorders in the combined five-site ECA household survey population (US-ECA) and in various homeless populations reported from 1980 to 1990

Study variable	US-ECA	Philadelphia	New York City	Boston	Los Angeles
Reference	Regier et al. 1988	Arce et al. 1983	Lipton et al. 1983	Bassuk 1984	Koegel et al. 1988
N	18,571	179	90	78	328
Sampling site	Households	Emergency shelter	Psychiatric emergency room	Shelters	Shelters, street
Male (%)	41.0	78.0	75.6	83.3	95.4
Diagnostic method	DIS[a]	Psychiatric exam	Psychiatric exam	Psychiatric exam	DIS[a] exam
DSM-III disorders					
No disorder	67.8	15.6	0[b]	NR	NR
Schizophrenia	1.3	37.4	72.2	30.3	13.1
Major affective	8.3	11.2	6.7	9.2	29.5
Dementia	1.3	5.0	NR	NR	3.4
Substance abuse	6.4	24.6	4.4	NR	69.2
Alcohol	3.3	20.1	NR	28.9	62.9
Drug	5.9	3.4	NR	NR	30.8
Mixed	NR	1.1	NR	NR	NR
Anxiety disorders	14.6	NR	NR	NR	17.6
Mental retardation	NR	2.2	NR	1.3	NR
Personality disorders	NR	6.7	12.2	21.0	6.1
Antisocial personality	2.5	1.1	NR	NR	20.8

household population, whereas the severe and disabling disorders predominated in samples of homeless persons. The rates of schizophrenia, dementia, mental retardation, antisocial personality disorder, substance use disorder, and of multiple coexisting disorders were particularly high in homeless populations (Fischer 1991).

Men in the homeless sample collected as part of the Baltimore ECA study were, for example, almost twice as likely to have a DSM-III mental disorder (American Psychiatric Association 1980) as were men of similar age living in households. The magnitude of difference between homeless men and household men was more than fourfold for affective disorders; threefold for schizophrenia, antisocial personality and cog-

Table 5–2, cont'd. Prevalence of selected DSM-III disorders in the combined five-site ECA household survey population (US-ECA) and in various homeless populations reported from 1980 to 1990

Study variable	U.S.	California	Baltimore	Buffalo	Baltimore
Reference	Rosenheck et al. 1988	Vernez et al. 1988	Breakey et al. 1989	Toro & Wall 1989	Fischer et al. 1986a
N	4,984	315	203	76	51
Sampling site	VA clinics	Shelters, street	Shelters, jail, soup kitchen	Shelter, street	Shelters
Male (%)	98.6	70.8	61.6	78.9	94.1
Diagnostic method	Psychiatric exam	DIS screener	Psychiatric exam	DIS, abbreviated	DIS[a]
DSM-III disorders					
No disorder	2.7	NR	15.7	27.4	21.6
Schizophrenia	12.3	11.0	10.5	1.4	2.0
Major affective	14.0	22.0	21.7	15.1	13.7
Dementia	2.2	NR	2.0	14.5	7.8
Substance abuse	NR	69.0	41.7	65.8	70.6
Alcohol	55.2	NR	34.6	52.1	NR
Drug	18.4	NR	16.8	37.1	NR
Mixed	NR	NR	NR	NR	NR
Anxiety disorders	2.3	NR	34.1	NR	39.2
Mental retardation	NR	NR	NR	NR	NR
Personality disorders	18.3	NR	42.0	NR	NR
Antisocial personality	NR	NR	14.4	37.1	15.7

nitive impairment; and twofold for substance abuse and anxiety disorders (Fischer et al. 1986b). Rates of mental disorder in a later Baltimore study of homeless persons remained high even in comparison to the low-income segment of the ECA household survey (Breakey et al. 1989, 1990). For example, the rate of schizophrenia was three times greater in poor (1.8%) than in domiciled subjects who were not poor (0.6%), but

Table 5–2, cont'd. Prevalence of selected DSM-III disorders in the combined five-site ECA household survey population (US-ECA) and in various homeless populations reported from 1980 to 1990

Study variable	U.S.	Pittsburgh	Detroit
Reference	Wright & Weber 1987	Davies et al. 1987	Mowbray et al. 1987
N	261	24	35
Sampling site	Clinics	SRO [hotels?]	State mental hospital
Male (%)	NR	00.0	63.0
Diagnostic method	Medical record	BPRS exam	Psychiatric
DSM-III disorders			
No disorder	0[b]	8.3	0[b]
Schizophrenia	36.0	20.8	28.6
Major affective	29.0	NR	11.4
Dementia	NR	NR	NR
Substance abuse	NR	NR	14.3
Alcohol	NR	33.3	NR
Drug	NR	4.2	NR
Mixed	NR	8.3	NR
Anxiety disorders	NR	4.2	NR
Mental retardation	5.0	NR	NR
Personality disorders	13.0	12.5	NR
Antisocial personality	NR	NR	NR

Note. ECA = Epidemiologic Catchment Area; DIS = Diagnostic Interview Schedule (Robins et al. 1981); NR = Not rated; BPRS = Brief Psychiatric Rating Scale (Overall et al. 1962)

[a] Lifetime rates displayed.

[b] Clinical samples of mentally ill individuals only.

was still substantially greater (11%) among the Baltimore homeless (Breakey et al. 1990).

Similarly, the rates of DSM-III disorders in a sample of homeless adults in Los Angeles exceeded those of the ECA household population for every disorder category. Homeless persons were 38 times more likely to be schizophrenic, 22 times more likely to have antisocial personality disorder, 6 times more likely to have affective disorders, 5 times more likely to be cognitively impaired, 4 times more likely to have anxiety disorders, and 3 times more likely to be substance abusers than adults who were not homeless (Koegel et al. 1988).

In addition to experiencing high rates of diagnosed psychiatric disorders, homeless persons also suffer nonspecific symptoms of emotional distress and demoralization at greater rates than the housed population. For example, the homeless sample in Los Angeles was 7.5 times more likely to report experiencing psychological distress at the time of the survey than was the Los Angeles ECA household sample (Farr et al. 1986). In Baltimore, the homeless sample was nearly 3 times as likely to suffer current emotional distress as the comparison sample of household men (Fischer et al. 1986b).

Homeless children experience developmental delays, emotional problems, and child abuse at greater rates than do children who are not homeless (Alperstein et al. 1988; Whitman et al. 1984). For example, Bassuk and her colleagues (1986, 1987, 1988) found that children in homeless families manifested developmental delays at rates more than 3 times that of children of poverty-class families who were not homeless. About half of the children aged 3–5 years were judged as needing psychiatric attention for anxiety and depression. Similarly, rates of psychiatric morbidity among homeless adolescents appear to exceed those in the general population. Yates and his associates (1988) determined that runaway patients of an adolescent ambulatory clinic in Los Angeles were 4.5 times more likely to have a mental health problem than nonrunaway youth; for example, 84% of runaways were currently depressed, compared with 24% of nonhomeless youth. In a sample of New York City homeless youth, mental health problems were estimated to affect between 70% and 90% of the subjects (Shaffer and Caton 1984).

Studies in Baltimore also demonstrated differences in mental health between older members of the homeless and household populations (Breakey et al. 1990). About half of homeless men and three-fifths of homeless women aged 50 and older had current symptoms of emotional distress. In contrast, in the ECA domiciled sample, only 12% of the older men and 16% of older women experienced emotional distress. More than one-quarter of the older homeless men and women showed signs of cognitive impairment, compared with 15% of the domiciled men and women aged 50 years and older.

Whether homeless people who are mentally ill differ from those who are not in terms of demographic characteristics is unclear. Homeless women are frequently described as more likely to be mentally ill than homeless men (Crystal 1984; Crystal et al. 1986; Ladner et al. 1986; Robertson et al. 1985; Rosnow et al. 1986; Schutt 1988; Schutt and Garrett 1986; Vernez et al. 1988; Wright and Weber 1987). For example, women in the New York City shelter system were observed to be about twice as likely as men to be identified as mentally ill (Crystal 1984; Crystal and Goldstein 1984). Women in Boston shelters were twice as likely as men to be assessed by staff as having psychological problems (McGerigle and Lauriat 1983).

Other studies, however, have found minimal gender differences in psychopathology among homeless people (Calsyn and Morse, unpublished paper; Crystal 1984; Solarz and Mowbray 1985). For example, homeless women in the Ohio statewide survey were slightly more likely than men to be judged psychiatrically impaired, but the difference was not statistically significant. The only significant gender differences observed were women's higher scores on the depression-anxiety scale and higher rates of impairment among persons living on the streets. The authors speculate that high proportions of homeless mothers in the sample might account for relatively low rates of impairment (Stefl and Roth 1986). Helfman (1986) found that homeless men in Wilmington, Delaware, were more likely than women to be assessed as in need of mental health services (51% and 33%, respectively), but psychiatric examination revealed no significant differences in the rate of major mental illnesses between homeless men (42%) and women (49%) in Baltimore (Breakey et al. 1989).

The data are also ambiguous regarding minorities. Vernez and his colleagues (1988) found that severely mentally ill homeless persons in California were somewhat more likely to be African American than white, but a number of studies have found higher rates among whites. For example, whites (59%) were considered in need of mental health services more often than African Americans (45%) or Hispanics (0%) in Wilmington, Delaware (Helfman 1986). The prevalence of mental illness was found to be greater among white clients of New York City shelters although the differences were small: about one-third of white clients were considered mentally ill compared to just under one-quarter of both African Americans and Hispanics (Crystal et al. 1986; Ladner et al. 1986). In the Health Care for the Homeless (HCH) population, the rate of mental illness was highest among whites (32%) and lowest among Hispanics (17%) (Wright and Weber 1987). A number of studies have failed to demonstrate substantial differences in the prevalence of mental disorder by race or ethnicity (Breakey et al. 1988; Koegel et al. 1988; Rosnow et al. 1985).

Age differences in the prevalence of mental disorder have been reported, with some studies finding higher rates of mental illness in older people, especially older women. In Milwaukee, homeless persons identified as mentally ill by virtue of previous psychiatric hospitalization or overt delusional, hallucinatory, or other symptoms were, on average, 7 years older than non-mentally ill individuals (Rosnow et al. 1986). However, no age differences were found between the psychiatric and nonpsychiatric groups of homeless clients of New York City public shelters (Crystal et al. 1986; Ladner et al. 1986). In the Los Angeles skid row study, age was unrelated to major mental illness (Koegel et al. 1988). In Boston, the mentally ill group tended to be younger than other groups (Mulkern et al. 1985). Wright and Weber (1987) observed differences in rates of mental illness by age and sex: rates were higher among younger men and decreased with age, but mental illness was much more common among women over age 30.

In Baltimore, more than one-quarter of older (50+ years) men and women showed signs of cognitive impairment compared to 10% or fewer of their younger counterparts. Rates of major mental illnesses were similar in older and younger men, but among women, they were much higher among older women. Three-fifths of women over 50 and four-fifths of women over 60 had a diagnosis, compared to fewer than half of women under 50 years old (Fischer and Breakey 1989).

Very young homeless persons are also at high risk. Homeless adolescents living on their own appear to have high rates of mental health problems (Solarz 1988). Emotional problems are also common among sheltered homeless children (Alperstein et al. 1988; Bassuk and Rosenberg 1988; Bassuk et al. 1986; Eldred and Towber 1986; Miller and Lin 1988; Paone and Kay 1988; Whitman et al. 1984).

Although nearly all research designs have been cross-sectional rather than longitudinal, one frequent implication in the literature is that prior experiences or comorbidities may influence a person's vulnerability to become homeless or to remain homeless. In addition to the presence of inappropriate or unavailable housing and mental health treatments, these factors may modify risk.

Out-of-home placement during childhood may be one such factor. For example, almost half of the former psychiatric patients in a New York City shelter sample had been placed away from their families as children (Susser et al. 1987). Nearly two-fifths of a Minneapolis sample of homeless adults had a history of such placement, and early placement was associated with long-term homelessness (Piliavin et al. 1988).

Mentally ill homeless persons also demonstrate long-standing difficulties in meeting social expectations. For example, mentally ill groups were less likely to be currently employed, to report past employment, or to have served in the military, compared with other homeless people (Crystal et al. 1986; Fischer et al. 1986a; Ladner et al. 1986; Rosnow et al. 1985; Vernez et al. 1988). Clinical researchers have noted that the disabling functional deficits of major mental illness may predispose some people to homelessness (Lamb and Lamb 1990).

Although social networks appear to be attenuated among the homeless population in general, mentally ill homeless persons show greater disaffiliation (Cohen et al. 1988; Rosnow et al. 1985). Common indices of social support include marital status, contact with friends and relatives, and sources of practical assistance. Helfman (1986) found that homeless persons who were married were less likely to be judged in need of mental health services than homeless adults who were single or divorced. In a California study, the homeless who had severe mental disorders were only half as likely to be currently married as were other homeless persons (Vernez et al. 1988). Rosnow and his colleagues (1985) reported that the homeless mentally ill group in Milwaukee were somewhat less likely to have ever married and identified fewer sources of support from friends and family than those having no discernible mental problem.

Homeless men on the Bowery aged 50 years and older with prior psychiatric hospitalizations did not differ from other homeless men of a similar age on various health and social indexes, but were significantly disadvantaged on measures of income, physical health, residential stability, and social support compared to a group of age-matched community men (Cohen et al. 1988). The homeless who were mentally ill in Buffalo reported less frequent family contact and named more professionals in their social networks than those who were not mentally ill (P.A. Toro and D.D. Wall, unpublished data, 1989). However, more than 90% of homeless adults in Minneapolis reported some contact with family members in the week prior to interview (Piliavin et al. 1988).

Comorbid Substance Use Disorders

The rate of comorbid substance use disorder among those with mental illness (often termed dual diagnosis) is substantial. Among mentally ill homeless adults in Baltimore, more than three-fifths of men and two-fifths of women also had an alcohol use disorder; more than one-fourth of men and one-fifth of women had concurrent drug use disorders (Fischer and Breakey 1991). In Milwaukee, nearly one-fifth of the mentally ill group also had an alcohol or drug problem, compared with almost half of the non-mentally ill group of homeless respondents (Rosnow et al. 1985). New York City shelter residents who were identified as the psychiatric group were roughly equally likely as other shelter residents to report substance abuse (about one-third) (Crystal et al. 1986; Ladner et al. 1986). Half of the homeless adults in Los Angeles identified as having schizophrenia or affective disorders were also chronic substance abusers (Farr et al. 1986). Vernez and his associates (1988) estimated that 22% of a sample of homeless individuals in three California counties were dually diagnosed for a mental disorder and a substance abuse disorder.

Half of homeless veterans with psychiatric problems also had concurrent alcohol abuse problems, and one-fifth had problems with drug abuse (Rosenheck et al. 1988). Toro and Wall (1989) found that the mentally ill group in a Buffalo sample of homeless people were more likely to receive a diagnosis of alcohol abuse than those who were not mentally ill.

Physical Health

A number of surveys suggest that chronically mentally ill persons have poorer physical health than the general population (Barnes et al. 1983; Koranyi 1979; McCarrick et al. 1986; Roca et al. 1987). The mentally ill homeless in a California study were $1\frac{1}{2}$ times more likely to perceive their health as fair to poor than the group that did not have mental disorders, and they had lower functional status as determined by their need for more help with instrumental activities of daily living (Vernez et al. 1988). More than half of the psychiatric group of New York City shelter residents reported current physical complaints, compared with one-third of the nonpsychiatric group, and the mentally ill group were $1\frac{1}{2}$ times more likely to report that health problems kept them from working (Crystal et al. 1986; Ladner et al. 1986). In the HCH client population, the mentally ill group had higher prevalence rates in almost every reported category of physical disorder than the non-mentally ill clients, with some of the greatest differences found in nutritional disorders (Wright and Weber 1987).

Crime and Victimization

Studies of homeless persons show that criminal activity and mental illness are correlated (Fischer 1988, in press; Snow et al. 1986). Ladner et al. (1986) found that nearly half of New York City shelter residents identified as mentally ill had histories of incarceration. Schutt and Garrett (1986) found that current legal problems were more frequent among homeless persons classified as mentally ill (30%), substance abusers (25% among drug abusers, 17% among alcohol abusers), and dually diagnosed (46%), compared with homeless persons with neither mental illness nor problems with substance abuse (less than 10%). Farr and colleagues (1986) reported that the chronically mentally ill homeless persons in their Los Angeles sample were about twice as likely as the non-mentally ill homeless to have been picked up by the police within the past year as well as to have spent time in jail. Among the homeless in Los Angeles County, involvement with criminal activities was associated with previous mental hospitalizations (Gelberg et al. 1988). In Minneapolis, about 15% of incarcerations were related to mental illness (Kroll et al. 1986). Arrest rates were found to be slightly higher among the mentally ill homeless men in Baltimore, and mentally ill women had rates of arrest nearly twice that of other homeless women (Fischer et al. 1989). In addition, diminished mental capacity of individuals may confer greater risk of arrest (French 1986).

Homeless persons with obvious disabilities, physical or mental, are at greater risk of victimization (Ball and Havassy 1984; French 1986; Muhlin 1986; Segal and Baumohl 1980). Solarz (1986) observed that the homeless who were former psychiatric patients were more likely to have been assaulted. Farr and colleagues (1986) found that chronically mentally ill persons among the Los Angeles homeless population were more likely to have been victimized (particularly assaulted) within the previous year and were more likely to report more than one type of victimization. Muhlin (1986) observed that shelter residents in New York who had mental health problems were more likely to be victims of theft and were apt to report fear of being harmed. Since there is evidence that homeless women may be more likely than men to be mentally disturbed, their risk of attack may be compounded (Ladner et al. 1986).

Course of Homelessness

The mentally ill group of homeless persons in Milwaukee had been homeless twice as long as other homeless people (Rosnow et al. 1986). Koegel and his colleagues (1988) found higher rates of schizophrenia and substance abuse disorders in the groups characterized by long-term and cyclical homelessness, whereas newly homeless individuals were slightly more apt to have affective disorders. In Wilmington, Delaware, homeless people who needed mental health care reported longer homeless stints than other homeless respondents (Helfman 1986).

Treatment

Because of concerns about the effects of deinstitutionalization, the extent to which homeless mentally ill people are in contact with the mental health service system has frequently been a topic of research. One consistent finding across many studies is that a large proportion of homeless mentally ill people report that they do not currently receive appropriate services. Studies of treatment utilization have generally relied upon self-reports, whose validity has been questioned by studies utilizing other informants (Drake et al. 1989; Lamb and Lamb 1990).

Nevertheless, participation in mental health treatment appears to lag substantially behind need (Farr et al. 1986; Fischer et al. 1986b). For example, more than one-quarter of homeless persons in Los Angeles reported experiencing psychiatric hospitalization in their lifetimes, but only 4% had been hospitalized within the past year. Approximately one-quarter of the homeless mentally ill respondents in another California study reported any prior psychiatric hospitalization; fewer than one-tenth had been hospitalized within the year, and one-fifth reported receiving outpatient mental health treatment in the past 6 months. Only 15% had taken medication for a mental problem during the preceding 6 months (Vernez et al. 1988). Younger homeless persons (under 40 years) in Chicago were more likely than the older group to report previous hospitalization for a mental problem. The association with age was more apparent among men than women (Rossi et al. 1986). Just under half of HCH clients meeting criteria for mental illness reported histories of psychiatric hospitalization, and little more than one-third of those with significant mental impairments were currently taking psychiatric medications (Wright and Weber 1987).

In Boston, three-fifths of the mentally ill group reported previous having had psychiatric hospitalizations, but the majority had not been hospitalized within the past 3 years (Mulkern et al. 1985). In Baltimore, three-fifths of homeless adults diagnosed with a major mental illness denied having been admitted to a psychiatric hospital. Of those with previous hospitalizations, nearly one-third experienced their first admission in childhood or adolescence, although 15% were not admitted until they were 40 years or older. The median time elapsed since first admission to research interview was 8 years, and for nearly one-quarter of the sample, treatment histories extended 20 years or more (Breakey, in press).

In a number of studies, homeless women have reported psychiatric treatment histories more often than men (Crystal 1984; Piliavin et al. 1988; Schutt 1988). In Baltimore, although rates of major mental illness by gender were similar, 65% of the women and 47% of the men diagnosed as having a major mental illness reported having had a prior psychiatric hospitalization (Breakey, in press). However, among those without a diagnosis of major mental illness or substance use disorder, 7% of men and 33% of women reported previous outpatient mental health care, and 13% of men and 22% of women reported a prior psychiatric hospitalization (Fischer, in press). In the Baltimore homeless study, older men (50 years and older) utilized mental health treatment services at about the same rate as the younger men, but the older women, despite their greater need, used treatment services at a somewhat lower rate than the younger women (Fischer and Breakey 1989). Although virtually all homeless women in a Washington, DC, shelter were deemed to need psychiatric evaluation and treatment, their prior treatment histories were insubstantial, consisting typically of short lengths of stay and little evidence of continuous care. Two-thirds of the sheltered women reported total treatment times of 0 to 15 days in a 5-year reporting period, and there were only two instances in which inpatient episodes exceeded 90 days (Depp and Ackiss 1983).

Whether mentally ill homeless people are more or less apt to use non-mental health services relative to other homeless groups is unclear. More than half of the severely mentally ill in a California sample reported making outpatient visits for physical health problems in the past 6 months, compared with fewer than one-third of the group that did not have mental disorders. In addition, the mentally ill group were between 1.8 and 4.5 times more likely to report treatment for substance abuse problems than were other homeless persons although their rates of abuse were similar (Vernez et al. 1988).

Conclusions

The epidemiological research conducted on mental illness among the homeless during the 1980s converges on several findings. Mental health problems are common among currently homeless populations. More specifically, severe and disabling mental disorders are 20 times more prevalent among homeless populations than among individuals living in impoverished households. Demographic characteristics may not differentiate homeless mentally ill persons from other homeless persons, but other characteristics do. Homeless mentally ill persons generally have long-standing histories of poor functioning, both socially and vocationally. Many also have a history of out-of-home placement as children. Mentally ill homeless persons have fewer social supports than other homeless persons. They also may be more likely to experience prolonged or recurrent homelessness. Like other homeless persons, however, those with mental illness have high rates of comorbid conditions, particularly substance use disorders. Finally, mentally ill homeless people report limited contact with mental health treatment, despite their apparent level of need.

References

Alperstein G, Rappaport C, Flanigan J: Health problems of homeless children in New York City. Am J Public Health 78:1232–1233, 1988

American Psychiatric Association: Diagnostic and Statistical Manual of Mental Disorders, 3rd Edition. Washington, DC, American Psychiatric Association, 1980

Arce AA, Tadlock M, Vergare MH, et al: A psychiatric profile of street people admitted to an emergency shelter. Hosp Community Psychiatry 34:812–817, 1983

Ball FLJ, Havassy BE: A survey of the problems and needs of homeless consumers of acute psychiatric services. Hosp Community Psychiatry 35:917–921, 1984

Barnes RF, Mason JC, Greer C, et al: Medical illness in chronic psychiatric outpatients. Gen Hosp Psychiatry 5:191–195, 1983

Bassuk E: The homeless problem. Sci Am 215:40–45, 1984

Bassuk EL, Rosenberg L: Why does family homelessness occur? A case-control study. Am J Public Health 78:783–788, 1988

Bassuk EL, Rubin L: Homeless children: a neglected population. Am J Orthopsychiatry 57:279–286, 1987

Bassuk EL, Rubin L, Lauriat AS: Characteristics of sheltered homeless families. Am J Public Health 76:1097–1101, 1986

Breakey WR: Clinical services for homeless alcoholics: implications of recent research and experience, in Homelessness: The National Perspective. Edited by MJ Robertson, Greenblatt M. New York, Plenum (in press)

Breakey WR, Romanoski A, Nestadt G, et al: Severe mental illness in the homeless. Paper presented at the annual meeting of the American Public Health Association, Boston, MA, November 1988

Breakey WR, Fischer PJ, Nestadt G, et al: Health and mental health problems of homeless men and women in Baltimore. JAMA 262:1352–1357, 1989

Breakey WR, Fischer PJ, Nestadt G, et al: Psychiatric morbidity in homeless and housed low-income people in Baltimore. Paper presented at the annual meeting of the American Public Health Association, New York, September-October, 1990

Calsyn RJ, Morse G: Homeless men and women: commonalities and a service gender gap. Unpublished paper. St. Louis, MO, University of Missouri Department of Psychology, no date

Cohen CI, Teresi J, Holmes D: The mental health of old homeless men. J Am Geriatr Soc 36:492–501, 1988

Crystal S: Homeless men and homeless women: the gender gap. Urban and Social Change Review 17:2–6, 1984

Crystal S, Goldstein M: The Homeless in New York City Shelters. New York, Human Resources Administration, 1984

Crystal S, Ladner S, Towber R: Multiple impairment patterns in the mentally ill homeless. International Journal of Mental Health 14:61–73, 1986

Depp FC, Ackiss V: Assessing needs among sheltered homeless women. Paper presented at the Conference on Homelessness: A Time for New Directions, Washington, DC, July 1983

Drake RE, Wallach MA, Hoffman JS: Housing instability and homelessness among aftercare patients of an urban state hospital. Hosp Community Psychiatry 40:46–51, 1989

Eldred CA, Towber RI: A One-Day "Snapshot" of Homeless Families at the Forbell Street Shelter and Martinique Hotel. New York, Human Resources Administration, 1986

Farr RK, Koegel P, Burnam A: A study of Homelessness and Mental Illness in the Skid Row Area of Los Angeles. Los Angeles, CA, Los Angeles County Department of Mental Health, 1986

Fischer PJ: Criminal activity among the homeless: a study of arrests in Baltimore. Hosp Community Psychiatry 39:46–51, 1988

Fischer PJ: Alcohol, Drug Abuse, and Mental Health Problems Among Homeless Persons: A Review of the Literature, 1980–1990. Rockville, MD, U.S. Department of Health and Human Services, 1991

Fischer PJ: Criminal behavior and victimization in the homeless: a review of the literature, in Homelessness: A Prevention-Oriented Approach. Baltimore, MD, Johns Hopkins University Press (in press)

Fischer PJ, Breakey WR: The elderly homeless: examples from the Baltimore Study, in Long-Term Care: Federal and State Perspectives for the 1990s. Proceedings of the Seventh Annual Conference of the Maryland Gerontological Association. Edited by Corinan R, Williams D, Rogers D. Baltimore, MD, Maryland Gerontological Association, 1989

Fischer PJ, Breakey WR: The epidemiology of alcohol, drug, and mental disorders among homeless persons. Am Psychol 46:1115–1128, 1991

Fischer PJ, Breakey WR, Shapiro S, et al: Baltimore mission users: social networks, morbidity, and employment. Psychosocial Rehabilitation Journal 9:51–63, 1986a

Fischer PJ, Shapiro S, Breakey WR, et al: Mental health and social characteristics of the homeless: a survey of mission users. Am J Public Health 76:519–524, 1986b

Fischer PJ, Breakey WR, Ross A: Criminal activity among the homeless. Paper presented at the annual meeting of the American Anthropological Association, Washington, DC, November 1989

French L: The victimization of the mentally deficient: a latent function of deinstitutionalization. Paper presented at the annual meeting of the American Society of Criminology, Atlanta, GA, October-November, 1986

Gelberg L, Linn LS, Leake BD: Mental health, alcohol and drug use, and criminal history among homeless adults. Am J Psychiatry 145:191–196, 1988

Helfman A: The Homeless and Mental Illness: A Field Study. Wilmington, DE, State of Delaware Division of Alcohol, Drug Abuse and Mental Health, Department of Health and Social Services, 1986

Koegel P, Burnam MA, Farr RK: The prevalence of specific psychiatric disorders among homeless individuals in the inner-city of Los Angeles. Arch Gen Psychiatry 45:1085–1092, 1988

Koranyi EK: Morbidity and rate of undiagnosed physical illnesses in a psychiatric clinic population. Arch Gen Psychiatry 36:414–419, 1979

Kroll J, Carey K, Hagedorn D, et al: A survey of homeless adults in urban emergency shelters. Hosp Community Psychiatry 37:283–286, 1986

Ladner S, Crystal S, Towber R, et al: Project Future: Focusing, Understanding, Targeting, and Utilizing Resources for the Homeless Mentally Ill, Elderly, Youth, Substance Abusers, and Employables. New York, Human Resources Administration, 1986

Lamb HR, Lamb DM: Factors contributing to homelessness among the chronically and severely mentally ill. Hosp Community Psychiatry 41:301–305, 1990

Lovell AM, Barrow SM, Struening EL: Between relevance and rigor: methodological issues in studying mental health and homelessness, in Homelessness: A Prevention-Oriented Approach. Edited by Jahiel R. Baltimore, MD, Johns Hopkins University Press (in press)

McCarrick AK, Manderscheid RW, Bertolucci DE, et al: Chronic medical problems in the chronically mentally ill. Hosp Community Psychiatry 37:289–291, 1986

McGerigle P, Lauriat A: More Than Shelter: A Community Response to Homelessness. Boston, MA, United Community Planning Corporation and Massachusetts Association for Mental Health, 1983

Miller DS, Lin EHB: Children in sheltered homeless families: reported health status and use of health services. Pediatrics 81:668–673, 1988

Morrissey JP, Dennis DL: NIMH-Funded Research Concerning Homeless Mentally Ill Persons: Implications for Policy and Practice. Washington, DC, Alcohol, Drug Abuse, and Mental Health Administration, 1986

Mowbray CT, Johnson VS, Solarz A: Homelessness in a state hospital population. Hosp Community Psychiatry 38:880–882, 1987

Muhlin GL: Pack of wolves or flock of sheep? Crime and victimization among New York City public shelter users. Paper presented at the annual meeting of the American Society of Criminology, Atlanta, GA, October-November 1986

Mulkern V, Bradley VJ, Spence R, et al: Homelessness Needs Assessment Study: Findings and Recommendations for the Massachusetts Department of Mental Health. Boston, MA, Human Services Research Institute, 1985

Overall JE, Gorham DR: The Brief Psychiatric Rating Scale. Psychol Rep 10:799–812, 1962

Paone D, Kay K: Immunization status of homeless alcoholics. Paper presented at the annual meeting of the American Public Health Association, Boston, MA, November 1988

Piliavin I, Sosin M, Westerfelt H: Conditions contributing to long-term homelessness: an exploratory study. Madison, WI, University of Wisconsin Institute for Research on Poverty, 1988

Regier DA, Myers JK, Kramer M, et al: The NIMH epidemiologic catchment area program: historical context, major objectives, and study population characteristics. Arch Gen Psychiatry 41:934–941, 1984

Robertson MJ: Mental disorder among homeless persons in the United States: An overview of recent empirical literature. Administration in Mental Health 14:14–27, 1986

Robertson MJ, Ropers RH, Boyer R: The homeless of Los Angeles County: An empirical assessment. Los Angeles, CA, University of California School of Public Health Psychiatric Epidemiology Program, 1985

Robins LN, Helzer JE, Croughan J, et al: National Institute of Mental Health Diagnostic Interview Schedule: its history, characteristics, and validity. Arch Gen Psychiatry 38:381–389, 1981

Roca RP, Breakey WR, Fischer PJ: Medical care of chronic psychiatric outpatients. Hosp Community Psychiatry 38:741–744, 1987

Rosenheck R, Phil PGM, Leda C, et al: Reaching out: the second progress report on the Veterans Administration Homeless Chronically Mentally Ill Veterans Program, December 28, 1988. West Haven, CT, West Haven VA Medical Center, 1988

Rosnow M, Shaw T, Concord CS: Listening to the homeless: a study of mentally ill persons in Milwaukee. Milwaukee, WI, Human Services Triangle, Inc, 1985

Rosnow MJ, Shaw T, Concord CS: Listening to the homeless: a study of homeless mentally ill persons in Milwaukee. Psychosocial Rehabilitation Journal 9:64–77, 1986

Rossi PH, Fisher GA, Willis G: The condition of the homeless in Chicago. Amherst, MA, University of Massachusetts Social and Demographic Research Institute, 1986

Schutt RK: Boston's homeless, 1986–87: change and continuity. Report to the Long Island Shelter. Boston, MA, University of Massachusetts, 1988

Schutt RK, Garrett GR: Homeless in Boston in 1985: The view from Long Island. Boston, MA, University of Massachusetts, 1986

Segal SR, Baumohl J: Engaging the disengaged: proposals on madness and vagrancy. Social Work 25:358–365, 1980

Shaffer D, Caton CLM: Runaway and homeless youth in New York City. Report to the Ittelson Foundation. New York, Ittelson Foundation, 1984

Snow DA, Baker SG, Anderson L, et al: The myth of pervasive mental illness among the homeless. Social Problems 33:407–423, 1986

Solarz A: Can you trust a homeless person? Another look. Paper presented at the annual meeting of the American Public Health Association, Las Vegas, NV, September-October 1986

Solarz A: Homelessness: implications for children and youth. Social Policy Report 3(4):1–16, 1988

Solarz A, Mowbray C: An examination of physical and mental health problems of the homeless. Paper presented at the annual meeting of the American Public Health Association, Washington, DC, November 1985

Stefl ME, Roth D: Homeless women and mental illness: comparisons with homeless men. Paper presented at the annual meeting of the American Public Health Association, Las Vegas, NV, September-October 1986

Susser E, Struening E, Conover S: Childhood experiences of homeless men. Am J Psychiatry 144:1599–1601, 1987

Tessler RC: What have we learned to date? Assessing the first generation of NIMH-supported research studies, in Homelessness and Mental Illness: Toward the Next Generation of Research Studies. Edited by Morrissey JP, Dennis DL. Rockville, MD, National Institute of Mental Health, 1990

Vernez G, Burnam MA, McGlynn EA, et al: Review of California's program for the homeless mentally disabled. Santa Monica, CA, RAND Corporation, 1988

Whitman BY, Spankel J, Stretch JJ, et al: Children of the homeless: a high risk of developmental delays. Paper presented at the annual meeting of the American Public Health Association, Anaheim, CA, November 1984

Wright JD, Weber E: Homelessness and Health. Washington, DC, McGraw-Hill, 1987

Yates GL, MacKenzie R, Pennbridge J, et al: A risk profile comparison of runaway and nonrunaway youth. Am J Public Health 78:820–821, 1988

Chapter 6

Why Clinicians Distance Themselves From the Homeless Mentally Ill

Linda Chafetz, R.N., D.N.Sc.

In public psychiatric services, particularly in the walk-in and crisis units serving the homeless, mental health problems are often complicated by the anger, resentment, and alienation engendered by extreme poverty and isolation. This distrust is felt not only by those whom Rossi and his co-authors (1987) call the "categorically homeless" but also by the larger group of the mentally ill who experience homelessness as a memory and an ongoing risk.

The responsibility for reaching out effectively to such clients clearly rests with staff, yet providers themselves may be overwhelmed by clinical problems, unprepared to deal with social and economic needs, and, finally, too demoralized to pursue what they perceive as lost causes. In this chapter, I focus on the problem of providing sensitive psychiatric services to homeless clients—specifically, the mutual withdrawal that occurs between disaffiliated, distrustful clients and their psychiatric caregivers.

The disappointing results of efforts to provide services to impoverished mentally ill persons would be discouraging under any circumstances. They represent a particularly sad turn of events for a community mental health movement based in the Great Society programs and antipoverty legislation of the 1960s (Bachrach 1978). However, despite the programs' early emphasis on the mental health of the poor, they did not address the specific therapeutic and support needs of the severely mentally ill. Mechanic (1987) suggests that an ideology

This chapter is adapted from Chafetz L: Withdrawal from the homeless mentally ill. Community Ment Health J 26:449–461, 1990.

of environmental causation, which de-emphasized treatment of severe disorders, may have actually contributed to their poverty, isolation, and marginalization.

Bridging the chasm of cultural and social differences that separate psychiatric providers and the homeless mentally ill may be one of the most important tasks in public psychiatric services today. Outcomes of programs meeting immediate needs of the homeless mentally will hinge on the quality of care provided and on the ability of providers to connect with clients. The history of psychiatry is replete with examples of policies that failed due to erosion of care at this level.

For example, Rothman (1971) linked the admission of the indigent insane to the 19th-century asylum with the decline of "moral management." As public hospitals admitted large numbers of "the manic, the furiously insane, and worst yet, the chronic," they witnessed attrition of sensitive attendants and loss of sensitivity among those who remained. Today, similar processes may be operating in public psychiatric services treating the indigent mentally ill. Signs include problems in recruiting and retaining talented clinicians and in maintaining morale among frontline providers.

To develop some understanding of these processes, I will begin by describing the factors that contribute to withdrawal from homeless clients and the forms of behavior that this retreat can assume. Describing the process is easier than proposing remedies, because both client and staff withdrawal are to some extent functions of factors beyond the control of psychiatric clinicians, in what Myerson and Herman (1987) call the "extratherapeutic system." However, to avoid making propositions for change would amount to a resigned acceptance of the status quo, perhaps akin to the "deep cynicism" mentioned by Rothman (1971). I conclude this chapter, therefore, by suggesting ways to support and direct clinicians working with the homeless, both through initiatives within services and through more formal training programs.

Reasons Caregivers Withdraw

The Resource Dilemma

A series of dilemmas confront personnel in public psychiatric settings, all of which may promote a pulling away from the severely mentally ill. The resource dilemma—that is, the shortage of goods and services available for clients with multiple problems—ranks first. This scarcity becomes most salient in the case of the homeless, who lack the most fundamental kinds of shelter and protection.

Regardless of the type or level of training, every psychiatric caregiver has been taught to some extent to conceive of care in terms of hierarchical needs, and to attend first to issue of comfort and safety. However, resources for comfort and safety of homeless clients, from clothes to bathing facilities, meals, and adequate housing, may be in short supply. Mental health professionals who identify the gamut of medical, psychiatric, and social needs, yet who work without access to a corresponding set of resources, may feel compelled to make "bricks without straw," unable to balance their own professional expectations against the realities of practice.

The Crisis of Belief

The immediate and urgent nature of the resource dilemma can make other issues appear almost frivolous by comparison. However, it is important to note that the resource shortage is attended by an equally important crisis of belief and values. Early community mental health centers were often charismatic organizations fed by the energy of a staff with strong beliefs in social and preventive psychiatry. If these beliefs did not provide a satisfactory framework for management of severe illness, their very existence provided cohesion, infusing hope and motivation into objectively difficult work situations.

Hopkin (1985) mentions this issue in a report on an emergency psychiatry setting in which rising acuity and recidivism rates served to discredit the prevailing crisis model. Staff began to lose faith in their treatment ideology as "the disparity between their values and their own observations" became apparent and undermined their earlier enthusiasm.

In contrast, a biomedical model addresses the acute psychopathology and medical comorbidity of severely mentally ill clients. However, it may not be sufficient to deal with the social concomitants of disability. In the case of the homeless, this narrow focus means that acute care is not connected to values and beliefs about eventual stabilization or rehabilitation. Thus, clinicians may work in the absence of a philosophy that gives meaning to daily work and that fosters belief in long-term outcomes.

The Absence of Reinforcers

In short-term, acute services, in which the contribution of acute care to long-term goals must often be assumed rather than observed, staff often function without the reinforcer of seeing the outcome of treatment. Emergency, walk-in, and brief inpatient services act as agencies of last resort for people in crisis, people at a low point in function at a moment when support systems have failed. While interventions in the acute area should logically influence long-term adaptation (for example, referral to appropriate support services for aftercare), clients who stabilize are least likely to reappear.

In contrast, recidivism and destitution reappear so often that they can take on almost a routine character and seem to be correlates of severe illness. This phenomenon was mentioned by Harding and others in 1987 and even earlier, in 1984, by Cohen and Cohen. These perceptions, based on experiences with skewed clinical samples, can induce profound skepticism about the possibility of change.

The Mind-Body Problem

Repeated exposure to the acutely ill induces more than a sense of futility. It presents objective stressors in the work situation, aversive conditions that can promote protective withdrawal over time. Poverty and isolation lend an edge of despair to serious symptomatology and can contribute to angry and even threatening or abusive behaviors that may require physical management.

Treating the problems of hygiene and self-care that street dwelling implies is considered unrewarding and unappealing by some psychiatric providers. In 1982, Baxter and Hopper described shelter providers' fears about contamination by their clients infected with lice, tuberculosis, respiratory ailments, and hepatitis. Even among medically trained providers, care of the homeless can elicit feelings of discomfort about exposure to contagion, odors, and infestation, feelings that undermine the provision of empathic care. The growing problem of AIDS has increased these concerns. Even the most accepting personnel may be dismayed by the magnitude of these clients' problems and the pressure they are under to deal with multiple, interacting needs in a limited time and with limited resources.

In sum, the clinician's experience involves continued contact with chronicity, recidivism, disadvantage, disturbing behavior, and the physical effects of homelessness. These conditions act as a series of shocks and disturbances in their own right and also raise uncomfortable questions about why some people are subject to so many forms of misfortune and about the efficacy of psychiatric intervention. To function under these conditions, to conduct "treatment as usual," providers practice a kind of defensive withdrawal that involves shifting their attention to aspects of the clinical situation that they perceive as somehow more tolerable or acceptable than the situation as a whole.

Symptoms of Withdrawal

Retreat to Biology

Mosher and Keith (1980) commented almost a decade ago that the ambiguous outcome data on psychosocial therapies could lead to a "why bother attitude." Medications undoubtedly have a central role in the management of major disorders, and physiological research on mental illness holds out great hope for the future. Nevertheless, a strictly biological orientation toward mental illness can be used to rationalize neglect of environmental and interpersonal issues and to justify one type of withdrawal from the severely mentally ill.

This stance is particularly perplexing when one considers the attention devoted to psychosocial care of the medically ill. The causes and treatment of illness are clearly physiological, but factors such as distress, support, motivation, and learning, nevertheless, are known to influence course of illness and outcome. Perhaps chronicity of illness distances providers and dampens enthusiasm for providing interpersonal care (Harding et al. 1987). Perhaps the "terrifying" aspect of schizophrenia and like disorders prompts this retreat (Minkoff 1987). When homelessness compounds chronic psychiatric illness, it may be comforting for the caregiver to attribute all suffering to the patient's physiological disorder and to withdraw from the expressive caregiving role. A clinical example illustrates this process.

Clinical Case

Ms. Smith, a 41-year-old woman with a history of bipolar affective disorder, was admitted to the locked inpatient psychiatric unit of a community hospital after the police brought her to the emergency service. Ms. Smith's symptoms clearly indicated a manic episode. She was also dirty, disheveled, and dehydrated after having spent what appeared to be at least several days wandering the streets. She was apparently evicted from a short-term hotel rental some weeks earlier and was known to a local shelter.

The admitting resident used the case as the basis for discussion with a group of students. Stressing the biological nature of the patient's illness and its deteriorating course, the resident pointed out the naiveté, even the futility, of directing attention at social or environmental factors. "We have many patients like this," he said. "We know almost nothing about them, and can only stabilize them with medications."

In fact, the medical record offered a great deal of information on Ms. Smith, whose was able, during the early years of her illness, to manage her treatment and to work full-time as an accountant, while contributing to the support of a child who lived with her former husband. Her manic episodes increased in frequency 8 years ago, making Ms. Smith dependent on disability payments for a subsistence-level income. The drop in her income level has affected her quality of life, a fact she resents strongly. During the past 5 years she has been obliged to obtain all services within public settings, which she describes as "humiliating." She has been hospitalized six times, usually for brief periods, and discharged each time with limited follow-up arrangements to various hotels.

Ms. Smith has experienced a course of illness with almost tragic overtones. The biological basis of her illness in no way negates her need for assertive support services. She may also require ongoing therapy to explore her desires and expectations. However, the process of discussing and planning goals may be painful and in no way assure a benign future course of illness. Under these conditions, a strictly pharmacological approach to treatment may have a defensive function for the caregivers.

Legalistic Retreat

In a 1980 article, Whitmer examines the role of mental health legislation in the criminalization of the deinstitutionalized mentally ill. He argues that stringent criteria for involuntary hospitalization contribute to neglect of difficult and potentially dangerous clients, who are essentially "forfeited" to the criminal justice sector. Whitmer describes severely disturbed individuals who cannot or will not accept the constraints of conventional programs, who cannot be compelled to comply with care, and who decompensate to the point of arrest and prosecution.

Although homeless clients do not universally fit this profile, the "young adult chronic" subgroup has some of its characteristics (Chafetz 1988; Schwartz and Goldfinger 1981; Segal and Bauhmohl 1980) and alert us, in a general sense, to the notion of client "forfeiture" as it occurs with the homeless. Because of the overwhelming nature of their problems, because they may be difficult to engage, homeless clients may be perceived by clinicians as too needy or too resistant to pursue with active outreach. An emphasis on their right to refuse treatment can provide a statutory rationalization for retreat from frustrating situations.

A vignette involving Mr. Jones, a young man with a diagnosis of paranoid schizophrenia, shows how legal preoccupation can mask this retreat.

Clinical Case

Mr. Jones arrived at a psychiatric emergency service requesting a sandwich. He appeared tense and irritable but insisted that he did not require treatment but was "just hungry." He reported that had no place to live and no source of income and described his home as the park.

Mr. Jones was well known to the service, which had functioned as his entry point to inpatient care in the past. In prior treatment episodes, his angry, forbidding behavioral style had often obscured paranoid delusions. Mr. Jones has previously acted upon these persecutory ideas, sometimes striking out at people in the treatment environment. This history of abusive behavior made staff reluctant to deal with him. A trainee was told by a staff member, "He looks pretty good today, he's fairly clean and well dressed. Since he doesn't seem to be gravely disabled, and since he isn't doing anything dangerous, maybe we can get rid of him."

Perhaps this remark reflected well-founded fears about pressuring Mr. Jones or increasing his agitation. However, the comments of the clinician also suggest the belief that a reasonably clean person cannot be gravely disabled (one criterion for involuntary civil commitment) and that persons who cannot be compelled to accept treatment should not be encouraged to consider it or to discuss possible sources of help with subsistence services.

No effort was made to establish enough contact with this client to evaluate the presence of an ambivalent desire for assistance. When Mr. Jones angrily refused to sign a consent for treatment, again claiming to be just hungry, attempts to explore his current status were abandoned. He was told that he was a voluntary patient and could leave and was escorted to the door.

Retreat to Environmentalism

It may seem paradoxical to suggest that one way to retreat from homeless clients is to emphasize the external factors, interpersonal and material, that influence behavior. Homelessness is an environmental issue, and the special problems of the homeless stem from the isolation they endure and the physical stressors of their life situations. Yet the mentally ill among the homeless are no less in need of psychosocial services than their counterparts in more stable housing. In fact, they may require a more interpersonally sensitive approach than less disaffiliated clients. A preoccupation with environmental concerns can, like a flight into legalisms, disguise a sense of inadequacy or an unwillingness to reach out to the client. Like a biological retreat, it can reinforce a sense of futility, a "why bother" stance.

Consider Mr. Green, a 40-year-old man who described himself as a long-term recipient of psychiatric services. He came to a walk-in clinic requesting housing assistance.

Clinical Case

Mr. Green said he arrived earlier in the week by bus from another city, with all his belongings in a duffel bag. He was robbed and assaulted near the bus station on the night of his arrival, and currently had no money, address, or viable social supports.

Distraught and tearful, Mr. Green complained of inability "even to pull myself out of this chair." The clinician was able to find an emergency bed for him, as well as information about obtaining public assistance. This clinician took satisfaction in his good rapport with emergency housing and social service providers. He strongly believed in dealing with subsistence issues practically and in not "over-psychologizing" social problems.

Mr. Green did not seem equally satisfied, and protested in an insistent tone that he was not ready to leave the service. When a dinner tray arrived, he asked the clinician to "help me cut this up." The provider, exasperated by the client's increasing demands, described Mr. Green as manipulative. In a later session, a supervisor pointed out to the clinician the extent of Mr. Green's helplessness and depression and of his own strong reactions to the client's dependence. Although the clinician had correctly identified the primacy of recent psychosocial stressors in this situation, he had withdrawn from the interpersonal demands they had created (Goldfinger 1983).

Reversing Withdrawal

The notion of mutual withdrawal, in which a client's withdrawal interacts with and is compounded by a therapist's avoidance, is a familiar issue in the care of the seriously mentally ill. Minkoff (1987) cites the draining effect of particularly needy or passive clients, the fear induced by psychotic processes, and the feelings of repulsion that clinicians may experience—but rarely acknowledge—in caring for physically unappealing clients. His review of the limited research on attitudes of professionals to the chronically mentally ill indicates that providers' reactions mirror those of the general public. He suggests that although formidable barriers to empathic care exist, only providers' attitudes make them appear insurmountable.

The attitudes of caregivers toward the homeless mentally ill have certainly affected the services they provide. The homeless mentally ill evoke a range of reactions related not only to their psychiatric disorders but also to their poverty, their isolation, and their social disaffiliation.

These reactions obstruct efforts to connect with impoverished clients and to humanize their care. The case of Ms. Smith, described earlier, provides an example. When providers state that nothing can be done for this type of patient, they fall into an all-or-nothing pattern and opt to ignore the possibilities for providing immediate care, for establishing trust, and for developing a preliminary rehabilitation plan, including advocacy for appropriate community supports.

Creating Meaning and Reinforcement

If providers' attitudes are to shift or change, it may be important to offer them the means to change, first of all in terms of information. Clinical personnel and students can benefit from experiences that take them beyond the spatial and temporal limits of the treatment setting. Providers in mainstream agencies encounter the homeless mentally ill at a moment of acute illness, when they are obliged (or legally compelled) to receive treatment in what may be unwelcoming or frightening surroundings. Clinicians are generally so accustomed to their own milieus that they fail to appreciate the impact of weapons or drug searches, locked doors, visible security personnel, and personal property inspections that are characteristic of entry to acute care settings. Few clinicians have any sustained experiences in shelters, flophouse districts, and other areas that their homeless clients inhabit and of the environmental stressors they experience there. Clinicians may be aware of their clients' noncompliance but be oblivious to the logistical problems the homeless encounter in connecting with providers of ongoing care (Goldfinger and Chafetz 1984). It is difficult for them to understand the sometimes frightening routes clients travel to treatment services, particularly when care is involuntary.

Off-site training and staff development activities can increase understanding of behaviors that previously appeared meaningless in all but symptomatic terms. They might also provide the opportunity to see homeless clients during periods of well-being, which could help foster the understanding that not all patients follow a downward functional spiral (or that homelessness is not always continuous and lengthy). Personnel might also come to appreciate the strengths of the homeless mentally ill, to acknowledge their ability to endure hardship and loneliness, and to recognize the adaptive value in some environments of characteristics such as anger and seclusiveness. For example, in the case of Mr. Jones, described earlier, an appreciation of the survival value of the client's suspicious and irate style might make his behavior, if no more comfortable, far more understandable, and reinforce efforts to find common ground with him.

More formal educational initiatives have the benefit of addressing groups whose attitudes have not yet been formed. As Minkoff (1987) comments with respect to care of the chronic mentally ill, it is easier to develop attitudes than to change ingrained ideas and beliefs. Much recent attention has focused on training members of the core disciplines as specialists in treatment of the chronically mentally ill. The emphasis of training would be to help providers develop strategies for clients' psychosocial rehabilitation.

Although these technologies are essential, it may also be important to enrich new curricula with areas of study that allow students to consider their work within a historical context and from a public health perspective. Relevant issues include problems of poverty and societal reaction that have historically influenced mental health policy, development of social welfare and mental health programs, successes and failures of prior reform efforts, preliminary outcomes of new service initiatives, and demographic trends that will affect service delivery in the future. It is crucial to prepare practitioners who understand that homelessness is not a problem of isolated individuals but a major social problem with important implications for health policy.

The Human Factor

Attitudes and reactions to homeless clients are not simply a function of information but also a result of affective factors that may not operate within the awareness of individual providers. Providers in public services seeing large numbers of the homeless mentally ill may indeed require some protection against the impact of the human misery they encounter on a daily basis. This ongoing contact with extreme poverty violates a sense of the world as just and predictable, threatening a sense of personal control and safety and setting defensive processes into motion to preserve what Perloff (1983) has called the illusion of invulnerability.

It is common to assign meanings to threatening events or conditions in order to resolve ambiguity about causation and to reestablish a sense of personal control. For example, to the extent that we need to believe in a just world, we may blame clients for causing (or deserving) their misfortunes (Alexander 1980; Lerner and Miller 1978). So, we may blame the homeless client for his or her fate in order to assign responsibility and meaning to chaotic and disturbing events. As Jonas (1986) states, poverty may be "the fault of the poor, or worse yet, a punishment for sin." Like any subjective reactions that influence care of the mentally ill, caregivers should be aware of their responses to poverty, residential instability, and social isolation or disaffiliation and should consider these responses critically. This effort implies the need for skilled and knowledgeable supervisors (Minkoff 1987).

Even with the best training programs and supervision, care of clients with multiple, severe, and interacting problems will continue to place special demands on providers. The task here, and one that falls to administrators, supervisors, and teachers, is to advocate for institutional resources that make comprehensive care feasible, including resources for nutrition and hygiene. It also means providing staffing levels that allow providers to devote adequate time and attention to the homeless.

Institutions must consider ways to reduce pressure on individual clinicians to divert difficult clients or to reduce their lengths of stay. Such demands create divided loyalties and ethical dilemmas that may eventually turn valuable clinicians to work in less conflicted situations. Skilled and committed providers will remain in stressful and demanding settings to the extent that they can perform according to their own expectations, receive the attention and support that they deserve, and, in short, find their work rewarding. Since the immediate results of their efforts will not be apparent, they have all the more need for administrative support and peer collaboration.

Beyond the Current Crisis

It might be argued that preparing clinicians to work with homeless clients in a sense supports the status quo and legitimizes the problem of homelessness itself. However, if all of the homeless mentally ill were issued acceptable housing tomorrow, the legacy of their experiences would endure and would constitute a clinical issue for those providing their psychiatric services. More than a decade has passed since Reich (1973) described care of the chronically mentally ill as a disgrace, since Reich and Siegel described New York's Bowery as a psychiatric dumping ground (1978), and since Segal and associates (1977) described Berkeley's enclave of young male vagrants.

Some younger adult patients cannot recall a time when disability was not linked to poverty and isolation; other community-based clients approach their middle or older years after long periods of inadequate and unstable housing. These people may share a profound sense of distrust of public services. Reaching out to alienated clients will continue to be an issue for providers in public psychiatric services, even as the phenomenon of homelessness recedes, as we hope.

New service initiatives appear to offer the means to extend effective community supports to the chronically mentally ill, including the subgroups that are more difficult to engage (Bond et al. 1984; Stein and Test 1980). Reports on residential programs also justify a great deal of optimism about developing effective, acceptable services (Lipton et al. 1988). These initiatives, like many service innovations in the past, benefit from the enthusiasm of providers involved in new programs, providers who are committed to work with the disadvantaged and the underserved. As new programs are reproduced on a broader scale and as service systems evolve to incorporate and work with them, the task may be to prepare and support providers who can maintain the momentum and continue to connect empathically with the chronically mentally ill and act as their advocates.

References

Alexander CS: The responsible victim: nurses' perceptions of victims of rape. J Health Soc Behav 21:22–33, 1980

Bachrach LL: A Conceptual Approach to Deinstitutionalization.Hosp Community Psychiatry 29:126–131, 1978

Baxter E, Hopper K: The new mendicancy: homeless in New York City. Am J Orthopsychiatry 52:393–408, 1982

Bond GR, Dincin J, Setze PJ, et al: The effectiveness of psychiatric rehabilitation. Psychosocial Rehabilitation Journal 7:6–22, 1984

Cohen P, Cohen J: The clinician's illusion. Arch Gen Psychiatry 41:1178–1182, 1984

Chafetz L: Recidivist clients: a review of pilot data. Arch Psychiatr Nurs 12:14–20, 1988

Goldfinger SM: The borderline patient, in The Practice and Management of Psychiatric Emergencies. Edited by Gorton J, Partridge R. New York, CV Mosby, 1983

Goldfinger SM, Chafetz L: Designing a better service system for the homeless mentally ill, in The Homeless Mentally Ill: A Task Force Report of the American Psychiatric Association. Washington, DC, American Psychiatric Association, 1984

Harding CM, Zubin Z, Strauss JS: Chronicity in schizophrenia: fact, partial fact, or artifact? Hosp Community Psychiatry 38:477–485, 1987

Hopkin JT: Psychiatry and medicine in the emergency room. New Dir Ment Health Serv 28:47–53, 1985

Jonas S: On homelessness and the American Way. Am J Public Health 76:1084–1085, 1986

Lanza ML: The relationship of vulnerability to victimization. Journal of Social Issues 39:41–61, 1987

Lerner MJ, Miller DT: Just world and the attributional process: looking back and ahead. Psychol Bull 85:1030–1051, 1978

Lipton FR, Nutt S, Sabatini A: Housing the homeless mentally ill: a longitudinal study of a treatment approach. Hosp Community Psychiatry 39:40–45, 1988

Mechanic D: Correcting misconceptions in mental health policy: strategies for improved care of the seriously mentally ill. Milbank Q 65:203–230, 1987

Minkoff K: Resistance of mental health professionals to working with the chronic mentally ill. New Dir Ment Health Serv 33: 3–20, 1987

Mosher LR, Keith SJ: Psychosocial treatment: individual, group, family, and community support approaches, in Special Report: Schizophrenia 1980. Schizophr Bull 127–158, 1980

Myerson AT, Herman GH: Systems resistance to the chronic patient. New Dir Ment Health Serv 33:21–24, 1987

Perloff LS: Perceptions at vulnerability to victimization. Journal of Social Issues 39:41–61, 1983

Reich R: Care of the chronically mentally ill: a national disgrace. Am J Psychiatry 130:911–912, 1973

Rossi PH, Wright JD, Fisher GA, et al: The urban homeless: estimating composition and size. Science 235:1336–1341, 1987

Rothman DJ: The Discovery of the Asylum: Social Order and Disorder in the New Republic. Boston, MA, Little, Brown, 1971

Schwartz SR, Goldfinger SM: The new chronic patient: clinical characteristics of an emerging subgroup. Hosp Community Psychiatry 32:470–474, 1981

Segal SP, Bauhmohl J: Engaging the disengaged: proposals on madness and vagrancy. Social Work 25:358–365, 1980

Segal SP, Bauhmohl J, Johnson E: Falling through the cracks: mental disorder and social margin in a young vagrant population. Social Problems 24:387–400, 1977

Stein LI, Test MA: Alternatives to mental hospital treatment. Arch Gen Psychiatry 37:392–397, 1980

Tudor GW: A sociopsychiatric nursing approach to intervention in a problem of mutual withdrawal on a mental hospital ward. Perspect Psychiatr Care 8:11–35, 1970

Whitmer GE: From hospitals to jails: the fate of California's deinstitutionalized mentally ill. Am J Orthopsychiatry 50:65–75, 1980

Chapter 7

Training Mental Health Professionals to Treat the Chronically Mentally Ill

John A. Talbott, M.D.

Given the striking interest in the public policy and service delivery issues relating to the care and treatment of the chronically mentally ill, it is surprising that there has been so little interest in the education and training of professionals who are expected to treat them. This oversight is probably the combination of a number of factors, including the traditional neglect of the public mental health sector by academia, the stigma and low status attached to those working in and training people to work in programs serving the chronically mentally ill, and the fact that little money earmarked for training has been directed toward training professionals to care for this patient population.

Interestingly, it seems that the literature gives more attention to training physicians to deal with the chronically mentally ill than it does to training other mental health professionals who work with the same population. This imbalance is probably due to a number of factors, among them that physicians may have the most to learn about treatment and care of this population, that physicians have been in the forefront of the recent surge of interest in the chronically mentally ill, or that other professional academic groups have fewer resources to expend in pursuit of altering training programs to meet the needs of this population.

In any event, in this chapter I will summarize the recent thinking and writing regarding training and educational programs geared to those who care for the chronically mentally ill. I will review what we know about who provides the bulk of care for this population; the curriculum content, experiential exposure, and attitudinal factors that constitute ideal educational programs; techniques for actually training persons to

work with the chronically mentally ill; and the problem areas encountered in training, such as burnout and countertransference.

Experience of Those Caring
for the Chronically Mentally Ill

Schwartz and associates (1981) conducted a survey of 75 psychiatrists
in the San Francisco area who had had long-term experiences caring
for severely disturbed patients in their residency training programs. Of
the 39% who responded, 82% had worked part-time or full-time in
public settings. Despite some methodological limitations, the study reported several findings of interest.

The psychiatrists had realistic goals about and familiarity with the
long-term course of chronic mental illness; were familiar with a comprehensive approach incorporating community supports, supportive
psychotherapy and medication; and regarded these patients as individuals. The research team found that the respondents were most satisfied
by small improvements in their patients' conditions, success in maintaining patients in the community, the positive aspects of the physi-
cian-patient relationship, and the opportunity to work with members
of a community support service team. They were least satisfied with
the frequent relapses of their patients, bureaucratic obstacles, the
patients' negative attitudes, devaluation of their profession's work by
society, and the lack of continuity of care.

The survey, albeit tentative and small in scope, did provide some
interesting and logical information that is of help in devising educational programs to train practitioners to care for the chronically mentally ill. However, it is important to note that because more than 50% of
the *psychiatric* care of the mentally ill is provided by nonpsychiatric
physicians, it is critical to include all physician training programs when
considering ways to provide training about the chronic mentally ill in
medical education (Goldberg et al. 1978). So much of the care of the
chronically mentally ill is carried out by family physicians or general
practitioners (in rural areas) and by general hospital emergency room
physicians (in urban areas) that the entire medical community must
become aware of the treatment and services needed by this population.

Educational Programs

Currently, most medical school curricula pay little attention to chronic
mental illness, and students are rarely or only briefly exposed to clinical work with this population—in striking contrast to their exposure to

severely and chronically medically ill patients. In addition, physicians in nonpsychiatric residencies are woefully lacking in such knowledge, and few continuing medical education programs concentrate on the chronically mentally ill.

Several themes common to all levels of education must be considered when implementing teaching programs directed to the care and treatment of the chronically mentally ill. I begin this section by discussing what educational efforts at every level should have in common. Later, I address the specific features of training that should be stressed at the various levels of education: medical school, residency, and continuing medical education. At each level, three areas of education—curriculum content, experience, and attitudes—are stressed. The current literature (Nielsen et al. 1981; Talbott 1980; Wilford 1981) suggests that these elements, while overlapping, are equally important and must be dealt with simultaneously.

Foremost among the goals of training programs for treatment of the chronically mentally ill is education about the special features of this patient population. It is critical that such patients receive a correct clinical diagnosis to ensure realistic, effective, and rational treatment planning (Minkoff 1987). A complete and accurate functional assessment is also necessary so that a similarly appropriate rehabilitation plan can be devised.

Most clinicians are primarily oriented toward those aspects of the patient's history and past medical records that relate to the medical condition. Frequently they place little or no emphasis on the patient's level of functioning (interpersonally, socially, and vocationally) and ability to perform the activities of everyday living. History of functioning, however, and current status often have much more bearing on the treatment and care plan than the traditional medical components of a past history and current status.

Another critical element in training physicians to best treat the chronically mentally ill involves the appropriate and effective use of psychoactive medication. Recent research has underlined the importance of providing medication appropriate to the phase of the patient's illness. Patients experiencing acute symptoms that interfere with their functioning may need more medication than patients who are attempting to master certain psychosocial tasks that demand coping skills (Segal 1978). Likewise, the dramatic differences between the psychopharmacologic treatment of schizophrenia and major affective disorders must be thoroughly understood, even by those who are used to dealing with mental illness psychopharmacologically on a daily basis.

The second major theme of all educational efforts relates to the role of the physician in the care of the chronically mentally ill. To date, most physicians have dealt with such patients either by isolating their medical condition from their broader psychosocial condition or by attempting to become all things to all patients. Neither approach achieves the maximum benefit. Physicians must appreciate the patients' medical and psychiatric problems in their larger social context. They must also realize that a range of disciplines and agencies is required to meet the many disparate needs of this group. Their role, then, must not be one of a medical specialist in isolation or a jack-of-all-trades but that of a medical specialist integrated into the larger human services network capable of meeting the needs of the mentally disabled person. Communication, referral, monitoring, and alertness to other problem areas are, therefore, critical.

As its third major theme, education of professionals who work with the chronically mentally ill must stress the need for a wide variety of professionals and paraprofessionals other than physicians to be involved in caring for this population. The host of services required by chronic patients living in the community is provided by a number of persons from a variety of disciplines—physicians, nurses, social workers, psychologists, activities therapists (e.g., occupational, recreational, and dance therapists), rehabilitation counselors and workers, educators, housing experts, and so on. Some of these therapists may assume a new role, almost a new profession or paraprofession, as case manager. The case management approach, which is generally unknown to others in medical practice, provides the cohesion that links the patient with the services needed (e.g., medical and psychiatric care, housing, income maintenance, and vocational and social rehabilitation).

The fourth theme needing emphasis at all levels of education concerns programs for the chronically mentally ill. Clinicians must be concerned with the patient's daily lives, yet generally they do not realize the wide range of programs required by chronic mental patients. Although they need not necessarily be familiar with the specifics of how all the patient's needs are met nor necessarily know all about the network of programs in a given community, they should know how to put the patient and themselves in contact with that network. They should also recognize that they are part of the network and of a bigger treatment team. Most programs in the network also function in teams, in which the members actively work together, each in different ways using particular skills to meet the patient's needs.

Finally, educational programs directed toward persons who will be dealing with chronic patients should emphasize that these patients require the provision of care by the array of services comprised by a community support system. They should also specify how the elements in this system work and relate to one another. The same range of personnel and programs available to the patient who is institutionalized—from cooks to radiologists and psychotherapy to vocational training programs—should also be accessible to a patient living in the community from his or her out-of-hospital support system.

Medical School

The most critical objective in the education of medical students is to modify current attitudes regarding chronic mental illness and the chronic mental patient. The current emphasis on acute treatment, acute medical facilities, and the surgical ("excision") model must be modified. Today's medical students must appreciate that the chronically mentally ill need long-term support and care and that exacerbations constitute only a small portion of their "patienthood." The emphasis of medical education must shift from the acute to the chronic, from the time-limited to the prolonged, from cure to care.

Medical students must be encouraged to understand the necessity for the breadth of the team involved in the optimum care of chronic patients. Most medical students typically come into contact with a nurse, perhaps a secretary or receptionist, and (if they are involved in electives in some areas) a specialty team. The psychiatric and psychosocial team is a much larger entity that requires special attention from the physician (e.g., in order to exchange information and develop treatment plans).

Teaching must reflect the multidimensional aspect of the patient's care. Didactic material should encompass not only the medical and psychiatric aspects of the treatment and care of the chronic patient but also the psychosocial and rehabilitation elements. Teaching should also involve persons from disciplines other than medicine, both in the classroom and in chronic care or community settings.

Opportunities for medical students to gain experience in chronic care and community settings is most important. We as teaching professionals recognize the great value that experiences outside the hospital have in the education of young physicians. Exposure to chronic patients, especially those involved in high-quality programs rather than those who are simply living in board-and-care homes or welfare hotels, would do much to set medical students thinking in an appropriate frame.

Nonpsychiatric Residency Programs

Nonpsychiatric residency programs represent another level at which a change in orientation could facilitate better care of chronic mental patients. Certainly those programs whose graduates deal with large numbers of chronic patients, such as internal medicine, general practice, family practice, and emergency medicine, should offer more teaching in and exposure to chronic mental illness. Even in other specialties, some additional instruction would be useful.

There is a special need to impart our current understanding concerning psychoactive drugs to nonpsychiatric residents. Topics should include their use, side effects, contraindications, and crossover effects as well as the problems of compliance and noncompliance. Nonpsychiatric residents should be made aware of the dilemma faced when a patient on long-term medication develops detrimental side effects (e.g., renal damage or tardive dyskinesia). Without the medication, the patient risks experiencing a recurrence of psychosis, regression, or other disabling symptoms; with it, the side effects may continue or worsen.

It would be useful for all medical specialists to have some actual contact with a mental health or community support team. This experience is critical in conveying the necessity of team operations and the wide variety of services needed by chronic patients as well as in helping to educate the physician about how to tap into supportive networks when he or she is in practice. The specialist must appreciate that he or she need not function alone or in isolation and that the other elements in the helping system are available. When they are not, the physician needs to know what gaps exist and (in the role of community leader) be cognizant of their existence, and also needs to understand the necessity of communicating with the team of persons and network of agencies dealing with the patient.

Psychiatric Residency Programs

There is an equal need for psychiatric training programs to attend to the problems of the care and treatment of the chronically mentally ill. Psychiatric training programs have for years concentrated predominantly on providing inpatient care of the acutely ill person with a history of moderately good functioning using mainly insight-oriented psychological therapies. To treat the chronically ill, poorly functioning person, the resident must be taught the reverse: to provide ambulatory care emphasizing rehabilitative and support system elements.

Woefully absent from most university residency programs is any exposure to the truly chronic patient in either an inpatient or a high-quality, community-based, team-run program. Any exposure that does occur takes place in the inpatient service of the university hospital isolated from any follow-up contact with a community support system— or perhaps as a grudging duty in a medication clinic in an outpatient department with little rehabilitative or community support connections, or for a token period in an overwhelmed and poorly run state hospital or community mental health center (CMHC). Prestige, quality, and investment do not seem connected with many chronic patient programs to which residents are exposed.

There is also a need for the resident to be involved in an important rather than a token role on an outpatient community team; in a low-intensity, low-contact setting; in an emergency crisis setting with exposure to chronic patients; and in consultation with community services. The resident must understand the variety, breadth, and scope of the skills of persons working in a variety of settings in the community care of chronic patients. He or she must also have the opportunity to work intensively and continuously with chronic patients throughout the residency program. Finally, residents must be assisted in the period of "transition to practice" from residency training, the most critical period of recruitment into positions caring for this population.

In addition, the residency curriculum usually emphasizes pharmacology but devotes too little time to the care and treatment of chronic patients and their special needs, to the elements of a community support system, and to the activities and responsibilities of all members of a community team. Likewise, it is necessary to improve the teaching of administration and systems approaches, legal issues, supportive psychotherapy, activities therapies, collaboration with patients and families, and knowledge of community care settings and agencies.

Seminars and courses that concentrate on psychopathology, disease entities, and treatment modalities all need alteration to include the elements of disability, functional assessment, and care of the chronically mentally ill over a long period of time. Such a focus should deal with the medical needs of such patients, the necessity for continuity of care and case monitoring, and the importance of a comprehensive spectrum of services. In all these endeavors the resident must receive high-quality teaching and supervision, not second-class treatment.

Finally, there is a critical need for attitudinal change, both by training directors and by general faculty. Interested residents have too few professional role models of clinicians dedicated to high-quality community care of the chronically mentally ill. Teaching about chronic illness tends to get shunted off to the side or at the end of courses, and exposure to such patients is perceived as unexciting, unimportant, or "unsexy." One mechanism for change is the involvement of training programs in the service programs that deal with chronic patients. Salary incentives may also help alleviate the paucity of high-quality persons entering this area. The residency program should also address the problem of passivity and dependency among patients and the psychiatrist's ability to tolerate these behaviors. It should also reinforce the fact that the chronically mentally ill person can react "neurotically" to the stress of chronic mental illness as we all would react to other stresses.

It is interesting to note that the first article detailing the curriculum, clinical experiences, and faculty supervision involved in residency training regarding the chronic mentally ill was only published in 1989 (Faulkner et al. 1989). The article also discusses in detail some of the barriers to instituting such programs.

Continuing Medical Education (CME) Programs

Although changes in the curricula of medical schools and residency training programs can be mandated by their respective faculties, changes in CME practices are less easily influenced, since physicians attend CME courses according to their perceived needs and current interests. Too little CME material is directed toward this patient population. However, it will be interesting to see if the "market" follows the increasing interest in the chronic patient. Certainly, there is a pressing need to update practicing physicians on the problems and treatment of the chronic mentally ill. Information about modern drug treatment, community support systems, rehabilitative techniques, and research relating to the prevention of chronicity all have their place in CME programs.

In addition, although many nonpsychiatric physicians have considerable contact with chronic patients in their offices or traditional medical settings (such as hospital wards or emergency rooms), they have little exposure to the newer, highly successful psychosocial rehabilitation programs located in the community or to comprehensive community mental health programs that serve the chronic patient. Exposure to such programs and services, either in an educational or in a consultative capacity, should greatly enhance practitioners' effectiveness in dealing with the chronically mentally ill.

A considerable amount of attention should also be given to the attitudes of the practicing physician toward the chronic mental patient. Physicians need to be helped to see persons with chronic mental illness in their total social context, to view their illness as but one part of a complicated skein of problems in life, and to assess the current symptomatology as part of the "whole patient."

There is also a need to retrain and update the training of psychiatrists practicing in chronic care settings, such as state hospitals and nursing homes. Although such efforts are not the primary responsibility of CME activities, they would not only upgrade physicians' skills in their current job but also permit them to become more involved in providing continuity of care for discharged patients and in developing community supportive care.

Implementation of Educational Strategies

To help implement the principles of education summarized above, several training programs have published descriptions of their programs. One of the most detailed is from the University of Oregon (Cutler et al. 1981), where residents spend part of their first year working in state hospitals, their third year working in CMHCs, and their fourth year working in a community support program. Thus, they gain exposure to patients in hospital, CMHC, and community programs. The didactic content covers community psychiatry, case management, planning of linkages, social network theory, deinstitutionalization, psychosocial rehabilitation, and interdisciplinary collaboration.

Another program, at the Massachusetts Mental Health Center, adapted a more traditional residency to better train residents to provide chronic care (White and Bennett 1981). This program tries to prepare the resident to assume multiple roles after graduation: primary clinician, consultant to a multidisciplinary team, medical back-up, and administrator. The program works by fostering the residents' involvement with psychosocial rehabilitation programs, nursing homes, vocational rehabilitation programs, and families, among others. In addition, didactic content dealing with the natural history of chronic conditions, maintenance medication, work with a multidisciplinary team, therapy with chronic patients, psychiatric rehabilitation, and alternatives to hospitalization is presented.

A final example is from St. Vincent's Hospital in New York (Mayo et al. 1982). There the resident has an experience with chronically mentally ill individuals as part of a preventive treatment program whose purpose is the rehabilitation and maintenance of this population. The unifying concept of the program is case management, and the resident functions as both consultant to and supervisor of the case manager. There is also a strong research component to the rotation.

In addition, the Western Interstate Commission for Higher Education (WICHE) has developed an elaborate training scheme for all mental health professions working with the chronically mentally ill (Davis 1981). This training scheme identifies the knowledge, skills or abilities, and attitudes and personality characteristics necessary to provide treatment in several key areas: psychiatric or mental health services, including medication, psychotherapy, crisis intervention, hospitalization, and case management; practical or rehabilitative services, including residential services, training in independent living skills, and vocational services; and community services, including natural support network services, advocacy services, and community development services. Together, the curriculum contains all the essential ingredients for programs that train people who will care for the chronically mentally ill, and it is an invaluable reference.

The reader is also urged to consult the recent National Institute of Mental Health (NIMH) conference report about clinical training for treating serious mental illness (Lefley 1990). The report describes national and local efforts to train social workers, psychologists, nurses, and rehabilitation specialists in the care of the chronically ill. It also addresses how to become involved with the patient's family. The report covers many of the same areas as were mentioned above, but they are discipline specific.

In addition to citing examples of how to train professionals to treat the chronically mentally ill, in the past I have spelled out (J.A. Talbott, unpublished paper, 1981) how *not* to train residents. Unsuccessful programs have no linkage with university departments (or have a relationship that involves no clinical responsibility), and rotations are token experiences. Courses are unrelated to the chronic mental patient, and there are separate tracks for those in university settings and those in public facilities. The role of the resident is either unclear, devalued, overburdened, or narrow in scope (e.g., confined to prescription writing).

Poor residency programs utilize teachers and supervisors who are only psychodynamically or psychoanalytically oriented or who will only supervise "good" therapy patients, or those who are "second-class" or burned out, or private practitioners with no public sector experience. The courses are only psychodynamically or psychoanalytically oriented and involve no systems or administrative content or functional assessment and rehabilitation. The role models are absent, weak, noncharismatic, "second-class," or burned out.

Research is sometimes only nonclinically oriented or unrelated to the clinical program, or it may be absent altogether in any affiliated public facility; residents are placed on teams supervised by a paraprofessional or no leader at all; services expose the resident only to institutional services, do not use community support programs or community agencies, and offer no family contact, outpatient department exposure, or home visiting–home care experience. Also, residents are overinvolved with programs serving the chronically mentally ill population early in their training (i.e., in their first or second years of residency) rather than after their identities as psychiatrists have begun to solidify.

Overcoming Negative Attitudes

A series of videotaped "trigger films" made by Robinowitz and associates (1982) as part of a joint project on the chronically mentally ill by the American Psychiatric Association (APA) and NIMH are a valuable adjunct to all training programs. The films present a variety of negative attitudes about work with the chronically ill. The films are intended to be followed by a discussion of the incident depicted. They include presentations of material about therapeutic pessimism regarding chronic mental illness (in this case, relapse in schizophrenia); use of only one mode of treatment (such as psychodynamically oriented psychotherapy); ways of dealing with families of the chronically ill; patients' compliance with medication; the process of advising a mentally ill spouse about divorce; physicians' refusal to do family therapy, make home visits, or accept chronic patients in a group; a decision to accept a job in the public sector; a supervisor who discourages residents who want to work with the chronically ill (e.g., in a psychodynamic way); a teacher who denigrates aftercare work with the chronically mentally ill, and negative attitudes about community care of the chronically mentally ill.

A Massachusetts Mental Health Center program has given special attention to countertransference attitudes. The faculty attempts to examine the place of hope in the presence of a poor prognosis, the role of rehabilitation versus treatment, the fear of precipitating psychoses, the importance of maintaining limited goals, and the tendency to find chronic patients "less interesting."

In addition, Stern and Minkoff (1979) have written about attitudes of workers in a community clinic that must be challenged in order for them to care effectively for the chronically ill. These include the notion that the clinic is not the appropriate place in which to treat chronic patients, that it must be all things to all people, and that it should "cure" people. The authors suggest shifting the emphasis of clinicians' attitudes from providing primary to tertiary prevention; from treating everyone to treating only the sickest patients; from gaining esteem from seeing only "good" patients to gaining esteem from seeing "difficult" patients; from valuing the ability to treat patients who can benefit from their treatment to valuing the use of new techniques; from valuing cure to providing care; and from hoping to return those patients who are doing badly to state hospitals to finding new resources for them.

Burnout among staff has also been an issue of concern for many years and is an ongoing challenge. Mendel (1979) suggests that burnout may be present when staff begin to blame and label the patients, become bored, complain, increase their frequency of meetings, and show signs of disorganization. It is agreed that burnout is caused by low staff-to-patient ratios, high numbers of schizophrenic patients, long hours, poor interactions between staff and patients, high frequency of staff meetings, few "time-outs" from the pressures of providing care, less sharing of work, higher education and rank, longevity in the field, decreased sense of success and control, decreased sense of closeness to patients, less humanistic views, and more time spent on administrative than on patient issues.

The solutions to burnout among staff flow directly from these causes. They include decreasing unrealistic expectations, not expecting personal needs to be met by patients, recognizing and discussing the problem of burnout openly, altering the case mix, allowing for more "downtime," participating in outside education, increasing the staff-to-patient ratio, decreasing the sequential number of hours of work, sharing patient care responsibilities, and improving work relations in as many ways as possible (Lamb 1979a, 1979b; Pines and Maslach 1978).

The Pew Project

Since 1989, the Pew Foundation has supported a national technical assistance effort to improve the care in the public mental health system by encouraging collaboration between state departments of mental health and university departments of psychiatry. The program is sponsored by five organizations: the APA, the National Association of State Mental Health Program Directors (NASMHPD); the American Academy of Child and Adolescent Psychiatry (AAACP); the American Association of Chairmen of Departments of Psychiatry (AACDP); and the American Association of Directors of Psychiatric Residency Training (AADPRT).

The project was an outgrowth of the Conference on State-University Collaboration sponsored by these same five organizations in June 1984 in Columbia, Maryland. The proceedings of the conference, *Working Together: State University Collaboration in Mental Health*, provided examples of fruitful and disastrous collaborative activities (Talbott and Robinowitz 1986).

The project consists of five elements:

1. A national office that coordinates all activities of the program (e.g., regional conferences, annual meeting workshops, consultations, and awards) as well as publishes a newsletter.
2. Regional invitational conferences for persons interested in improving the public mental health system, attended by both state and university representatives and held in various parts of the country over

the 3-year period of the grant. The goal of these conferences is to present working models of state-university collaboration, to examine specific needs of different groups, to suggest initiatives for change, and to initiate formation of collaborative information and support networks to reinforce efforts leading to change. These meetings have had relatively high faculty-to-attendee ratios and have emphasized interactive and experiential approaches. The project's steering committee and faculty members work with project staff to prepare generic background and resource materials for all attendees as well as to develop appropriate materials for follow-up.

3. An ongoing consultation process (rather than one-time visits) with state, regional, or other governmental mental health administrators and university leaders. Such consultations involve one to three individuals: a state representative, a university representative, and an education or training expert who "bridges" state and university efforts (as is the case in the state-university collaborations in Maryland and Oregon). The amount and intensity of on-site consultation varies according to consultees' program needs and resources. Telephone and written communication continues between visits, and the number of consultants involved in the ensuing visits is determined by program needs and directions.

4. Intensive hands-on training workshops at the annual national meetings of the five parent organizations involving both skill development and information dissemination. Their goals are to train individuals involved in these efforts, promote dissemination of information about these activities, and encourage new collaborative efforts.

5. Presentation of annual awards annually to exemplary programs that have improved or expanded their state-university collaboration. The awards are presented at the annual Hospital and Community Psychiatry Institute and are profiled in a special section of the journal *Hospital and Community Psychiatry.*

The Future

As with so many areas involving the chronically mentally ill, an analysis of the literature reveals that the trick no longer is isolating what needs to be done but doing it. We know the principles underlying good training programs, what works and doesn't work in translating these principles into actual training situations, and what attitudes need to be overcome to deliver both good training and good service programs. We must now use this knowledge to realize our intentions.

References

Cutler DL, Bloom JD, Shore JH: Training psychiatrists to work with community support systems for chronically mentally ill persons. Am J Psychiatry 138:98–202, 1981

Davis M: From Dependence to Independence: Staffing Community Program for the Chronically Mentally Ill. Boulder, CO, Western Interstate Commission on Higher Education, 1981

Faulkner LR, Cutler DL, Krohn DD, et al: A basic residency curriculum concerning the chronically mentally ill. Am J Psychiatry 146:1323–1327, 1989

Goldberg D, Babigian HM, Locke BZ, et al: Role of non-psychiatrist physicians in the delivery of mental health services: implications from 3 studies. Public Health Rep 93:240–245, 1978

Lamb HR: Roots of neglect of the long term mentally ill. Psychiatry 42:201–207, 1979a

Lamb HR: Staff burnout in work with long-term patients. Hosp Community Psychiatry 30:396–398, 1979b

Lefley HP (ed): Clinical Training in Serious Mental Illness: Proceedings of the National Forum for Educating Mental Health Professionals to Work With the Seriously Mentally Ill and Their Families (DHHS Publ No ADM-90-1679). Washington, DC, U.S. Government Printing Office, 1990

Mayo J, Babel R, Carvello R: Planning for the future in psychiatric training: the place of the chronic care program. Compr Psychiatry 23:1–8, 1982

Mendel WM: Staff burnout: diagnosis, treatment and prevention. New Dir Ment Health Serv 2:75–83, 1979

Minkoff K: Beyond deinstitutionalization: a new ideology for the postinstitutional era. Hosp Community Psychiatry 8:945–950, 1987

Nielsen AC, Stein LI, Talbott JA, et al: Encouraging psychiatrists to work with chronic patients: opportunities and limitations of resident education. Hosp Community Psychiatry 32:767–775, 1981

Pines A, Maslach C: Characteristics of staff burnout in mental health settings. Hosp Community Psychiatry 29:233–237, 1978

Robinowitz C, Lurie HJ, Quick SK: Improving Psychiatric Supervision (videotape). Washington, DC, American Psychiatric Association, 1982

Schwartz S, Krieger M, Sorensen J: Preliminary survey of therapists who work with chronic patients: implications for training. Hosp Community Psychiatry 32:779–800, 1981

Segal SP: Attitudes toward the mentally ill: a review. Social Work 34:211–217, 1978

Stern R, Minkoff K: Paradoxes in programming for chronic patients in a community clinic. Hosp Community Psychiatry 30:613–617, 1979

Talbott JA: Medical education and the chronic mentally ill. Journal of the National Association of Private Psychiatric Hospitals 11:58–63, 1980

Talbott JA, Robinowitz C (eds): Working Together: State-University Collaboration in Mental Health. Washington, DC, American Psychiatric Press, 1986

White HS, Bennett, MD: Training psychiatric residents in chronic care. Hosp Community Psychiatry 32:339–343, 1981

Wilford BB (ed): Physicians and Chronic Patients: Potentials for Community Based Care. Chicago, IL, American Medical Association, 1981

Section II:

Treatment and Rehabilitation

Chapter 8

Clinical Care of Homeless Mentally Ill Individuals: Strategies and Adaptations

Ezra Susser, M.D., M.P.H.
Elie Valencia, J.D., M.A.
Stephen M. Goldfinger, M.D.

Homeless individuals with severe mental illnesses are a diverse group whose symptoms and disabilities span a broad range of severity and chronicity (Lamb 1984; Susser 1990; Susser et al. 1989; World Health Organization 1980). Nevertheless, clinicians have found that there are some useful general principles that can be applied to work with this population (Bachrach 1987; Barrow et al. 1987; Breakey, in press; Cohen 1988, 1990; Drake and Adler 1984; Goldfinger and Chafetz 1984; Martin and Nayowith 1989; Morse and Calsyn 1986; Susser et al. 1990). Effective clinical interventions with the homeless mentally ill population frequently require substantial alteration in the initiation, scope, focus, and timing of clinical work (Bachrach 1987; Goldfinger and Chafetz 1984). In this chapter, we focus on areas that differentiate work with this group from work with domiciled psychiatric patients.

The order of our comments roughly approximates the chronology of emerging issues for those working with individuals staying in shelters or in public spaces. We identify and discuss four basic stages: 1) introduction of services into the community, 2) outreach, 3) provision of treatment and other services during the time that individuals remain homeless, and 4) support in the transition to housing.

In each stage, there is a critical feature that differentiates this type of work from most other forms of outpatient health care. In stage 1, the introduction of services, the locales are nonclinical and socially marginal. In outreach, stage 2, the persons to be treated are not seeking care.

The authors thank Andrea White, M.S.W., and Dorrett Johnson, R.N., for their contributions to this chapter.

In stage 3, treatment, a central goal is housing, and in stage 4, transition to housing, care must be transferred from shelter or outreach team to the appropriate community services.

These critical features have many implications for psychiatric care.

Introduction of Services

Clinical teams often work with the homeless mentally ill in public and private shelters, parks, streets, subways, bus and train terminals, and other public spaces. They enter these settings without any invitation from the potential recipients of services who live there. In fact, their presence may be unwelcome to many of these persons. Therefore, they must search for ways to introduce themselves neatly into the social fabric. The appropriate strategy must be predicated on an examination of the prevailing subculture, including attitudes toward mental illness and its treatment, behavioral norms, and the nature of social networks. Often, deviations from traditional approaches are needed.

A transitional hotel in one large city provided accommodations for homeless mentally ill women, many of whom had been living in bus terminals and other public spaces. In the hotel, mental illness and treatment for it were highly stigmatized (Cohen 1989). When the on-site clinical team recruited a psychiatric consultant, his presence was initially seen as intrusive and threatening. Thus, the women were unlikely to present voluntarily for psychiatric treatment, and referrals by staff could have been seen as a humiliation and have been resented.

In order to reshape the interaction between the psychiatrist and the community, the clinical team used a weekly bingo game. Run by the psychiatrist, the bingo game became a source of amusement and curiosity. Its friendly and nonthreatening atmosphere made it the best attended activity in the hotel. Allowing for an alteration of roles, the psychiatrist now became a guest to be treated with hospitality rather than an interloper to be feared (Susser, in press). The approach was successful. Once the psychiatrist became a familiar and accepted figure in the hotel, women who had avoided him at first began to seek treatment, and staff could be assured that referrals would not cause shame.

In another setting, a large municipal men's shelter, a quite different subculture prevailed (Gounis and Susser 1990). The mostly young African American and Latino men had extensive ties to family and others in the surrounding community. Mentally ill individuals often belonged to clearly defined subgroups that controlled different parts of shelter life (e.g., Latinos, African Americans, Cuban immigrants, gay men, etc.). Within each subgroup, a few individuals had a large influence on defining attitudes toward service utilization within the shelter.

Soon after the establishment of an on-site mental health program in the shelter, it became apparent that one of the keys to establishing contact with the mentally ill men was to identify and gain the endorsement of these influential individuals. To do so, the on-site program extended itself somewhat beyond the usual purview of a mental health program by advocating for the improvement of shelter conditions, forming "rap groups," and offering limited job training for healthy men. As a result, the program established credibility with several men who had wide respect in the shelter. Indeed, these men eventually became a major source of referrals of mentally ill men to the program.

This type of adjustment can also be a critical preliminary step to providing good health care in other settings—for instance, in non-Western cultures (Paul 1955). Indeed, services to homeless individuals might be considered analogous to cross-cultural treatment interventions. Distinct subcultures emerge in shelters and street life (Baxter and Hopper 1981; Cohen and Sokolovsky 1989; Gounis, in press; Lovell, in press; Morrisey et al. 1985; Susser and Gonzalez, in press). Only by observing, analyzing, and accommodating the prevailing values, social structure, and population expectations can services be effectively introduced.

Outreach

Outreach teams for the homeless mentally ill identify persons in need of treatment and enter into some relation with them. This approach is unusual in the health care field, except in the context of public health concerns such as the control of infectious diseases. Generally, treatment contacts are initiated by (or on behalf of) the sick person, rather than by a team of professionals seeking "cases" in the community. The distinction is not lost on the homeless, who sometimes regard outreach teams as intrusive and somewhat suspect. The use of outreach teams by municipalities to "clear" public spaces such as train stations tends to reinforce these suspicions. Nonetheless, outreach to the homeless mentally ill is appropriate and, indeed, essential. Without outreach, many of these persons would simply be left destitute and untreated.

Most outreach teams are assigned to public spaces such as parks, city blocks, and bus stations, where they approach people who appear to be homeless and mentally ill. The team offers food, clothing, or other assistance as a basis for the initial contacts. Some creative outreach workers take additional steps. They note the daily activities that are meaningful to an individual and use them to establish an ongoing relation. For example, an outreach team trying to contact a woman who had been living in bus terminals for years noticed she had a fondness and talent for making clothing out of pieces of cloth. Although this woman refused to accept any food or clothing from the team, she was willing to accept the raw materials for her work—pieces of cloth—on a regular basis.

In another case, a man living in a park was observed reading a bundle of newspaper while sitting on a bench. At first, he was quite hostile to any approach by the outreach team. Regular weekly delivery of newspapers was arranged, and he came to look forward to it. Later, the outreach team itself delivered the newspapers.

Other teams contact the homeless mentally ill as they pass through institutions such as drop-in centers, soup kitchens, shelters, and jails. An outreach team in a supportive institution can use this context to facilitate its work. For instance, in a good drop-in center homeless persons find a sort of sanctuary: a place to sit quietly or to talk and be heard out respectfully and a place to form social ties safely. They are also offered food, access to showers, clothes, coffee, and use of a telephone. This setting provides a meaningful context for the initial contact between clinician and client (Segal and Baumohl 1985).

On the other hand, an outreach team that operates in a relatively hostile institution—such as a jail or a municipal shelter—has to develop the proper context itself. This is often done by creating its own sanctuary within the institution. In New York City municipal shelters, for instance, on-site mental health programs use their allocated space to offer, among other things, daily respite from an overcrowded and dangerous environment (Gounis and Susser 1990).

Some of the best teams include homeless persons as team members or adjuncts. They tend to be more knowledgeable about the social context and to be perceived as less threatening than other staff. In some street outreach teams, homeless team members may make the first contact with clients and later introduce the clients to the team clinicians. In another strategy in a large men's shelter, mentally ill men in the psychiatry program regularly take notice of shelter residents who seem withdrawn or bizarre and persuade them to see the clinical team.

Efforts to screen homeless individuals for mental disorders and assess their need for treatment, if necessary, tend to take place in short contacts, over weeks or months. It is impractical to routinely conduct lengthy evaluation interviews as in outpatient clinics, because many clients do not tolerate this type of assessment. Programs develop other ways to assess clients. In one large men's shelter, a clinical team offers small paid jobs, such as making a delivery or a purchase, to men who seem appropriate candidates for the psychiatric program but who are not yet in treatment. These clients are often willing to be accompanied to coffee shops, grocery stores, and other community settings. Thus, their behavior is observed in a range of circumstances. At the same time, much relevant history is elicited in conversation.

One can allow clients to set a gradual pace in accepting treatment for mental problems. Development of trust is crucial, and it takes time. One might spend a good deal of time with people who are not actually enrolled in a program; and even some who are enrolled may be receiving assistance in only a few concrete areas (such as getting clothes and food). Later, once a modicum of trust has been established, some of them will accept medications or other recommended treatments. The process of reaching some agreement with the client about the level of clinical intervention can be quite delicate and requires therapeutic skill.

If a person is seriously disabled with mental illness, at some point one must choose among strategies to proceed to treatment even if the person is not eager to be treated (Susser et al. 1990). Attending to clients' medical problems can serve in building a relationship and later be used as a vehicle for providing psychiatric services. Although many homeless individuals demonstrate little interest in mental health care (Ball and Havassy 1984) or actively avoid it, they frequently will accept medical attention when it is offered. Many in the population believe mental health care makes them feel more uncomfortable, but they tend to associate medical attention with feeling better, particularly if they are experiencing pain or discomfort. Therefore, offering to provide foot care, cold medications, or help with lice infestations may be a first step toward being viewed as someone who can provide help and relief (Goldfinger 1990).

Clients who are more comfortable with treatment for medical than for "mental" problems tend to be more receptive to psychiatric treatment when it is framed in medical terms. For instance, one might introduce psychiatric care by (rightly) explaining that some medical problems affect feelings and behavior. Treatment would then proceed with a focus on the aspects of care that most resemble ordinary medical care (e.g., medication).

Not all clients prefer the medical approach. Some reject treatment for medical problems and medication, but seek therapy and accept the psychiatric patient status with ease. These clients might be enlisted in a joint effort to solve specific problems in their lives. They may agree to monitor symptoms and even to accept episodic hospitalizations.

Even the most "resistant" (Goldfinger and Chavetz 1984) clients might be willing to talk to a mental health professional, even a psychiatrist, as long as they are free to define the nature of the conversation. They will then be able to avoid areas that they are afraid to discuss (such as psychotic symptoms) and may also avoid formal assessment and treatment until they are more comfortable. Although some professionals regard such casual chatting as time-consuming and frustrating, it can be an essential first step toward developing rapport. Chatting regularly with a psychiatrist involves an implicit recognition of a need for treatment; trust can develop over time, making other interventions possible.

From these various starting points, one can generally proceed to more comprehensive treatment in a gradual way. One learns to choose the best moments to insist on introducing a further treatment. Some mentally ill individuals, however, cannot be persuaded to enter either treatment or supportive housing. In these cases, assistance in survival, even some form of rehabilitation, can still be offered in the given context. There may be room for advocacy on a limited basis, such as in obtaining access to shelter, food, and clothing. It may be possible to elaborate on simple daily activities, such as sewing or reading the newspaper, to the point that they can generate income or social networks. Even if one can do no more than reinforce and facilitate the activities that provide structure and meaning in a person's life, one may be significantly improving that person's chances of survival and quality of life, while laying the groundwork for a further relation in the future.

Some individuals who refuse treatment are so severely ill that they cannot care for themselves. Involuntary hospitalization might be the only feasible option. The process of hospitalization offers many opportunities to establish a relationship with a patient (Kanter 1991). Patients may feel a new appreciation for the outreach worker who accompanied them through the arduous and frightening process of involuntary admission. By bringing news and gifts to and from patients, the outreach worker can help to maintain (and at the same time learn about) the patients' social network. Years later, patients may remember the outreach worker's frequent visits and well-chosen gifts.

Treatment and Other Services

The point at which outreach merges into treatment is hard to define (Intergovernmental Health Policy Project 1987). Indeed, the principles of outreach are applied throughout the treatment phase as new interventions are introduced. A good rule of thumb is that a client who is formally enrolled in a program and who is willing to discuss treatment goals with the clinical team is in the treatment phase.

Some of the treatment approaches used with the homeless mentally ill differ little from those used with domiciled patients. As noted earlier, our focus is on the differences. In work with the long-term homeless, the primary difference is that housing is almost always a central focus in treatment.

A long preparatory phase might be needed before housing becomes a real alternative. For instance, an individual might need to achieve a minimal level of hygiene, control of severe symptoms, and an entitlement income. Also, it may take months until a client feels comfortable in discussing housing in any realistic fashion. Nevertheless, from the start, one is constantly laying the groundwork for a housing placement.

An analogy may be made to outreach work. In outreach, one does not discuss treatment on the first contact, but one is constantly searching for ways to introduce it; similarly, in treatment, one is always preparing the client to obtain housing.

In the preparatory phase, clinical teams usually rely on some form of case management. There is substantial agreement that case management that includes assessment, planning, linkage, monitoring, advocacy, and follow-up must play a central role in the ongoing care of homeless mentally ill clients (Goldfinger 1990; Intagliata 1982; Sullivan 1981; Turner and Shifren 1979). What has been found most useful is a clinical model of case management, involving a primary relationship between the case manager and the client (Deitchman 1980; Harris and Bergman 1987; Kanter 1989; Lamb 1980). This model of case management combines the provision of "hard goods and services" with what some see as the logical extension of supportive psychodynamic psychotherapy (Frances and Goldfinger 1986).

Clinicians working with this disenfranchised group have also effectively used radical approaches in advocacy, client education, peer support, and training in community living skills (Susser et al. 1990). Such interventions must be tailored to the context. A group of residents of a women's shelter categorized the skills needed to be a good panhandler. These included understanding the neighborhood, "sizing up" potential givers, and having a convincing story. Clients then applied these skills in negotiating for carfare from the shelter staff; they "sized up" the worker who provided it and showed the worker the necessary appointment slips. Later, the same skills were used in applying for welfare, a task that became less foreboding when broken down to a set of familiar practices, now used to obtain money from a different channel.

Once the client is ready to discuss housing options, a housing group might be used to set the treatment plan. Information on housing is presented, the skills required to live in each type of housing are specified, and prior experiences are discussed. Thus, group members develop a keener sense of their preferences, their capabilities, and their options before making a choice. For individuals who do not like to attend groups or cannot tolerate them, the same principles can be applied in individual treatment.

The process of adjusting hopes and expectations can be difficult. A client might initially envision him- or herself in a two-bedroom apartment and view others in the same program as capable of living only in a special facility for the disabled. He or she may regard any supportive residence as a dead-end alternative. It is usually helpful to reframe the present options as a beginning rather than an ending.

Clients may be encouraged to visit several potential residences and to reject any and all that make them feel uncomfortable. The program then tries to identify and discuss with the clients the reasons for their discomfort. In the process, the clients' housing needs become more clearly defined. For instance, a mentally ill man living in a bus terminal was ready to accept the help of an outreach team in finding housing. However, he was vague about what housing meant to him and what type he would accept. As a first step, he visited a supportive residence that seemed appropriate to the team. It became clear from his reactions to the visit that he was not interested in this residence or any other housing that would curtail his independence. He wanted to continue much of his present life—and in particular to spend his days in the bus terminal—but with the added resource of a room. The team then directed its efforts to finding such accommodation and arranging for supportive services to be available to him there.

In choosing a residence, a client considers many factors, including cost, access to stores and to transportation, tolerance for rules such as a curfew, and the level of on-site services. Two features are crucial to many clients but are easily overlooked by staff. One is the proximity to the client's social network, including the networks formed while the client was homeless. The second is stigma. Many clients find it hard to accept housing for the disabled. In New York City, Boston, and elsewhere, there has recently been some success in creating supportive residences that are not identifiable as facilities for the disabled (Hellman 1988). In particular, single-room-occupancy hotels with on-site services have been found to be acceptable to a broad range of homeless mentally ill persons (Lipton et al. 1988; Susser et al. 1990).

Homeless individuals are generally willing to consider offers of permanent housing, but a few long-term homeless people are so adapted to their environment that they persistently reject any offers of housing. A man with paranoid schizophrenia living in one municipal shelter never leaves the premises. He sleeps on the floor in the shelter hallway. Despite his disabilities, this man is highly skilled in shelter living. He buys protection from other residents. He uses the showers and takes meals at precisely the times that one is least likely to be victimized. For years he has spent his days in the shelter mental health program but has outright refused all offers of housing. The shelter appears to satisfy a range of needs. He has access to food, clothing, and a day program.

He can observe a lively social scene without having to take part in it. He is known to most and cared for by some. In short, he is part of a community—and one that is not restricted to the mentally ill. As in other such cases, it is difficult to assess whether his preference for the shelter is entirely due to his psychiatric condition. Perhaps he suspects that he will not find a comparable niche elsewhere.

Treatment of the mentally ill who are newly or episodically homeless, as opposed to treatment of the long-term homeless, may be considered a form of secondary prevention of homelessness. The approach resembles crisis intervention. One works with family and social networks to identify the origins of the present crisis, to limit deterioration as relations become more strained, and, finally, to reach an accommodation to the situation (Gounis et al. 1987). An effort is made to provide the clients' social network with feasible alternatives for handling conflicts that may lead to homelessness. Even a modest amount of psychoeducation and support for the family can make a difference. Most programs have not recognized the significance of early intervention, however, and focus primarily on helping the long-term homeless.

The difficulty of [providing] treatment needs to be emphasized. In our observation, typically only a minority of the clients who enroll in a program reach the point of housing placement. Further, many of the individuals who do find housing become homeless again—in one study, 41% within 18 months (Caton et al. 1990). Premature placement, inappropriate placement sites, lack of available concomitant psychiatric and rehabilitation services, and termination of ongoing case management and other supports are frequent contributors to this unfortunate outcome.

Transition to Housing

Specialized services for the homeless mentally ill are, by definition, time-limited. Once placed in housing, however, the formerly homeless individual generally remains mentally ill and vulnerable to another episode of homelessness. Therefore, transferring care from programs for the homeless to other community resources at or around the time of housing placement is a critical step. This step may be considered analogous to the transfer of care from hospital to community services at the time of hospital discharge.

The appropriate timing and nature of the transfer of care are controversial. Many programs for the homeless transfer care rather abruptly at the time of housing placement, often because they are required to do so by their funding agency. We disagree with this approach. Clients feel vulnerable at this time, and their need for support is at a peak. In addition, the patterns of behavior and support systems required to maintain housing stability are not yet present. An abrupt and complete transfer of care at such a time is perilous.

Some clinical programs have extended services into the critical transition period. One such program, Critical Time Intervention (CTI), has been initiated by two of the authors (E. Susser and E. Valencia) as a clinical trial aimed at reducing the recurrence of homelessness after placement in housing. CTI is presently being tested in men with schizophrenia in a north Manhattan municipal shelter. It is a time-limited intervention using a straightforward approach that could be replicated with ease.

For up to 9 months after a client leaves the shelter, the CTI team assists him in establishing durable patterns of medication compliance, money management, and (when appropriate) control of substance abuse. For instance, a system of medication compliance can involve, in addition to the client, a clinician in the outpatient clinic, a family member, and a local pharmacist, each taking a limited role in monitoring and reinforcing compliance. The members of this network have access to one another. The medication compliance system is tested "in vivo" and modified if necessary during the transition period.

The CTI team is also equipped to teach social skills that promote housing stability. This step is most important for people who have been homeless or who have been living in institutions for long periods, or perhaps for all their adult lives. The individual might learn to seek advice from a designated person before he responds to a "housing crisis" (e.g., a complaint by the landlord about his behavior).

The potential role of kin in establishing stable support systems is given special focus in the CTI experiment; family members, after all, tend to outlast other supports. The team aims to define clearly limited—even though crucial—long-term roles for family members. There is no implication that the family is in any way to blame for the person's homeless condition.

Conclusion

In spite of the diversity of settings in which clinical teams work with the homeless mentally ill and the variation in the training and preferences of the clinicians, some common themes prevail when working with this population. One has to introduce oneself into a marginal locale, determine who is to be treated there, arduously recruit them into treatment, find them housing that they will accept, and establish a durable system of support to prevent future homelessness. Each of these steps is truly a challenge that calls on the clinician to experiment.

In meeting these challenges, clinicians in this field have in some ways been forced to move ahead of the mainstream of community psychiatry. Thus, they learn how to introduce clinical services in a way that is most acceptable to a community; spend time with clients and learn intimately about their lives in the community; find ways to interest even the most hard to reach in treatment; and develop interventions to promote stability in housing (as perhaps might also be done by mental hospitals for discharged patients).

Except in the best model systems in community psychiatry, such as the Dane County system (Stein and Test 1985) or the Continuing Care Program at the Massachusetts Mental Health Center (Hellman 1988), clinicians are rarely given the opportunity to do these things. It is our hope that not only the homeless mentally ill but also other mentally ill persons will benefit from the advances in this field.

References

Bachrach LL: Issues in identifying and treating the homeless mentally ill, in Leona Bachrach Speaks: Selected Speeches and Lectures. Edited by Bachrach LL. San Francisco, CA, Jossey-Bass, 1987, pp 43–62

Ball FIJ, Havassy BE: A survey of the problems and needs of homeless consumers of acute psychiatric services. Hosp Community Psychiatry 35:917–921, 1984

Barrow SM, Hellman F, Plapinger J, et al: Preliminary Findings from an Evaluation of Programs for the Mentally Ill Homeless. New York, New York Psychiatric Institute, June 1986 (revised 1987)

Baxter E, Hopper K: Private Lives/Public Spaces: Homeless Adults on the Streets of New York City. New York, Community Service Society, 1981

Breakey W: Mental health services for homeless people, in Homelessness: A National Perspective. Edited by Robertson M, Greenblatt M. New York, Plenum (in press)

Caton CLM, Wyatt RJ, Grunberg J, et al: A follow-up of chronically homeless mentally ill. Paper presented at the annual meeting of the American Psychiatric Association, New York, May 1990

Cohen MB: Interaction and Mutual Influence in a Program for Homeless Mentally Ill Women. Unpublished doctoral dissertation. Florence Heller School for Advanced Studies in Social Welfare, Brandeis University, Waltham, MA, 1988

Cohen MB: Social work practice with homeless mentally ill people: engaging the client. Social Work 34:505–512, 1989

Cohen N (ed): Psychiatry Takes to the Street. New York, Guilford, 1990

Cohen N, Sokolovsky S: Old Men of the Bowery. New York, Guilford, 1989

Deitchman WS: How many case managers does it take to screw in a light bulb? Hosp Community Psychiatry 31:788–789, 1980

Drake RE, Adler DA: Shelter is not enough: clinical work with the homeless mentally ill, in The Homeless Mentally Ill: A Task Force Report of the American Psychiatric Association. Edited by Lamb HR. Washington, DC, American Psychiatric Association, 1984, pp 141–152

Frances A, Goldfinger SM: "Treating" a homeless mentally ill patient who cannot be managed in a shelter system. Hosp Community Psychiatry 37:577–579, 1986

Goldfinger SM: Homelessness and schizophrenia: a psychosocial approach, in Handbook of Schizophrenia, Vol 4. Edited by Herz I, Keith SJ, Docherty JP. New York, Elsevier Science Publishers, 1990, pp 355–385

Goldfinger SM, Chafetz L: Designing a better service delivery system for the homeless mentally ill, in The Homeless Mentally Ill: A Task Force Report of the American Psychiatric Association. Edited by Lamb HR. Washington, DC, American Psychiatric Association, 1984, pp 91–108

Gounis K: Temporality and the domestication of homelessness, in The Politics of Time (Monograph Series, Vol 4). Edited by Rutz H. American Ethnological Society (in press)

Gounis K, Susser E: Shelterization and its implications for mental health services, in Psychiatry Takes To The Streets. Edited by Cohen N. New York, Guilford, 1990

Gounis K, Conover S, Susser E, et al: First-timers at the Franklin Men's Shelter: a program to prevent shelterization of newly homeless men. New York, New York City Department of Mental Health, 1987

Harris M, Bergman HC: Case management with the chronically mentally ill: a clinical perspective. Am J Orthopsychiatry 57:296–302, 1987

Hellman SJ: The continuing care service. New Dir Ment Health Serv 39:73–87, 1988

Intergovernmental Health Policy Project: Consensus Conference on Outreach Services for Homeless Mentally Ill People. Washington, DC, George Washington University, 1987

Intagliata J: Improving the quality of community care for the mentally disabled: the role of case management. Schizophr Bull 8:655–674, 1982

Kanter J: Clinical case management: definition, principles, components. Hosp Community Psychiatry 4:361–368, 1989

Kanter JS: Integrating case management and psychiatric hospitalization. Health Soc Work 16:35–42, 1991

Lamb HR: Therapist-case managers: more than brokers of services. Hosp Community Psychiatry 31:762–764, 1980

Lamb HR (ed): The Homeless Mentally Ill: A Task Force Report of the American Psychiatric Association. Washington, DC, American Psychiatric Association, 1984

Lipton FR, Nutt S, Sabatini A: Housing the homeless mentally ill: a longitudinal study of a treatment approach. Hosp Community Psychiatry 39:40, 1988

Lovell A: Seizing the moment: power and temporal in street life, in The Politics of Time (Monograph Series, Vol 4). Edited by Rutz H. American Ethnological Society (in press)

Martin MA, Nayowith S: Creating community: groupwork to develop social support networks with homeless mentally ill. Social Work with Groups 11:79–93, 1989

Morrisey JP, Dennis D, Gounis K, et al: The Development and Utilization of the Queens Men's Shelter. Albany, NY, Bureau of Evaluation Research, New York State Office of Mental Health, 1985

Morse G, Calsyn RJ: Disturbed homeless people in St. Louis: needy, willing, but underserved. International Journal of Mental Health 14:74, 1986

Paul B (ed): Health, Culture and Community: Case Studies of Public Reaction to Health Programs. New York, Russell Sage Foundation, 1955

Segal S, Baumohl J: The community living room. Social Casework 66:111–116, 1985

Stein LI, Test MA: The evolution of the training in community living model experience. New Dir Ment Health Serv 26:7–16, 1985

Sullivan JP: Case management, in The Chronic Mental Patient. Edited by Talbott JA. New York, Human Sciences Press, 1981, pp 119–131

Susser M: Disease, illness, sickness: impairment, disability, and handicaps. Psychol Med 20:471–473, 1990

Susser E: Working with people who are homeless and mentally ill: the role of a psychiatrist, in Homelessness: A Preventive Approach. Edited by Jahiel R. Baltimore, MD, Johns Hopkins University Press (in press)

Susser I, Gonzalez A: Sex, drugs, videotape: the prevention of AIDS in a shelter for homeless men in New York City. Med Anthropol (in press)

Susser E, Struening E, Conover S: Psychiatric problems in homeless men: lifetime psychosis, substance abuse, and current distress in new arrivals at New York City shelters. Arch Gen Psychiatry 46:845–850, 1989

Susser E, White A, Goldfinger S: Some clinical approaches to the homeless mentally ill. Community Ment Health J 26:459–476, 1990

Turner J, Shifren I: Community support systems: how comprehensive? in Community Support Systems for the Long-Term Patient. Edited by Stein L. San Francisco, CA, Jossey-Bass, 1979

World Health Organization: International Classification of Impairments, Disabilities, and Handicaps. Geneva, World Health Organization, 1980

Chapter 9

Outreach Intervention Models for the Homeless Mentally Ill

Neal L. Cohen, M.D.
Luis R. Marcos, M.D., Sc.D.

Rapid growth in the number of homeless mentally ill across the country during the 1980s has led advocacy groups and the media to focus attention on the inadequacies of the community mental health care system (Barbanel 1988; Hemphill 1989). The seriously mentally ill are most vulnerable to the disorganizing effects of stressors associated with homelessness, poverty, drug abuse, and a dysfunctional service system. Life in the community is far more complex and less easily controlled than is life in an institution. People are free to stay away from clinic appointments, to reject medications, and to refuse mental health services.

Therefore, programs designed to meet the needs of seriously mentally ill persons must be shaped to fit the unique needs of the target population and service system in their communities (Bachrach 1988). They must be able to reach into their neighborhoods and homes to make a continuum of services accessible for those who most need them (Sullivan and Cohen 1990).

One service component that is essential for the maintenance of a comprehensive and integrated system of community care services for the chronically mentally ill—and one that is often missing—is the interdisciplinary mobile crisis intervention and outreach team (Cohen and Sullivan 1990; Primm and Houck 1990; Witheridge 1990). This chapter describes the goals and characteristics of outreach intervention models, in particular the Homeless Emergency Liaison Project (HELP), established in New York City in the early 1980s. Project HELP emphasizes outreach with access to hospital treatment through involuntary commitment.

The Outreach Intervention Model

Outreach teams work to fill a gap in mental health services by providing the services that no one else provides, at times on an urgent basis. Differences in the specific mission of these outreach teams will dictate the model of intervention and the staff composition necessary to work within the program model.

For example, an outreach team whose function is primarily providing emergency psychiatric intervention may be staffed with an emphasis on medical personnel, whereas an outreach team emphasizing case management services may emphasize social work capacity. Similarly, the model of intervention in crisis-oriented teams emphasizes rapid assessment and triage decision making rather than the relationship-building work and client-monitoring functioning of case management teams.

In any of these service models, the outreach team is unique in its effort to step into the "total ecology" of the person and to assist those agencies that can be mobilized to maintain adequate supports for individuals living in the community. The work is extremely labor intensive, often involving two or more staff members' spending entire days with one individual. The teams must be flexibly designed to provide those services that a particular group or individual is missing.

Therefore, neither a crisis intervention nor a case management model alone comfortably fits the range of services usually required by the population of seriously and chronically mentally ill persons who are homeless. Services for chronically disaffiliated people must include community housing with accessible social and mental health services, crisis beds, drop-in centers, and treatment and rehabilitation services, all addressing the diversity of biopsychosocial needs. Among the most effective service systems are those that enlist an outreach team to provide linkage to a vast network of service components in a manner that has eluded the organization of traditional community-based mental health programs (Cohen 1990).

The outreach team aims to build a relationship in which even the most fragile and disaffiliated homeless persons may feel trust and respect from the team members. The approach should be nonthreatening and respectful of the individual's place in the community, even though he or she is homeless. The initial outreach encounter sets the tone for what the individual may continue to expect from the outreach team. Giving a homeless person a warm cup of coffee, a sandwich or piece of fruit, or an item of clothing makes the offer of assistance seem relevant and understandable. Often, the outreach team using this approach may spend months dropping off items of food or clothing for a homeless person who may say little, if anything, to them.

Although the task may appear simple and repetitive, clinicians who do this work well must possess a variety of skills and have the capacity to be flexible about their roles in the team. Clinical staff may sometimes question whether food preparation or delivery is an appropriate component of their job description. Viewing the team's work at a surface level, however, means missing the complexity and dynamics of the relationship to the homeless individual.

Having a specific expertise derived from a limited, discipline-oriented training and perspective is inadequate to perform the many tasks facing the outreach team. The most successful approach blends diverse perspectives into a holistic systems view directed at the total person and the set of problems in need of solution.

The homeless mentally ill are a diverse group of people who differ in as many characteristics as they share. Diagnosis, chronicity, social networks, work history and skills, level of functioning, and current symptomatology all vary widely among this population. The resistance of many to treatment services is partially derived from a fear and distrust of institutions and the professionals associated with them. As a result, gaining the trust of homeless mentally ill persons is basic to the work of all program models. Without any cooperation from the homeless person in making a clinical assessment, the outreach worker will be able to judge only the most obvious aspects of the person's level of functioning and relationship to the immediate environment.

Outreach teams have more success engaging mentally ill persons into mental health care if they have knowledge of the physical setting as well as the network of social systems with which an individual interacts. When the population is also homeless, that knowledge is frequently very limited and may be limited to data on the individual's location (whether inside or outside; protected or unprotected; alone or with others) and degree of protection from adverse weather conditions. The social and physical ecology of a homeless person's location is clinically vital information for formulating a meaningful plan for the provision of the most essential services relevant to that individual's life in that community.

To establish the individual's level of functioning and service needs, the outreach team scrutinizes the condition of a homeless person's clothing to make inferences about the individual's orientation, judgment, and adaptiveness. Specifically, clean clothes that cover the body suggest a vastly different level of organization than tattered clothes that expose body parts to cold temperatures. The presence of severely torn clothing that exposes genitals or breasts may signify a serious impairment in reality testing. Similarly, the quantity and organization of a homeless person's belongings also provide clues to his or her level of functioning and adaptation to street conditions.

Physical appearance and behavior provide information on an individual's health status. Edematous lower extremities may reflect impaired cardiac functioning; a productive cough may indicate the presence of a tuberculosis infection. Many medical problems are exacerbated by exposure to extremes of heat and cold, contaminated food, and inadequate personal hygiene (Tsemberis et al., in press).

The crises that homeless mentally ill persons face are often related to the most basic issues of survival, such as exposure to severe cold or hot weather, inability to obtain food and clothing, deteriorated medical status, and increasingly impaired judgment that prevents them from making even the most simple social decision. All outreach teams must be able to provide the necessary linkage with medical and psychiatric treatment, on either a voluntary or involuntary and inpatient or outpatient basis. Emergency room care must be accessible, whether through municipal ambulance transport or in the van or station wagon of the outreach team.

Immediate medical or psychiatric care at an emergency room may be lifesaving but also may trigger the need for follow-up management of problems that are difficult to supervise when a homeless person remains living on the street. The crisis intervention–oriented team may not need to intervene urgently after assessing a homeless mentally ill person but will need to provide the case managers with clinical guidelines for contacting the team again when further deterioration in the person's medical or psychiatric status is noted.

Outreach team service models addressing the needs of the homeless mentally ill should adapt to characteristics of the target population to be served. In New York City, the network of municipal shelters has become a long-term institutional arrangement for many thousands of men afflicted with a wide range of disabilities; a majority of these men have been found to have histories of heavy substance abuse, psychiatric disorder, or both (Susser et al. 1989). Services to the residents of these shelters need to be linked to off-site resources, including housing, mental health services, job training, and detoxification programs (Gounis and Susser 1990). Therefore, knowledge of service systems and treatment planning for persons with dual diagnoses of mental illness and chemical dependency is vital to the work of outreach teams with shelter residents.

The powerful influence of the social ecology and institutional context within which homeless persons survive also has an impact on clinical work with these populations. Gounis and Susser (1990) and Grunberg and Eagle (1990) describe the pervasiveness of demoralization among long-term shelter residents who have developed patterns of behavioral passivity and dependency like the ones so prevalent among patients of long-term stay hospitals. This phenomenon, known as shelterization, acts as a barrier preventing mental health workers from engaging homeless persons.

The prevalence of young, violence-prone, substance-abusing males in the municipal shelter system in New York City has been partially responsible for the migration of many fragile, older, severely and chronically mentally ill persons from shelters to life in the streets. These individuals frequently report that they believe the streets are safer than the predatory environment of the shelters. A psychopathology featuring social withdrawal, apathy, and psychomotor retardation was found to be commonplace among many homeless mentally ill persons who preferred life on the streets to institutional alternatives, such as shelters, group homes, long-term care facilities, and so on (Cohen et al. 1986).

The presence of severe deficit symptomatology and deterioration in functioning highlights the difficulty in engaging and treating this population of homeless mentally ill (Cohen and Sullivan 1990). In New York City, for example, attention to the clinical and survival needs of this subpopulation of the homeless mentally ill has been accomplished through the establishment of Project HELP, which emphasizes outreach with access to hospital treatment through involuntary commitment. Some of the political, legal, ethical, and clinical issues that have been raised by this initiative will be examined here.

Project HELP

The vulnerability of many homeless mentally ill and the role for mobile psychiatric outreach services was recognized in New York City in January 1982, when a 61-year-old, chronic mentally ill woman was found dead in the cardboard box on a New York City street that had been her home (Cohen et al. 1984). The woman had been living in the box for more than 8 months, ever since her public assistance benefits had been revoked due to "failure to appear for recertification." After rebuffing the efforts of various agencies to relocate her, she died of hypothermia just hours before a court order was obtained directing her removal to a hospital for evaluation.

Project HELP was developed shortly thereafter through the collaboration of several city agencies to provide rapid transport of such individuals to a hospital facility in the face of a life-threatening emergency. Project HELP is staffed by an interdisciplinary team consisting of psychiatrists, nurses, and social workers. Operating 7 days a week, the team's van cruises the borough of Manhattan, where the majority of the homeless are known to live, and accepts referrals on a telephone hotline. The psychiatric staff was empowered under Section 9.37 of the New York State Mental Hygiene Law to order police officers to involuntarily transport homeless mentally ill persons who were at "imminent risk of danger to self or to others" to a designated psychiatric emergency room. The initial targets were the most seriously impaired homeless mentally ill, who had formerly been able to "die with their rights on" (Treffert 1985) by defying the efforts of social service and health care systems to engage them in treatment voluntarily.

The project's target population was found to be readily identifiable even in New York City's crowded streets. Primary visual indicators of the need for these outreach services included an extremely dirty and disheveled appearance; torn, dirty, or multilayered clothing; clothing that was grossly inappropriate to the weather conditions (e.g., layers of heavy coats and woolen hats in midsummer or scanty, tattered clothes in midwinter); and a collection of belongings in bags, boxes, or shopping carts. Primary behavioral indicators include walking in traffic, urinating or defecating in public, lying on a crowded sidewalk, and remaining mute and withdrawn.

Typically, many of those approached by the Project HELP team flee or refuse to become engaged in any way. They may pull a blanket or rug more tightly over their heads or crawl deeper into their boxes. Those who refuse services in such a manner are evaluated as thoroughly as possible. If an individual flees, mobility is assessed as an indication of medical status. Evaluations may also include a check of storekeepers in the area to obtain information about the individual's behavior and food intake.

One of the original premises of Project HELP was the need for aggressive outreach services in response to extremes of weather conditions. It was assumed that cases of hypothermia among the homeless could be prevented by a mobile psychiatric unit with the ability to facilitate treatment for those patients unable or unwilling to use existing services. Project HELP became operational as the winter of 1982–1983 approached. With extended forecasts predicting an unusually bitter winter, it was assumed that Project HELP would move a significant number of patients out of the cold. The onset of winter weather, however, revealed the adaptive capabilities of the typical Project HELP patient to a life-endangering environment. During inclement weather, many street people move into subway stations and to other locations that offer some warmth.

In the first $2\frac{1}{2}$ years of its operation (November 1982 through May 1985), the Project HELP outreach teams worked within a strict interpretation of the mental hygiene law in New York State, which requires that involuntary transport of mentally ill persons be based on clear evidence of dangerousness to self or others. As a result, of 1,600 homeless persons evaluated during this time period, only 48 (3%) were transported involuntarily for psychiatric evaluation to the emergency rooms of public general hospitals.

Clinical Case

Maria, a 67-year-old, Hispanic female was assessed by Project HELP in the hallway of her former apartment building. She had refused to pay more than $25 per month for her apartment and also had refused to pay for any utilities for several years. She paid a resident of the building to allow her to use toilet facilities. She slept sitting up in a corner of the staircase. Her limited diet consisted of fast foods, which she could eat only when she was certain the bathroom would be available. She was garbed in layers of clothing covered by several large garbage bags, regardless of the season.

Maria refused all efforts at providing services for her because of her fixed delusion that anyone from whom she accepted anything would turn into a horse with an iron heart. She refused all offers of aid. She would, however, allow her temperature and pulse to be taken. During a period of particularly hot weather, she continued to wear her layers of woolens covered by plastic bags. When her pulse became thready and when she continued to refuse any offers of assistance, Maria was involuntarily transported.

On January 22, 1985, the mayor of New York City declared a cold weather emergency for the first time in the history of the city. The announcement initiated a new public policy whereby when the temperature or wind chill factor dropped to 5°F, the police were authorized to determine whether homeless individuals had any realistic recourse to shelter from the bitter cold weather. In the absence of available shelter, the police officers were instructed to offer voluntary transport to a city shelter. If the individual refused, transport to a municipal general hospital emergency room for medical and psychiatric examination on an involuntary basis was authorized. This policy was reinstated in New York City on November 4, 1985. This time, however, the cold weather emergency became effective whenever the temperature dropped to 32°F. As a result, scores of homeless persons were brought to municipal hospitals (Purnick 1985).

These policy initiatives were accomplished without changing the state laws governing the involuntary removal of individuals to hospitals. Instead, public policies and administrative processes were altered to permit a more flexible interpretation of existing legal statutes that reflected the shift toward *parens patriae* and police powers (Marcos and Cohen 1986). As a result, the Project HELP team transported 140 individuals to psychiatric emergency rooms between November 1985 and April 1986 (6 months), compared to the 48 who had been designated for involuntary transport during the first $2\frac{1}{2}$ years of operation.

Increasing public awareness and outrage regarding what was seen as the inhumane quality of life of the homeless mentally ill who refuse treatment services brought about renewed political pressure to relax the laws that regulate involuntary psychiatric treatment (Marcos et al. 1990). On several occasions in the early 1980s, the courts of New York and other states interpreted the mental hygiene law to permit the involuntary hospitalization of the mentally ill who presented a threat of harm to themselves as a result of their failure to meet their essential needs for health or safety (Cohen and Marcos 1990). Thus, less restrictive case law has supported the notion that dangerousness does not have to be based solely on patients' active efforts to harm themselves, and that it is lawful to commit mentally ill individuals whose neglect of essential needs or refusal to care for themselves presents a real threat to their well-being.

Toward this goal of broadening the criteria for the involuntary treatment of psychiatrically impaired homeless mentally ill persons, on October 28, 1987 the mayor of New York City expanded the mission of Project HELP. Staff were authorized to involuntarily remove from the city streets severely mentally ill individuals who neglected their essential needs for food, clothing, shelter, and medical care; those who, by reason of their mental illness, lacked the capacity to comprehend the need to protect themselves from obvious danger; and those who were, in the view of most observers, at risk of physical harm within the reasonably foreseeable future (New York City Health and Hospitals Corporation 1987). These criteria remain in force today.

Patients who meet these criteria are transported to Bellevue Hospital's psychiatric emergency room for further evaluation and, if indicated, are admitted to a newly created 28-bed, short-term intensive care psychiatric inpatient unit. Once the specialized unit reaches capacity, additional Project HELP patients are sent to other psychiatric units of the hospital. Each patient is examined by a psychiatrist on the street, another psychiatrist in the emergency room, and a third psychiatrist within 48 hours of admission to the inpatient unit. The three psychiatrists must concur independently on the need for involuntary hospitalization in order for the patient to remain in the hospital.

Following the acute phase of hospital care, these patients are provided access to a variety of community-based and institutional settings specifically developed or modified for this initiative. One program component is a 70-bed inpatient unit at Creedmoor Psychiatric Center, a long-term-care state facility located in the borough of Queens. This service is for patients who are deemed in need of extended institutional psychiatric care. Also, the city established a 30-bed rehabilitation transitional living program staffed by Bellevue Hospital clinicians at a municipal shelter for men. This setting serves as a temporary discharge alternative for improved patients for whom no other community setting is readily available.

Clinical Case

Joyce, a 40-year-old African American woman, was the first person brought to the hospital under the new policy initiative (Cournos 1989; Marcos, in press). The outreach team found Joyce in her usual street location, in the fashionable Upper East Side area of Manhattan, where she had remained for over a year. Wearing lightweight clothing, she was poorly clad for the cold weather. Her hair was visibly infested with lice, matted, and unkempt. She was dirty and disheveled; the area around her smelled of urine and feces. As usual, she became loud, angry, and threatening as the team approached. She was suspicious of passersby and the team members but demonstrated no clear evidence of delusions or hallucinations.

She denied having any problems and appeared unaware of being in a precarious situation. Concerned citizens in the neighborhood had reported that Joyce had been running into traffic and behaved threateningly to certain passersby without evidence of having been provoked. She was involuntarily transferred to Bellevue Hospital after the psychiatrist diagnosed her as suffering from chronic schizophrenia, paranoid type, and determined that she posed a danger to herself in the reasonably foreseeable future.

It is noteworthy that on several occasions prior to the new initiative, the outreach team and police had transported Joyce to a nearby municipal hospital for emergency room evaluation. In each instance, the emergency room psychiatrist released her on the grounds that she did not meet the dangerousness threshold for involuntary hospitalization (substantial risk of imminent physical harm to self or to others). The failure of emergency room psychiatrists to admit Joyce prior to the initiative of October 28, 1987, demonstrates that the risk of physical harm to many of the homeless mentally ill is not easily recognized when psychiatric assessments are conducted in a context divorced from the harsh realities of those individuals' lives on the streets.

The outreach team has the unique vantage from the street to examine the homeless person's risk of self-harm due to neglect of essential needs. Good communication with hospital staff who are receptive to information not immediately discernible in the emergency room is essential to the integration of data necessary to make critical treatment decisions (Cohen et al. 1990).

In carrying out the policy mandate of the project, the outreach team functions as an emergency room on the streets for the estimated 2,000 to 3,000 street-bound homeless individuals who are severely mentally and physically ill but who consistently resist support and treatment. The Project HELP outreach workers collaborate with a number of community outreach programs that may be able to detect serious deterioration in functioning among homeless persons followed in their case loads.

This policy represents the first governmental initiative to involuntarily remove from the streets and hospitalize homeless mentally ill individuals who, due to neglect of their essential needs, are considered a danger to themselves in the reasonably foreseeable future. Previously, police intervention was considered only at times when an individual displayed behavior indicative of dangerousness to self and the threat of death was deemed substantial or imminent. This more restrictive threshold for involuntary commitment had resulted in increasing frustration among service providers, law enforcement personnel, and average citizens—who, confronted with growing numbers of severely mentally ill homeless individuals living on the streets, could no longer understand or tolerate what they perceived as government neglect of the seriously ill.

The New York City program has been the focus of intense media attention, both locally and nationally. Although the media generally reflected widespread public support for the initiative, critics have denounced the policy. Civil libertarians, especially the American Civil Liberties Union, portrayed the new policy as a real threat to the civil liberties of fragile and victimized individuals. Critics of the city administration described the program as an attempt to conceal the overwhelming problems in the city's response to the homeless problem—dangerous conditions in the city shelters and lack of affordable housing for poor and working-class families. Other critics rejected the program as motivated by a desire to clear fashionable neighborhoods of unsightly and disturbing homeless people (Marcos 1989).

Patient Characteristics

The authors examined the records of the 298 mentally ill homeless individuals who were brought to the Bellevue Hospital emergency room between October 28, 1987, and October 27, 1988, after being examined by Project HELP in the streets. The time period represented the first year of the program under its expanded mission (Marcos et al. 1990). Review of patient records provided demographic data, psychiatric histories, data on duration of homelessness, and psychiatric and medical diagnoses.

Of the 298 mentally ill homeless, almost two-thirds ($n = 196$) were men, and almost one-half ($n = 143$) were white. Their ages ranged from 16 to 80 years (mean, 40 years). Most were either single ($n = 228$, or 76.5%) or separated or divorced ($n = 50$, or 16.8%). Of the 178 persons who responded to questions about their education, the average level of schooling completed was 11th grade. The vast majority (79.4%) were born outside New York City, including 20.6% who were born in foreign countries. Of the patients who provided such information, 92.1% had histories of at least one previous psychiatric hospitalization, and 65.8% had been homeless for more than 1 year. As many as 33.6% of the patients said that they had been homeless for more than 5 years.

Patients were given ICD-9 primary diagnoses of schizophrenia (80.1%), affective disorders (7.7%), organic brain disorders (5.4%), and other psychiatric disorders (6.7%) (World Health Organization 1978). Most patients ($n = 217$; 73.1%) suffered from at least one medical condition in addition to a primary psychiatric diagnosis. The most common physical conditions, present in at least 20% of the patients, included peripheral vascular disorders, anemias, infestations, and diseases of the respiratory system, particularly tuberculosis. In addition, 103 (34.7%) of the patients had a secondary diagnosis of substance abuse.

The 298 individual patients accounted for 340 emergency room visits to Bellevue Hospital. Thirty-seven patients were evaluated more than once in the emergency room, and some were rehospitalized during the 1-year study period. In 286 of the 340 visits (84.1%), the patients were transported to the hospital involuntarily; 328 visits (96.5%) resulted in hospitalization, 315 (93%) of which were involuntary. Hospitalizations, medical treatments, and transfers to state psychiatric centers for extended care were challenged subsequently by the patients in 131 court hearings. In the great majority of these hearings ($n = 114$, 87%), the court upheld the hospital psychiatrists' recommendations. The patients' average length of stay at Bellevue Hospital was 61.3 days (range, 2 to 228 days).

Discharge dispositions for the 340 visits to Bellevue Hospital were obtained from clinical records. Half of the patients were transferred to a state psychiatric center for extended care. This proportion is substantially higher than the 8% rate at which the adult psychiatric inpatient population in New York City public hospitals were transferred to state facilities during the same time period (Office of Mental Hygiene Services, New York City Health and Hospitals Corporation 1988). Other dispositions included discharge to the care of relatives or self (19.1%), to community residences with different levels of support (17.1%), to the transitional shelter program (6.2%), and to nursing homes and other health care facilities (3.8%). In 12 cases (3.5%), patients left the hospital without consent.

Follow-up information was obtained by calling patients or their aftercare placement agencies at 3-month intervals. The last follow-up calls were made during October 1989, 2 years after initiation of the program. A total of 188 of the 298 patients (63%) either were contacted directly or their location was confirmed through their aftercare setting. Of this group, at the time of the follow-up contact, 80 patients (43%) were hospitalized in either a psychiatric facility or a health-related facility. Eighty-three patients (44%) were living in the community in settings such as residences, adult homes, single-room-occupancy hotels, and the transitional shelter program or living with relatives or by themselves. Two patients (1%) were known to be dead, and 23 patients (12%) were known to be back living on the streets.

Discussion

Project HELP benefits the homeless mentally ill through the use of a crisis intervention and outreach model that provides for the assessment of a fragile, disaffiliated, and severely psychiatrically impaired population. Social service agencies, courts, and health care providers are continually frustrated by these patients' refusal of services and determination to stay on the streets. The severely impaired judgment that accompanies the delusional thinking of many of these individuals has resulted in such tragic consequences as vast medical deterioration or death. We hypothesize that the program's emergency intervention prevented life-threatening progressive physical or psychiatric decompensation for many seriously mentally ill homeless patients. The finding that at least 28% of Project HELP's patients were living in the community and 27% were receiving institutional care 2 years after the intervention suggests the program has had a positive impact on the target population. Despite differences in patient samples and methods, other recent pilot studies on hospitalization and posthospitalization care of the homeless mentally ill reveal comparable outcomes (Bennett et al. 1988; Drake et al. 1989).

It is noteworthy that some form of contact was made at 3-month intervals with 63% of this group of patients for up to 2 years following the initial inpatient care episode. Despite the known difficulties in monitoring the seriously and persistently mentally ill, patient tracking systems, interagency clinical and administrative linkages, and outreach capacity for case management services can enhance continuity of information in this population and lead to improved care (Bachrach 1981; Mechanic and Aiken 1987).

The large proportion of patients transferred to a state psychiatric center for extended care (50%) reflects a subset of homeless with severe psychiatric impairments in need of long-term institutional psychiatric care (Marcos et al. 1990; Sargent 1989). This population of homeless mentally ill patients appears to manifest different psychopathology than do many of the 628 homeless mentally ill persons evaluated at Bellevue Hospital's emergency room independently of the program during the same time period. Specifically, fewer patients in the latter group carried a diagnosis of schizophrenia (50.3%), more of them were male ($n = 517$, 82.3%), and on average they were younger (mean age, 34.7) (Office of Mental Hygiene Services, New York City Health and Hospitals Corporation 1989).

In an earlier study, Cohen and colleagues (1986) reported a level of psychopathology among a cohort of the Project HELP patient population equal to or greater than that of the most recidivistic chronically mentally ill inpatients at Bellevue Hospital. The homeless patients transported by Project HELP revealed a unique constellation of florid psychotic symptomatology that coexisted with negative or deficit symptoms, including social withdrawal, dependency, apathy, and psychomotor retardation. The presence of a symptom complex with severe deficit symptomatology in association with florid psychotic symptoms and deterioration in functioning highlights the difficulty in engaging and treating the population of homeless mentally ill. Even when neuroleptic medications can be given, severe isolation and withdrawal often persist, blocking the patient's engagement in therapeutic services.

Clearly, the homeless mentally ill are characterized by a wide spectrum of psychiatric impairment ranging from substance abuse, personality disorders, dementias, major affective disorders, and the schizophrenias. In addition, because of a range of functional adaptational abilities, some homeless mentally ill cope marginally with their life on the streets, while others are gravely disabled, disorganized individuals who are at the greatest risk of danger to themselves or to others.

Our findings suggest that the multiply disabled homeless mentally ill require aggressive outreach interventions and, if necessary, involuntary hospitalization. The outreach strategy of this program is to observe a fragile, disenfranchised population—people at severe risk—so that they can be rapidly transported for treatment should further deterioration occur. The presence of significant negative or deficit symptoms requires an active monitoring program that in times of crisis can initiate involuntary treatment. Although it is necessary to develop a more comprehensive system and treatment structure for these patients, the Project HELP team fills a serious service gap.

The crises these patients face are often related to the most basic issues of survival, including exposure to severe, cold weather, inability to obtain appropriate food and clothing, deteriorated medical status, and increasingly impaired judgment that prevents even the most simple social interactions. Solutions proposed to care for the mentally impaired homeless must address these essential survival issues. Clearly, outreach—even outreach with the capacity to make involuntary hospital commitments—must be only a small part of a continuum of services tailored to the specific needs of the population.

Many styles of outreach interventions are appropriate to the needs of a diverse group of homeless mentally ill individuals. In New York City, outreach approaches to the homeless mentally ill vary in the type of direct services provided and the linkage with other service providers for housing, entitlements, and psychiatric or medical care (Barrow et al. 1989). Ideological factionalism regarding the causes of homelessness has influenced the design of program models and treatment plans for the homeless mentally ill. For example, some outreach workers believe that mental illness must be treated before housing needs can be met and appropriately utilized (Drake and Adler 1984). But many homeless advocates insist that stable housing be provided before special needs of the homeless mentally ill are addressed.

Ideological entrenchment, however, cannot take the place of good assessments of individual patient needs and connections to accessible and relevant services, which are so necessary considering the wide diversity of subgroups of homeless, including those homeless with psychiatric impairments. Models of outreach intervention need to be tailored to the realities of service system accessibility in the community in order to maintain responsiveness to the individual's needs. Those homeless mentally ill who are the most visible victims of the era of deinstitutionalization are greatly in need of outreach approaches to connect and reconnect them to community services. In all instances, the work is labor-intensive and requires a commitment to establishing linkages among a continuum of service providers, especially if the larger service system is fragmented and poorly coordinated.

References

Bachrach LL: Continuity of care for chronic mental patients: a conceptual analysis. Am J Psychiatry 40:46–51, 1981

Bachrach LL: On exporting and importing model programs. Hosp Community Psychiatry 39:1257–1258, 1988

Barbanel J: Slaying in cathedral spurs scrutiny of mental health care. New York Times, September 16, 1988, p B1

Barrow SM, Hellman F, Lovell AM, et al: Effectiveness of Programs for the Mentally Ill Homeless: Final Report. New York, New York State Psychiatric Institute Community Support Systems Evaluation Program, 1989

Bennett MI, Gudeman JE, Jenkins L, et al: The value of hospital-based treatment for the homeless mentally ill. Am J Psychiatry 145:1273–1276, 1988

Cohen NL (ed): Psychiatry Takes to the Streets. New York, Guilford, 1990

Cohen NL, Marcos LR: Policy, law, and involuntary emergency room visits. Psychiatr Q 61:197–204, 1990

Cohen NL, Sullivan AM: Strategies of intervention and service coordination by mobile outreach teams, in Psychiatry Takes to the Streets. Edited by Cohen NL. New York, Guilford, 1990, pp 63–79

Cohen NL, Putnam J, Sullivan AM: The mentally ill homeless: isolation and adaptation. Hosp Community Psychiatry 35:922–924, 1984

Cohen NL, Hardesty A, Putnam J, et al: Homeless mentally ill: issues of clinical measurement. Paper presented at the annual meeting of the American Psychiatric Association, Washington, DC, May 1986

Cohen NL, Tsemberis S, Barron C: Homeless mentally ill patients who are dangerous. Paper presented at the annual meeting of the American Psychiatric Association, San Francisco, CA, May 1990

Cournos F: Involuntary medication and the case of Joyce Brown. Hosp Community Psychiatry 40:736–740, 1989

Drake RE, Adler DA: Shelter is not enough: clinical work with the homeless mentally ill, in The Homeless Mentally Ill: A Task Force Report of the American Psychiatric Association. Edited by Lamb HR. Washington, DC, American Psychiatric Association, 1984

Drake RE, Wallach MA, Hoffman JS: Housing instability and homelessness among aftercare patients of an urban state hospital. Hosp Community Psychiatry 40:46–51, 1989

Gounis K, Susser E: Shelterization and its implications for mental health services, in Psychiatry Takes to the Streets. Edited by Cohen NL. New York, Guilford, 1990, pp 231–255

Grunberg J, Eagle PF: Shelterization: how the homeless adapt to shelter living. Hosp Community Psychiatry 41:521–525, 1990

Hemphill C: Mentally ill waiting for days for beds in the city's hospitals. New York Newsday, January 4, 1989, p 3

Marcos LR: Media power and public mental health policy. Am J Psychiatry 146:1185–1189, 1989

Marcos LR: Taking the mentally ill off the streets: the care of Joyce Brown. Int J Mental Health (in press)

Marcos LR, Cohen NL: Taking the suspected mentally ill off the streets to public general hospitals. N Engl J Med 315:1158–1161, 1986

Marcos LR, Cohen NL, Nardacci D, et al: Psychiatry takes to the streets: the New York City initiative for the homeless mentally ill. Am J Psychiatry 147:1557–1561, 1990

Mechanic D, Aiken LH: Improving the care of patients with chronic mental illness. N Engl J Med 317:1634–1638, 1987

New York City Health and Hospital Corporation: Program for Strengthening Services to the Homeless Mentally Ill in Need of Psychiatric Hospitalization. New York, New York City Health and Hospital Corporation, September 9, 1987

Office of Mental Hygiene Services, New York City Health and Hospitals Corporation, New York, 1988

Office of Mental Hygiene Services, New York City Health and Hospitals Corporation, New York, 1989

Primm AB, Houck J: Costar: flexibility in urban community mental health, in Psychiatry Takes to the Streets. Edited by Cohen NL. New York, Guilford, 1990, pp 107–120

Purnick J: Police to round up homeless when a cold wave grips city. New York Times, October 23, 1985, p B8

Sargent M: Update on programs for the homeless mentally ill. Hosp Community Psychiatry 40:1015–1016, 1989

Sullivan AM, Cohen NL: The home visit and the chronically mentally ill, in Psychiatry Takes to the Streets. Edited by Cohen NL. New York, Guilford, 1990, pp 63–79

Susser E, Struening EL, Conover S: Psychiatric problems in homeless men. Arch Gen Psychiatry 46:845–850, 1989

Treffert DA: The obviously ill patient in need of treatment: a fourth standard for civil commitment. Hosp Community Psychiatry 36:259–264, 1985

Tsemberis S, Cohen NL, Jones R: Conducting psychiatric assessments on the street and other unorthodox settings, in Intensive Treatment of the Homeless Mentally Ill. Edited by Katz SE, Nardacci D, Sabatini A. Washington, DC, American Psychiatric Press (in press)

Witheridge TF: Assertive community treatment: a strategy for helping persons with severe mental illness to avoid rehospitalization, in Psychiatry Takes to the Streets. Edited by Cohen NL. New York, Guilford, 1990, pp 80–106

World Health Organization: Mental Disorders: Glossary and Guide to Their Classification in Accordance With the Ninth Revision of the International Classification of Diseases. Geneva, World Health Organization, 1978

Chapter 10

In Search of Pumpkin Shells: Residential Programming for the Homeless Mentally Ill

Richard R. Bebout, Ph.D.
Maxine Harris, Ph.D.

> Peter, Peter, pumpkin eater,
> Had a wife and couldn't keep her,
> He put her in a pumpkin shell,
> And there he kept her very well.—Mother Goose

The pressing need for decent, affordable, and adequately supported housing alternatives for the homeless mentally ill defies easy answers. No magical solution—no universal "pumpkin shell" in which all might live very well—has emerged. Nevertheless, hundreds of new housing initiatives, many stimulated by McKinney Act dollars, have appeared since the American Psychiatric Association's task force on the homeless mentally ill published its recommendations nearly a decade ago. At that time, the task force called for the establishment of "an adequate number and ample range of graded, stepwise, supervised community housing settings" (Talbott and Lamb 1984, pp. 5–6).

In spite of the proliferation of housing programs, the field lacks conceptual clarity. Unnecessarily politicized debate about the relative importance of supported housing and residential treatment and about whether housing opportunities should be segregated or mainstreamed reflects not only legitimate philosophical differences but also the absence of a well-articulated framework for describing and evaluating housing and residential services. Although there have been a few systematic attempts to develop standardized taxonomies of community residential programs (Arce et al. 1982), in practice, terms such as halfway house, quarterway house, and even three-quarterway house (Campbell 1981) have no consistent denotative meaning across jurisdictional lines.

However, despite disagreement about many of the parameters of residential care, some important empirical questions have at least been asked, if not yet answered. Forthcoming research findings promise to refocus the field's attention on solutions informed by hard data to complement an ever-expanding clinical knowledge base.

Virtually all mentally ill adults can be considered at risk for homelessness, although some, called the hidden homeless (Pepper 1985), exhibit chronic patterns of residential instability, cycling between marginal placements while never being literally homeless. The effectiveness of any service system for persons who are seriously mentally ill and homeless is limited by the breadth of resources an individual case manager or resource manager can reliably access on a client's behalf (Talbott and Lamb 1984). Clinically managed, functionally integrated housing programs are needed to meet the diverse needs of mentally ill persons who experience homelessness, at least episodically.

One system of residential services, the residential continuum model, deserves renewed attention. This model incorporates a range of options that differ on several dimensions simultaneously. In this chapter, we examine the advantages and disadvantages of this model for the homeless mentally ill. We start by exploring the characteristics and attitudes that are essential to successful implementation of residential continuum, more important even than the constituent programs. Then, we describe specific programs that we helped develop and manage at Community Connections, Inc., a private nonprofit mental health agency in Washington, DC (Harris and Bergman 1988).

Many aspects of that program may not be replicable or appropriate for program planners in other settings; strategic elements are transferable, however (Bachrach 1988). Finally, we introduce several dimensional constructs in the hope of developing a common language for understanding the tremendous diversity apparent in residential programs across the country.

Of Straw or Brick? The Residential Continuum Model

"Then I'll huff and I'll puff and I'll blow your house in." Well, he huffed, and he puffed, and he puffed and he huffed, but he could NOT blow the brick house down.—The Three Little Pigs

Continuum Characteristics

The concept of the residential continuum represents an organizational structure capable of subsuming a variety of discrete housing alternatives. Although component programs—including an array of supervised, congregate living arrangements as well as semi-independent apartment units—are functionally differentiated, a residential spectrum is unified under a single administrative and clinical authority. The spectrum model is a clinical entity rather than a physical one; conceptualizing housing services as more than bricks and mortar has numerous practical implications.

Integration of housing and clinical services. Consensus now exists about the need to link housing and clinical services, but a variety of models for implementing this goal have been developed (Wittman 1989). One method of linking housing and services is through contractual arrangement so that beds or slots are obligated to the service agency, but no commitment is made to a given consumer. A second method of combining services is through highly structured, multicomponent programs. Here, services may be bundled in such a way as to require an individual to accept a standard, all-or-nothing package. Although some components may be quite attractive and well-suited to an individual's needs, others may be contraindicated.

Alternatively, multicomponent service programs that are more lightly structured offer a menu of services available à la carte. Clients, in partnership with case managers, can then select a more individualized service plan. Here, an array of residential programming is situated under the same umbrella as case management services. Both exist within a larger agency charged with overall responsibility for providing integrated and comprehensive mental health services. The chief advantage of this practice is to allow the client to continue to receive clinical services despite changes in residence. Commonly, services are terminated when a resident either fails or graduates from a given residential program. Too often residential services are delimited by the buildings that house either the residents or the program.

The marriage of treatment services to housing provides for high levels of integration at both the programmatic and the clinical levels. Administering housing and clinical services jointly prevents factions from responding to a difficult client by saying, "Not my problem." Treatment and residential services work in tandem, seeing themselves as a functional unit rather than as two separate entities potentially at odds with one another.

Administratively, barriers are too easily created when parallel systems exist, even if they are linked contractually. Responsibility becomes diffuse, and coordination between distinct systems that do not regard themselves as part of a functional unit can become increasingly cumbersome and time consuming. The existence of a single organizational entity, on the other hand, helps to assure clients (and case managers) of continuous access to a range of suitable alternatives with a minimum of bureaucratic interference.

Fluidity.   The residential spectrum model permits clients to enter the continuum at multiple points. Participants need not move along the continuum in a preordained fashion. Although critics have characterized the typical continuum for having rigid expectations that residents will enter at a single point and proceed along a uniform path, "much like the progression through grades in school" (Ridgway and Zipple 1990, p. 21), nothing inherent in the model requires such a practice. To the contrary, emphasis is placed on individualized planning within broad guidelines.

The metaphor of a railroad tunnel seems to capture the traditional view of a continuum—the train enters at one end and must go out the other. In contrast, a fluid continuum is more appropriately likened to a subway system that can be entered or existed at any stop, although some transfer points and routes are more heavily traveled than others. To require clients to move along a uniform pathway is to ignore the tremendous heterogeneity that exists among the homeless mentally ill. It assumes that everyone can, or wants to, reach a common level of adjustment or the same "final destination."

Flexibility.   Typically, clients move through the residential spectrum toward increasing independence and decreasing levels of supervision. However, allowances are made for movement back toward the more restrictive end of the continuum as needed. Seriously mentally ill persons who have been homeless are often uncomfortable assuming the role of patient and are reluctant to accept the need for medication and other forms of treatment. Most have received little information about the nature and course of their illnesses. Many are members of a younger generation that has had limited contact with formal treatment systems.

Because of the nature of their illnesses and because they receive treatment only intermittently, the homeless mentally ill are prone to relapses and often progress unevenly toward age-appropriate life goals, such as independent living. One homeless person may accept supervised accommodations initially while progressing gradually toward independent living, a second may refuse supervision only to experience continued residential instability, and a third may lose several rooming house placements or apartments before accepting increased supervision, assistance with money management, or shared living arrangements. Consequently, flexibility in the operation of a residential continuum is essential if the goal is to accommodate the special needs of the homeless mentally ill who often are young and have dual diagnoses.

Linear models of development have an inherent difficulty inasmuch as either implicitly or explicitly, movement in one direction is regarded as regression and movement in the other as progress. Both staff and clients must be assisted in "unlearning" such traditional, linear notions of growth and change. Workers should become sensitized to the power of language to refocus attention to issues of achieving "fit" or matching the client with appropriate housing arrangements and away from universal standards for success and failure.

Success at the programmatic level must be redefined more broadly as well to include variables other than numbers served, percent of patients moved to permanent housing, and decreased system dependency. Sometimes, increased service utilization represents a necessary and healthy intermediate step before a movement toward greater independence. The goals of stability and client acceptance of an appropriate level of support and supervision seem more appropriate indicators of program success than independence per se or immediate decreases in the consumption of services.

Responsiveness. Residential progress and transfers throughout the continuum must be monitored carefully because moves, even those labeled positive, are stressful and may trigger periods of destabilization. One mechanism for assuring integration and regular communication between housing support staff and the primary clinician or team is through a weekly residential rounds forum. Meetings should be attended by case managers, clinical supervisors, and housing support staff in order to assure maximum integration and a rapid and flexible response to the changing needs of clients.

Symptomatic changes are frequently detected by an apartment coordinator or by live-in residential counselors before deterioration is noted by the clinical team. Case management contacts are often task oriented and, like office-based psychiatric evaluations, can serve a structuring and organizing function for clients. As a result, the client's current level of acute symptomatology and distress may be obscured, even if the client is not intentionally underreporting psychotic symptoms in order to avoid medication increases or a loss of independence. Residential staff, on the other hand, are often positioned to observe changes unobtrusively through frequent but casual in-home contact with clients and consequently can target difficulties or problematic placement very early. To be maximally effective, interventions must be planned and implemented jointly by professional level case managers and paraprofessional support staff.

Component Programs

The seven discrete levels of residential care described below constitute a core group of residential alternatives that might be considered for inclusion in any planned continuum. Although the levels of care represent major anchor points along the continuum, an infinite number of refinements are possible. Emergency shelter facilities, often considered the first tier in a three-tiered taxonomy (Baxter and Hopper 1984), are excluded from the present discussion. Comments are restricted to transitional accommodations (tier 2) and long-term supportive residences in the community (tier 3).

The continuum of agency-managed housing that is currently employed at Community Connections, Inc., in Washington, DC, is presented in Table 10–1 together with a summary of the hypothetical continuum, or residential spectrum model, outlined by Pepper (1985). There are striking parallels between the two models in spite of minor differences in the number of persons served at each level of care and other surface characteristics. That these models were conceived and developed independently constitutes a form of convergent validity.

Table 10–1. Residential components of Community Connections and comparable elements of Pepper's hypothetical residential spectrum

Community Connections	Pepper spectrum[a]
1. Crisis residences (14 beds; 3 days to 4 weeks)	Crisis residence (10 beds, 1 to 3 weeks)
2. Transitional residence (12 beds)	Supervised residence (14 beds)
3. Therapeutic residences (8 beds each for a total of 16)	"Developmental" or "Growth" House (14 beds)[b]
4. Supervised residence (8 to 12 beds for a total of 30 beds)	"Supportive residence" (14 beds)
5. Training apartments (12 beds; time-limited, preparatory setting; 3 to 4 on-site contacts weekly	Supervised Apartments (14 beds; daily staff visits for monitoring, support)
6. Clustered apartments (80 to 150 beds in units for 1 to 4 persons; weekly contact; leased by agency)	Supportive apartments (14 beds; 1 to 2 contacts weekly; agency or individually leased)
7. Satellite apartments (20 to 50 beds; monthly on-site contact; individually leased)	Open community living
8. District of Columbia Community Residence Facility (CRF) system	Resident Congregate Care for Adults (RCCA) (NY State)

[a] From Pepper 1985.
[b] From Pepper and Ryglewicz 1985.

Neither model should be regarded as a prototype or a prefab housing solution. However, there is significant overlap in their philosophies and strategies, and the methodology can be readily adapted to accommodate the specific population characteristics and unique needs of target groups served by other agencies. The development of a continuum should ideally reflect proactive planning that takes into account the specific characteristics of the region and population to be served, including age and diagnostic makeup; in practice, program components are more commonly created in piecemeal fashion.

Crisis residential services. A crisis residential program provides temporary residential placement for clients experiencing acute crises while living in the community. The length of stay may range from as short as 3 days to upwards of 4 to 6 weeks in some settings. Crisis residential services are usually provided to a maximum of 6 to 8 residents in home-like settings that feature intensive, round-the-clock staffing by professional or paraprofessional residential counselors (Desmond et al. 1991), although some models provide crisis support in scattered-site, family settings (Stroul 1987). Screening, treatment and discharge planning, and supervision of live-in staff are generally provided by a multidisciplinary team, including professionals from nursing, psychology, social work, and psychiatry working either on a full-time or part-time consulting basis.

A primary goal of the crisis residential program is to provide high levels of supervision and support to persons in an emotional or psychiatric crisis that might otherwise result in a rehospitalization. Temporary removal from the person's permanent living situation and placement in the therapeutic setting provides relief from stressful life events while minimizing the disruptiveness and sense of failure often associated with hospitalization. Although some work or day treatment activities may be suspended for a brief time during the acute phase of the crisis, other parts of the individual's normal routine continue throughout.

Crisis residential programs have a number of specific applications for working with the homeless mentally ill and persons who exhibit persistent residential instability. First, crisis programs can serve a preventive function if the mission of the program is expanded to include the resolution of not only psychiatric crises per se but also residential crises, such as a temporary loss of housing that might rapidly result in the person becoming homeless or psychiatrically destabilized.

Second, crisis programs can supply invaluable assessment data. Whereas the response to medication and residential history of long-term patients referred from hospital settings is well known, dangerously little may be known by the referring shelter worker about a homeless person. He or she may be actively psychotic and unable or unwilling to accurately report details of his or her treatment history. Within the crisis residence, staff can conduct thorough, ongoing assessments to be used in evaluating the appropriateness of subsequent residential options. In addition to collecting biographical and treatment data, these evaluations should address an individual's need for and capacity to tolerate structure and supervision.

Third, crisis residences may serve as a gateway to the rest of the residential continuum for homeless mentally ill persons preparing to relocate from the streets or an emergency shelter setting. In contrast to the flexible, streamlined admissions procedures that typify crisis programs, a lengthy certification process may be required by many similarly structured longer-term settings. The delay may discourage homeless persons from applying.

Finally, crisis programs can function as a "step-down" following a brief psychiatric admission or an inpatient stay for detoxification of persons who are homeless and who have dual diagnoses.

Therapeutic residential services.   Group houses that offer aggressive rehabilitation services in the context of a time-limited, intensively staffed program are also needed. Growth- or treatment-oriented services may be driven by a variety of theoretical perspectives, but each reflects an explicit developmental demand. For example, a house might feature a moderately long stay, perhaps 9 to 12 months, and emphasize the use of skill remediation and behavioral strategies, such as contingency contracts, as an adjunct to other traditional case management strategies. Alternatively, a house in which stays were longer could employ psychodynamically oriented individual and group psychotherapy approaches over a 12- to 24-month stay. The aim would be to establish a safe holding environment.

Such programs can serve clients who in the past might have benefited from long-term, intensive inpatient treatment but who present no significant behavior management problems, such as dangerousness, that would warrant hospitalization. For homeless persons who have either rejected long-term inpatient treatment or who have been poorly tolerated by traditional settings, these homes may provide a unique opportunity to enjoy manageable "dosages" of change-oriented treatment for an extended period.

Transitional residences.   Transitional residential services place heavy emphasis on careful assessment to identify and address specific behavior patterns that have interfered with successful community adjustment and that have contributed to residential instability. One important objective of such programs is to become better at matching the discharged patient with existing housing options based on the individual's need for supervision and level of contact seeking (socioemotional demands). In the District of Columbia, transitional residences frequently house clients who are referred at the conclusion of a lengthy inpatient stay and who are not yet in complete remission. Many have significant residual symptoms or exhibit skill deficits related to institutional dependency. The transitional residence affords staff ample opportunity to determine when residents have reached "baseline" and to make judgments about their capacity to benefit from more aggressive, growth-oriented rehabilitation services.

Although transitional housing can serve a useful purpose, the homeless mentally ill often exhibit certain resistance to such placements. The modal resident in a transitional residence may be quite symptomatic. Because being labeled "crazy" on the street is not only undesirable but also dangerous, homeless persons actively resist this identification. Consequently, transitional housing must seek to avoid practices that require patients to play the role of patients or that promote the phenomenon of "shelterization," a term used by Grunberg and Eagle (1990) to describe a process of adaptation to shelter life characterized by diminished social responsiveness, self-neglect, and increased passivity and dependency on shelter staff. In particular, rules that are reminiscent of shelter life and that diminish the sense of being at home and feeling a sense of belonging must be modified. For example, houses that might otherwise expect residents to be involved in daily, off-site activities may find it necessary to suspend those demands at least temporarily.

Supervised residential services. At long-stay supervised residences, the level of structure and support is about the same as or slightly less than that provided in other clinically managed group residences. However, length of stay is unlimited, and there are minimal expectations regarding movement toward more independence. Although some clients might require less intensive supervision over time, for others the residence is expected to be a semipermanent arrangement. Recreational activities with relatively few demands and opportunities for socialization in a homelike environment are emphasized over treatment- or training-oriented programming. Consistent with this philosophy, the staffing plan might call for a permanent staff person to live at the residence rather than having temporary staff rotate onto the residence on a shift basis in order to promote stability. Such settings are often appropriate for homeless mentally ill persons who in the past have fled more aggressive treatment programs or high-demand environments but who accept tangible supports such as prepared meals.

Training apartments.   A small number of units designated as training apartments constitute the most carefully supervised level of apartment living. Daily on-site contact and individualized training sessions can be provided by carefully supervised preprofessionals or professionals known as skills trainers. Training apartments are devoted to assessing and increasing apartment readiness. Length of stay is limited, typically to between 3 and 6 months. Training efforts are designed to remedy deficits in the skills of menu planning, food preparation and storage, shopping, money management, routine cleaning and household maintenance, conflict resolution, and leisure planning.

When staff disagree among themselves or staff and a program participant disagree about the client's readiness for apartment living, placing the client in a training apartment is frequently an appropriate compromise solution. A training apartment may be an ideal setting for a homeless mentally ill individual who is not well known to the sponsoring agency, especially if he or she reports having had a series of apartment placements that were aborted for reasons that are poorly understood. Training apartments provide an excellent opportunity to evaluate skills and to remedy obvious deficits in a safe setting and can play a key role in interrupting the cycle of homelessness.

Clustered apartments.   Another, more independent level of apartment living is offered by clustered apartments. Situated in townhouses and small apartment buildings in which two or more units are leased by the agency, clustered apartments should be located within a small radius of the responsible agency in order to assure staff and clients easy access to one another. In clustered apartments, paraprofessional support staff supervised by the mental health clinic play an important role as an adjunct to outreach efforts by case management staff. For example, apartment support staff conduct weekly house meetings that focus on problem solving, household maintenance, and conflict resolution between roommates or neighbors. They can work in conjunction with primary case managers to obtain food stamps and housing subsidies (when available) and to coordinate the timely payment of rents and utilities.

Apartment staff might also sponsor weekly group food shopping trips and make themselves available for consultation at the store for budgeting and menu planning at the request of the client. Clients who are known to spend money allotted for food on alcohol or drugs or who otherwise misuse funds can be asked to submit receipts as part of an overall plan of compliance monitoring. Such plans must be developed in close collaboration with the clinical teams, perhaps during weekly residential case reviews or in a similar forum. The availability of attractive, semi-independent apartments is obviously a major "hook" to encourage homeless mentally ill persons to accept ongoing psychiatric and support services.

Satellite apartments. Located at scattered sites further from the agency, satellite apartments represent the most independent end of the continuum. On-site meetings can be held less frequently, perhaps once or twice a month rather than weekly, and clients may no longer want or need to participate in agency-sponsored shopping trips. Although the agency may routinely be the lease holder for the apartment units, residents should be encouraged to consider the apartments they sublet home. In rare cases, they may assume total responsibility for payment of rents and utilities and for negotiating repairs or other minor disputes with landlords. Although many homeless mentally ill persons aspire to this level of independence, only a small minority reach this end of the continuum.

Critical Dimensions of Housing Environments

A small but growing number of studies have explored the relationship between facility characteristics and residential outcomes. A few focus on objective administrative and organizational features, such as facility size, cost of care, staffing ratios, funding sources, and type of ownership (Nagy et al. 1988). Others, discussed below, attempt to analyze less tangible aspects of the social environments. Rather than generate an exhaustive list of discrete variables relevant to residential outcomes, we have identified a limited set of dimensional constructs from the literature on milieu factors: structure, interpersonal intensity, degree of self-sufficiency, length of stay, and orientation toward growth or maintenance. This set of factors represents an effort to look beneath the surface characteristics of housing types to provide a foundation for the classification and future discussion of the present range of housing alternatives.

Structure. Sadly, structure—which Lamb (1980) called "the neglected ingredient in community treatment"—can be counted among the significant casualties of the past 3 decades of deinstitutionalization. In the effort to rid service delivery system of the destructive aspects of institutional care, numerous practices and procedures that might have retained their usefulness have also been discarded. Too often community service planners have eschewed the need for structure, order, and containment.

Sometimes these policies are intended to champion civil liberties but too often they merely reflect political or economic realities. Direct care staff sometimes share a distaste for imposing contingent demands on clients and a fantasy that it is possible to avoid exercising unilateral forms of authority.

Ironically, facilities that superficially appear to be the most permissive and that attempt to operate without clearly defined rules and clear, graded responses to behavior considered misconduct may ultimately be experienced as intolerant or arbitrary because their only response to misconduct is to discharge the resident. Responsible community programming demands that we develop creative ways to infuse residences of all types with structure in a variety of forms.

The literature on residential services commonly attaches at least three meanings to the notion of structure. First, structure in its most basic and restrictive form refers to locked doors and other security features. Although statutes vary tremendously across state and municipal lines with respect to the permissibility of locked doors and even the use of physical restraints, these tools need not be the exclusive province of large institutional settings. Safety and security considerations are particularly important for housing planners working with the homeless mentally ill, who are more likely than their domiciled counterparts to have been the victims of violent crime. Additionally, homeless persons are perhaps more likely to resort to violence, because they have used aggressive behavior as a way of coping with the dangers that pervade life on the streets and in emergency shelter settings (Grunberg and Eagle 1990) and because their psychoses are often inadequately treated.

Rule systems represent a second facet of structure. Rule systems may range from a minimum of clearly articulated expectations, perhaps addressing only curfews or sanctions against fighting or drug use, to elaborate and finely tuned behavior management programs. Limits on visitation or privileges for off-site excursions, controlled access to cash, and formal contracts, even "riders" on lease agreements, stipulating participation requirements or consequences of rules violations all constitute structuring techniques whose primary purpose is to govern resident conduct.

Third, structure can assume the form of regular, scheduled activities sponsored by the facility operators. Examples include consistent mealtimes and medication calls; brief house meetings with a problem-solving focus; resident participation in completing household chores, planning menus, and cooking; recreational activities, such as informal game nights, theater trips using dotted or discounted movie tickets, or Friday night video viewings. Such activities function to occupy leisure time and to enhance self-esteem. All three aspects of structure—safety and security, rules systems, and activity programming—function to render the environment safe and predictable.

Interpersonal intensity. The level of socioemotional demands or interpersonal intensity is also a salient element of residential environments. Residential sites that are high on the dimension of socioemotional demands typically feature either a familylike atmosphere or a milieu therapy model for a small number of residents. Active participation in groups is frequently required, meals are served family style, and attendance on outings is expected. Although such settings offer much support, the level of interpersonal intensity may become overwhelming and can lead to regressive reactions among borderline patients or fight-or-flight responses among persons with paranoid or schizoid adaptations, a group that is probably disproportionately represented among the homeless segment of the mentally ill population.

Low-intensity environments must also be available for persons who avoid contact with other people. Allowed sufficient interpersonal "space," individuals who require a great deal of privacy and separation in order to successfully manage their symptoms and to function optimally may gradually increase their level of social participation.

Self-sufficiency. Residential settings also differ with respect to the degree to which clients are expected to be self-sufficient in the management of their day-to-day lives, including finding transportation, attending to grooming and personal hygiene, preparing meals, administering psychotropic medications, and maintaining a schedule of regular activities. Determining the appropriate level of hands-on assistance to give to an individual is complicated by the fact that persons with psychotic-spectrum illnesses frequently possess the instrumental skills needed to perform any singular activity of daily living but are unable to tolerate multiple demands simultaneously (Drake et al., in press). Stress intolerance and residual symptoms of schizophrenia may render the individual incapable of initiating or completing routine aspects of self-care without patient and repeated prompting. The disparity between the clients' ability and performance frequently causes helpers to attribute their failure to care for themselves to laziness or willful refusal, which can be toxic and threaten a residential placement.

Sometimes, the opposite—doing too much for the client—occurs as well. Providing too much assistance can have a crippling effect, causing atrophy rather than stimulating the gradual recovery of function. A range of levels of instrumental assistance and expectations for self-sufficiency among and within residential settings is needed in order to adequately serve the whole spectrum of mentally ill adults.

Length of stay.   Although debate continues about whether transitional or preparatory settings or permanent homes are more appropriate placements for the homeless mentally ill, it is likely that each arrangement has distinct advantages and can play a role in a total system of care. Transitional placements provide superior opportunities to conduct formal diagnostic evaluations for persons who are just off the streets or who have been inadequately treated. Persons who might otherwise deteriorate in spite of increased case management supports can receive intensive supports on a temporary basis. Although aggressive case management can frequently avert the need for a residential transfer, temporary removal from a failing placement may be necessary. Placing clients in respite programs and transitional residences with lengths of stay from 3 to 6 months may at times be more cost-effective methods of crisis resolution than simply stepping up contact with the clients in their permanent residences.

The existence of additional supports in preparatory settings, such as the training apartments described above, may lead clinicians to accept applications for apartment placement from individuals who might otherwise be considered poor candidates for semi-independent living. The heightened monitoring and support available in such settings permit staff to make riskier placement decisions. By explicitly defining a placement as a trial visit for evaluation purposes, a clinician may rapidly terminate the stay if necessary and return an individual to a higher level of care without causing the client or the referring case manager to regard the decision as a breach of contract.

For persons capable of living independently, semi-permanent arrangements have obvious advantages, including their ability to provide stability, a sense of ownership, and the experience of being rooted. Desirable, permanent housing also promotes client motivation and compliance with other treatment demands. When only permanent apartments are available, however, progress toward independence can sometimes be delayed unnecessarily because of the degree of certainty program coordinators might otherwise require before approving apartment placement. Such judgments are based on a variety of factors, including the clinical and economic cost associated with failed placements.

Conversely, a disorganized homeless person is sometimes more willing to accept a structured, supervised placement because it is explicitly defined as temporary. Whereas the prospect of a long-term placement in an intensively supervised setting might cause a client to flee, a time-limited respite stay or "vacation" might represent an acceptable, face-saving alternative.

Orientation toward growth. A comprehensive system of residential services must incorporate both growth-oriented and maintenance-oriented settings. Too often, service planners mirror the prevailing attitudes of the larger society by overvaluing aggressive rehabilitation and treatment programs and vigorously rejecting the need for low-demand environments. They may expressly denounce stabilization and maintenance goals.

On the other hand, interviewers (Lamb 1979) and clinicians frequently encounter individuals who are themselves keenly aware of their inability to tolerate social or vocational demands. Some report making a deliberate choice to actively limit exposure to pressure of any kind in order to avoid decompensation. Such "adaptation by decompression" (Lamb 1981, p. 20) must be embraced by service planners as a legitimate need for some, perhaps many, mentally ill people, at least for long intervals in their lives. Effective planning requires that we recognize the legitimate roles of asylum and rehabilitation at different times in the same individual's lifetime.

There is an inherent risk in mixing these models within specific program sites, however. For some individuals, high-expectancy environments stimulate an appropriate wish for independence but for others such environments represent a false hope of achieving beyond the level of which they are capable. Prolonged exposure to inflated expectations and subtle internal and external pressures to change may precipitate a crisis among highly disabled residents, even when providers are sensitive enough to distinguish between opportunities for growth and demands for growth.

Relationships among factors. Further research is needed to determine the relationships among these dimensions. Some factors may be conceptually and statistically independent. For example, some research evidence suggests that the level of structure in a residential setting is relatively independent of the amount of socioemotional support or stimulation available (Coulton et al. 1985). Other factors, such as an orientation toward growth or maintenance and the degree to which housing arrangements are considered transitional or permanent, seem intuitively related. Both growth and transition imply change and reflect expectations for significant movement.

A variety of schemes for classifying residential settings can be generated by grouping settings based on the degree to which each of several factors is present. For example, an environment that makes few demands for interpersonal involvement (low socioemotional setting) or for self-care (low self-sufficiency setting) but that makes continued residency contingent on medication compliance and the designation of a representative payee to manage funds (high structure setting) may be ideal for persons who are highly symptomatic or who avoid intimacy. Some combinations may be especially therapeutic, others may be toxic, and still others simply may not exist naturally.

The interactive effects of client characteristics and milieu factors seems critical to our understanding of chronic residential instability among the mentally ill (Kruzich and Kruzich 1985). Further research is needed in order to construct a fuller, textured image of housing settings and contextual factors that influence residential and treatment outcomes.

The degree of homogeneity and heterogeneity of the client population is a variable that cuts across the other dimensional factors discussed already and also deserves research attention. Some programs are defined by a narrow mission statement or treatment approach and consequently limit participation based on age, diagnostic grouping, or symptom severity. Others define themselves more broadly. Programs with exclusionary policies may serve a sector of the population well but may have difficulty maintaining their boundaries because of financial pressures or shifting trends in the larger population from which referrals are drawn. In the natural histories of highly specialized programs, competent and specifically trained staff often experience confusion and job dissatisfaction as the program's mission changes. On the other hand, programs accepting "all comers" may be so diffuse that their effectiveness in addressing any single service need is greatly reduced. Ascertaining the level of homogeneity that is best suited to a program's specific aims, therefore, presents a challenge for both researchers and program planners.

Of Crooked Men and Crooked Houses: Myths and Mistakes

There was a crooked man, and he walked a crooked mile,
He found a crooked sixpence against a crooked stile,
He bought a crooked cat, which caught a crooked mouse,
And they all lived together in a little crooked house.—Mother Goose

Although the residential continuum appears to be a viable model for linking housing and support services, in practice, unwanted outcomes may occur due to myths and misconceptions about residential movement. Four recurring conceptual problems or faulty assumptions that may interfere with the successful operation of housing initiatives are explored below.

The Goal of Permanency

The conventional wisdom about eliminating homelessness among the mentally ill places a premium on providing permanent, independent living arrangements that may be inappropriate. The mobility and transient nature of this population must be taken into account when planning an array of housing alternatives (Bachrach 1984). Many homeless and mentally ill adults exhibit a widely recognized pattern of cycling between short-stay facilities. Brief stays in supervised living arrangements are punctuated by repeated attempts at independent living and numerous decisions to relocate. In response to feelings of boredom, dissatisfaction, or despair, many mentally ill persons resort to what Lamb (1981, p. 28) called a "geographical solution," perpetually moving in an enactment of the magical belief that problems can be outrun or left behind.

Available data indicate that significant levels of residential impermanence persist even after homeless persons have been successfully engaged in case management services. Harris and Bachrach (1990) report a median tenure for residential stays of just 3.8 months for a sample of homeless women receiving aggressive case management services, some for 2 or more years. Commenting on a kind of restlessness and perpetual motion evident among many homeless, Harris and Bachrach argue that "for at least some homeless mentally ill individuals, giving them the freedom to move about among residential settings may be instrumental in keeping them involved in a treatment program and off the streets" (p. 254). These findings raise questions about the priority ordinarily given to the availability of independent and permanent residences and suggest that program planning principles that flow from assumptions about permanency may require substantial revision.

Client-Centered Programming

Program administrators, clinicians, and advocates often fail to make an essential, but subtle, distinction between "client-centered" and "client-driven" programming. Client-centered principles compel planners to incorporate consumer preference to the extent possible but also to exercise sound professional judgment about the feasibility of stated objectives. In contrast, client-driven approaches imply that programs attempt to honor client opinions or requests almost irrespective of known clinical realities.

For example, consumer surveys show that all homeless individuals, independent of the presence or absence of obvious mental illness, express pronounced preferences for independent apartment settings over supervised or congregate living arrangements (Goering et al. 1990). Yet caseworkers point to the need for higher levels of supervision and support than is practical in the context of apartment living. As a solution, residential service providers can affirm an individual's values and preferences without gratifying specific ill-fated demands or adopting the client's time frame for achieving the goal of independent living.

The potential folly of client-centered programming is illustrated by a survey by Goering and colleagues (1990) of housing preferences among homeless women. The women reported a widespread unwillingness to live with the mentally ill or those with histories of substance abuse or criminal activity. The authors commented, "Ironically, if taken at face value, these opinions could result in admission criteria for a housing project that would exclude most of the women interviewed" (p. 793).

The Peter Principle and the Myth of Linear Change

A variant of the oft-cited Peter Principle seems to apply to residential services. Misapplication of the linear continuum model frequently results in the promotion of individuals to the level of their residential incompetence. Well-intended clinicians frequently respond to relatively brief periods of stability by advocating that their client be afforded the opportunity to attempt the next level of residential care. Rather than interpret the newfound stability as evidence that the client has reached an appropriate level of supervision, case managers argue optimistically for providing increased independence. This phenomenon may be attributed to what Lamb called the tendency by our society toward "basic moral disapproval . . . of dependency, of a passive inactive lifestyle, and of a person's accepting public support instead of working" (Lamb 1981, p. 22).

Sometimes the impetus toward an excessively independent living arrangement appears in fact to originate with the client, but at other times it seems to reflect an inability by staff members to tolerate extended dependency in their clients. Those same values and attitudes, because they have also been internalized by the client, are sometimes the source of enormous pain.

Clinical Case

A 31-year-old schizophrenic male with a history of serious alcohol abuse reported that he had left home and lived on the streets for several years during which time he had been hospitalized three times. He refused periodic invitations to live with a relative, who would have required that he work and contribute to household maintenance, expectations he felt unable to meet. After enrolling in a case management agency with supported housing, the man initially lived in a low-demand, supervised residence that featured prepared meals and minimal expectations for participation in group activities. His psychiatric condition stabilized very rapidly, and he experienced more complete symptom remission than at any other time since the onset of his illness in his early twenties.

After approximately 4 months, the case manager, who was in his early thirties, reopened discussions about apartment living and soon thereafter referred the client to a supported apartment. After a brief period of relative quiet, he deteriorated quickly. His serum lithium levels suggested that medication compliance had slipped, beer cans were found outside his apartment, and his roommate reported that he was cooking hot dogs by holding them under hot running tap water. The case manager initially increased his on-site contacts, offering hands-on assistance with food shopping, meal preparation, and cleaning, but little improvement was noted. Supervision revealed a very strong identification by the case manager and an intense wish to see his client succeed. Once the case manager was able to recognize the client's need for continued support and supervision, the client quickly accepted a recommendation for a staffed group home with surprisingly little resistance.

The Myth of a Paradigm Shift

The residential continuum model described here has been challenged recently by advocates of the supported housing movement. They have argued that a paradigm shift is under way that will replace the continuum model with the supported housing model—an extension of the psychosocial rehabilitation model that emphasizes self-determination, consumer choice, individualized habitation plans, and the creation of permanent homes in normalized, mainstream environments (Ridgway and Carling 1987; Ridgway and Zipple 1990). Its proponents are critical of the residential continuum model for its reliance on staff-controlled, transitional preparatory settings and medical-model treatment philosophies, and for perpetuating unhealthy and debilitating social role expectancies such as the "patient role."

Although these criticisms may be legitimately applied to ill-conceived or poorly implemented programs, the concept of a continuum itself need not be abandoned. Given the overwhelming need for a comprehensive national response to the problems of homelessness and residential instability among the mentally ill, it seems wise to incorporate the broadest possible range of models. And, in light of the absence of systematic, well-controlled studies of residential service models, it seems premature to assume that emerging models are mutually exclusive.

Fields (1990) suggests instead that supported housing be considered one element in a comprehensive matrix of residential alternatives. In our judgment, supported housing may represent only a relatively narrow segment on the continuum. Probably only a minority of mentally ill adults can benefit from mainstream, low-cost housing or tolerate the role demands of normalized settings. The achievements of those individuals who recover the capacity to live independently or to work productively are cause for celebration. For others, those values are persistent and painful reminders of the rugged individualism of a culture that perpetually consigns them to live on the fringes. A true paradigm shift would entail sweeping social change and new, more inclusive definitions of societal participation—a shift from goals of assimilation that perpetuate existing social templates to goals of accommodation that place the burden of change on the culture rather than the individual.

Conclusions

Clinically managed housing networks for persons with serious and persistent mental illnesses can be an effective strategy for addressing the needs of persons who have experienced either chronic or episodic homelessness. A range of housing solutions must be made available if we are to meet the diverse and changing needs of persons recovering from both psychotic-spectrum illnesses and homelessness. Many of today's homeless belong to a class of "never institutionalized" mentally ill adults (Bachrach 1984). As a consequence, those treating them in the community grapple with a level of denial about psychiatric illness not usually found among formerly institutionalized persons. Many such persons have had frequent but very brief hospital stays that have done little to educate them about the nature, course, and treatment of their illnesses. That is not an argument for reversing the trend away from unduly lengthy institutional stays, but the impact that contemporary policies and practices have had on matters of socializing people into the "patient role" and on compliance medication regimens and treatment cannot be overlooked.

Community service planners face additional challenges in connection with the youthfulness and associated alcohol and substance abuse evident among today's homeless mentally ill, features that make them less likely to accept, and to be accepted by, traditional residential service settings. Admissions and discharge policies must become increasingly inclusive. In order to embrace the unique challenges posed by those homeless persons with the dual disorders of psychosis and substance abuse conditions, some liberalization of rule structures seems indicated (Kline et al., in press).

Research attention must be paid to comparing the relative strengths and weaknesses of various residential care models, and especially strategies for linking housing and services. It may prove helpful to turn to other fields to guide the development of effective research and clinical models. Within gerontology, for example, there are a number of models for residential programming for the aged; careful study may reveal less than obvious parallels to the housing crisis that exists currently in the mental health services community (Newman 1991). Findings from studies of structural and milieu factors that impact on residential outcomes (Coulton et al. 1985; Nagy et al. 1988) should be replicated and used as a foundation to increase our acuity in matching persons to existing environments and in designing new residential settings to better meet the needs of the homeless mentally ill.

As the nation struggles to eliminate homelessness among the mentally ill and to create viable systems of care in this "postdeinstitutional" era, innovative residential services will play a rapidly expanding role. To be truly responsive to the needs of the homeless mentally ill—the young, the old, those with addictive disorders in addition to debilitating psychoses, men and women with partners or with children, even those with crooked cats, all of them—housing must be redesigned to conform to their needs rather than requiring them to fit themselves into our houses. Crooked is in the eyes of the beholder.

References

Arce AA, Vergare MJ, Adams R, et al: A Typography of Community Residential Services: A Task Force Report of the American Psychiatric Association. Washington DC, American Psychiatric Association, 1982

Bachrach LL: The homeless mentally ill and mental health services: an analytical review of the literature, in The Homeless Mentally Ill: A Task Force Report of the American Psychiatric Association. Edited by Lamb HR. Washington, DC, American Psychiatric Association, 1984

Bachrach LL: The chronic patient: on exporting and importing model programs. Hosp Community Psychiatry 39:1257–1258, 1988

Baxter E, Hopper K: Shelter and housing for the homeless mentally ill, in The Homeless Mentally Ill: A Task Force Report of the American Psychiatric Association. Edited by Lamb HR. Washington, DC, American Psychiatric Association, 1984

Campbell M: The three-quarterway house: a step beyond the halfway house toward independent living. Hosp Community Psychiatry 7:500–501, 1981

Coulton CJ, Fitch V, Holland TP: A typology of social environments in community care homes. Hosp Community Psychiatry 36:373–377, 1985

Desmond M, Bergman H, Harris M: Development of a model for crisis residential services. T.I.E.-Lines 8:3–4, 1991

Drake RE, Osher FC, Wallach MA: Homelessness and dual diagnosis. Am Psychol (in press)

Fields S: The relationship between residential treatment and supported housing in a community system of services. Psychosocial Rehabilitation Journal 13:105–113, 1990

Goering P, Paduchak D, Durbin J: Housing homeless women: a consumer preference study. Hosp Community Psychiatry 41:790–794, 1990

Grunberg J, Eagle PF: Shelterization: how the homeless adapt to shelter living. Hosp Community Psychiatry 41:521–525, 1990

Harris M, Bachrach LL: The chronic patient: perspectives on homeless mentally ill women. Hosp Community Psychiatry 41: 253–254, 1990

Harris M, Bergman H: Capitation financing for the chronically mentally ill: a case management approach. Hosp Community Psychiatry 39:68–72, 1988

Kline J, Bebout RR, Harris M, et al: Models of treatment for homeless, dually diagnosed adults. New Dir Ment Health Serv (in press)

Kruzich JM, Kruzich SJ: Milieu factors influencing patients' integration into community residential facilities. Hosp Community Psychiatry 36:378–382, 1985

Lamb HR: The new asylums in the community. Arch Gen Psychiatry 36:129–134, 1979

Lamb HR: Structure: the neglected ingredient of community treatment. Arch Gen Psychiatry 37:1224–1228, 1980

Lamb HR: Maximizing the potential of board and care homes. New Dir Ment Health Serv 11:19–33, 1981

Nagy MP, Fisher GA, Tessler RC: Effects of facility characteristics on the social adjustment of mentally ill residents of board-and-care homes. Hosp and Community Psychiatry 39:1281–1286, 1988

Newman S: Evaluation research. Paper presented at National Conference on Housing Initiatives for Homeless People With Alcohol and Other Drug Problems. Sponsored by the National Institute on Alcohol Abuse and Alcoholism and the Interagency Council on the Homeless, San Diego, CA, March 1991

Pepper B: Where (and how) should young adult chronic patients live? The concept of a residential spectrum. T.I.E.-Lines 2:1–6, 1985

Pepper B, Ryglewicz H: The developmental residence: a "missing link" for young adult chronic patients. T.I.E.-Lines 2:1–3, 1985

Ridgway P, Carling PJ: Strategic Planning in Housing and Mental Health. Boston, MA, Center for Psychiatric Rehabilitation, Boston University, 1987

Ridgway P, Zipple AM: The paradigm shift in residential services: from the linear continuum to supported housing approaches. Psychosocial Rehabilitation Journal 13:11–31, 1990

Stroul BA: Crisis Residential Services in a Community Support System. Rockville, MD, National Institute of Mental Health, 1987

Talbott JA, Lamb HR: Summary and recommendations, in The Homeless Mentally Ill: A Task Force Report of the American Psychiatric Association. Edited by Lamb HR. Washington DC, American Psychiatric Association, 1984

Wittman FD: Housing models for alcohol programs serving homeless people. Contemporary Drug Problems 16:483–504, 1989

Chapter 11

The Need-for-Treatment Standard in Involuntary Civil Commitment

Virginia C. Armat
Roger Peele, M.D.

The hundreds of thousands of psychiatrically ill living in this nation's streets, jails, and other unsuitable settings dramatize a terrible failure in modern society—our inability to obtain psychiatric treatment for our mentally ill. The senseless abandonment of a need-for-treatment standard in involuntary commitment has gratuitously impaired the welfare of the seriously mentally ill. We review here the events that have contributed to this tragedy in order to argue for reintroducing a need-for-treatment standard in involuntary commitment as a way of halting the epidemic of neglect, including homelessness, among the severely and chronically mentally ill.

Rise and Fall of the Concept of Need For Treatment

The 19th Century

By the first half of the 19th century, a thesis called moral therapy had originated in Europe that posited that mental illnesses derived from exposure to certain degrading but alterable conditions in the community. Treatment, therefore, required removing the patient from such settings—jails and almshouses, for example—and placing them in more salubrious, so-called moral settings, or asylums, where they were expected to be cured. In the 1840s, moreover, Dorothea Dix launched a revolution on behalf of the mentally ill based on humanitarian grounds as well as her own belief in moral treatment. The success of Dix's crusade saw the building of comfortable public psychiatric hospitals in mostly rural surroundings across the nation. By the middle of the century, public support of the need—whether moral or simply protective—for psychiatric treatment was widely accepted.

One of Dix's most appealing arguments, of course, was that asylums were a good financial investment because they would cure mental illness, especially if treatment began promptly (Isaac and Armat 1990). Unfortunately, as we shall see, her argument appeared more than a century too soon—coming so far ahead of any truly effective treatments—to have hope of validation. Yet, public support of the need for treatment held steady for a century before plummeting in the 1960s and 1970s.

In the latter half of the 19th century, moral therapy lost favor for a number of reasons. Many patients did not respond even to "moral," comfortable, small-scale settings—raising doubts about the "cult of curability." (Discharge rates did fall through the period, but readmission rates remained high, suggesting the cure rate was not what it may have seemed.) In any case, the approach fared best in small settings with a supportive climate: moral theorists had considered 200 beds the optimum size for asylums (Isaac and Armat 1990). The large influx of patients admitted after the Civil War, as well as their heterogeneity, destroyed the intimate environment envisioned by the architects of moral therapy.

And finally, the second half of the 19th century and the start of this one saw the beginning of an organic model—sometimes called "the medical model"—the idea that mental illness resulted from brain pathology. This framework left little conceptual room for "milieu" approaches. Physicians interested in a link between mental illness and brain pathology embraced the organic, or medical, model as "scientific" and therefore more legitimate. Thus, Alois Alzheimer began uncovering the common symptoms of the dread brain disease that bears his name.

In the last century, the view that psychiatric treatment could be misused also began to take hold. This change in attitude emerged notably in the case of Mrs. Elizabeth Packard, who in 1860 successfully challenged her commitment by her husband to a psychiatric hospital in Illinois. She also successfully campaigned for laws requiring a jury trial to determine whether the person should be committed. When the jury trials proved a humiliating experience for many patients and relatives, the pendulum swung toward more informal, private, and (ironically, perhaps) less fair—because less scrutinized—procedures in the early part of the 20th century. Mrs. Packard's efforts, and continuing abuses, engendered mistrust in the commitment process in this country that fuels today's anticommitment climate. It should be recalled, however, that legal challenges to physicians' opinions about the need for commitment are not usual in most other nations of the world.

And, also, even though there was little belief in the curability of mental illness from the 1860s through the mid-1950s, there was no substantial erosion of the perception of the need for treatment or for asylums in the form of public psychiatric hospitals. In the Depression and during World War II, however, financial support for these huge institutions did decline, while their populations grew.

In fact, by the late 19th century, many psychiatric hospitals were overcrowded, understaffed, and underfunded. They would remain that way despite calls for reform decade after decade. Psychiatry enjoyed great success in World War II: toward the war's end, the vast majority of military psychiatric casualties were returned fit to their units. But this contrasted with the despicable conditions prevailing for ordinary patients in the public institutions. In 1948, Albert Deutsch's *Shame of the States* provided a devastating exposé of the inhumanity in many (not all) public psychiatric hospitals. Growing public outrage built strong antihospital sentiment that became more urgent in the ensuing decades because of several factors.

The Fifties

In the 1950s, there were four key developments. First, the number of patients in public mental hospitals in the United States peaked at 559,000 in 1955, increasing the pressures on the states to find a solution. For example, New York that year devoted 38% of its budget to pay for 90,000 resident patients (Isaac and Armat 1990). As Daniel P. Moynihan (1988), senator from New York, said, "Mental illness was seen as perhaps the most pressing problem New York state faced."

Second, also in that year, Congress authorized the creation of the Joint Commission on Mental Illness and Health with an appropriation of more than $1 million. The National Institute of Mental Health (NIMH), the American Psychiatric Association (APA), the Mental Health Association, and other organizations had lobbied for this legislation in a post-Dix crusade for reform.

Third, the advent of electroconvulsive therapy (ECT) in the 1930s, together with the introduction of psychoactive medications in the 1950s, gave hope of truly effective treatment for the first time since the halcyon days of moral therapy. ECT proved notably helpful for depression, and the new medications could actually blunt the more florid signs and symptoms of psychosis. This development not only spurred reform but also created the misleading impression that medication alone would suffice for the psychiatrically ill, a falsehood that has fostered neglect of patients' multiple other needs.

Fourth, antihospital reformers claimed that "labeling" patients as mentally ill, and the institutions themselves, produced psychopathology in the patients—an "institutional neurosis" (Barton 1959; Goffman 1961).

In 1958, the call for reforming public psychiatric hospitals yielded to demands for a scorch-and-burn policy that would simply abolish such hospitals. As the president of the APA, Harry Solomon (1958), put it:

> I do not see how any reasonably objective view of our mental hospitals today can fail to conclude that they are bankrupt beyond remedy. I believe, therefore, that our large mental hospitals should be liquidated as rapidly as can be done in an orderly and progressive fashion. (p. 3)

The Sixties

In 1960, three disparate developments began to undermine the public perception of the need for psychiatric treatment. The first was the Supreme Court decision in *Shelton v. Tucker*, a case not involving the psychiatrically ill but one that would ultimately pave the way for the concept of providing the least restrictive setting for the mentally ill. The high court's opinion stated:

> Even though the government purpose be legitimate and substantial, that purpose cannot be pursued by means that broadly stifle fundamental personal liberties when the end can be more narrowly achieved. (p. 257)

Second, Morton Birnbaum (1960), a primary care physician and a lawyer, published an article in the *American Bar Association Journal* entitled "The Right to Treatment." In it, he argued "that if an inmate is being kept in a mental institution against his will, he must be given proper medical treatment or else the inmate can obtain his release at will in spite of the existence or severity of his mental illness" (1960, p. 503). His concept inspired, in part, such pivotal court decisions as *Rouse v. Cameron* and *Wyatt v. Stickney*, which directed institutions to provide treatment to their patients. (The cases, however, did not contain actual decrees of that right, which is the subject of another story [see Isaac and Armat 1990].) Institutions found the best way to meet these requirements was often by reducing the number of patients served in order to provide adequate treatment to those who remained—a far cry from Birnbaum's dream of increasing access to treatment.

Third, Ronald D. Laing published *The Divided Self* (1960). Little was noted of Laing's ideas initially, but over the 1960s he popularized the radical—and specious—idea that development of a psychiatric illness was a sane approach—"a rational strategy"—to "an insane world" (p. 39).

In 1961, other events further eroded the case for psychiatric treatment. The Joint Commission published a seven-volume report called Action for Mental Health. Among its many recommendations were calls for public hospitals to limit the number of beds to 1,000 and for clinics to be established for every 50,000-person catchment area. Although the report was not antipsychiatry, it reinforced the climate urging reform.

Also in 1961, Gerald Caplan, an English-trained psychoanalyst, published *An Approach to Community Mental Health*. Caplan drew on milieu- or Freudian-based psychiatric approaches and championed both primary and secondary prevention based on psychoanalytic explanations of the cause of psychiatric illnesses. His views convinced some community mental health centers (CMHCs) in the middle and late 1960s that mental health workers should treat the community as a whole.

Making a more "psychiatrically well" society would mean treating illness in the community and thus forestall the need for hospitalization, nay, even the occurrence of severe mental illness! This philosophy harked back to moral therapy shibboleths of the early 19th century, which attributed mental suffering to the corrupting influences of their milieu or community.

The same year saw publication of Thomas Szasz's *The Myth of Mental Illness* (1961). The book's dismissal of mental illness as a harmful metaphor and false premise attracted few professionals but a number of influential legal activists. Followers of Szasz and Laing would form the antipsychiatry movement, which maintained that involuntary treatment was not legitimate because there was no illness to treat or that the symptoms were environmentally caused.

Asylum by Irving Goffman (1961) advanced the concept that some signs and symptoms of psychiatric illness stem not from illness but from being in institutions. "Deculturation" was his term for the effects of "institutionalism" on patients. The better the institution, he said, in the sense of offering a more structured program, the more likely hospitalization there would result in deculturation.

In 1963, Congress passed three laws that revolutionized the treatment of the psychiatrically ill. In that year, President John F. Kennedy signed into law legislation providing for federal funding of CMHCs and improvement grants for public mental hospitals. The Community Mental Health Centers Act of 1963 derived to some extent from testimony that community services would evolve as an alternative to institutional care and treatment. However, no evidence in the form of double-blind studies or other research was presented in support of such suppositions. As Wyatt and DeRenzo (1986) pointed out, the homelessness and neglect of the mentally ill since then can be traced in part to just such lack of research, or "sciencelessness."

In the same year, the psychiatrically ill became eligible for federal Aid to the Disabled, the precursor to Supplemental Security Income (SSI) and Social Security Disability Insurance (SSDI). These programs grant federal payments to thousands of mentally ill patients for the purpose of assisting them in living outside institutions. The guidelines for SSI and SSDI do not, of course, deny the existence of mental illness, and these programs often enhance the quality of life of the psychiatrically ill; but they have contributed to a false confidence in the extent to which patients are taken care of by such entitlements.

Also in 1963, the Senate approved model legislation setting forth new involuntary commitment standards. The model established dangerousness to self or others as the sole standard of commitment and eliminated need-for-treatment criteria; it also separated the need for involuntary commitment from competency. "The model bill that the Senate drafted in 1963 specified that the mentally ill patient would lose no civil rights on commitment, and the District of Columbia adopted it in modified form in 1964," according to Isaac and Armat (1990, p. 118). In the District of Columbia and most states, there had been a presumption of incompetency for patients committed involuntarily. Separating the two meant that it was rare that clinicians attempted to achieve a court finding of incompetency in any area. Yet this distinction was adopted in state after state, laying the foundation for court decisions in the late 1970s regarding the right to refuse treatment.

Ironically, this reform had been intended to encourage treatment by destigmatizing commitment, which had formerly deprived mental patients of their civil rights. That is, a patient considered committable had also been considered incompetent—that is, unfit to write a will, marry, dispose of property, vote, or even drive a car. With the reform, as one witness told the Senate hearings, a patient would no longer need fear what hospitalization would "do to his employment record, to his general position in the community" (Isaac and Armat 1990, p. 118). Another witness averred that mental hospitals could be "looked upon as treatment centers for sick people in the same sense that general hospitals are" (Isaac and Armat 1990, p. 118). In fact, the senators' approach in the end made care *less available* by restricting the numbers of people committed—to those who were dangerous—and by insinuating that there was a legal basis for involuntarily committed patients to be considered competent to refuse treatment.

In 1964, federal regulations associated with the 1963 Community Mental Health Centers Act called for the centers to provide the following services:

1. Inpatient services
2. Partial hospitalization services
3. Outpatient services
4. Twenty-four-hour emergency services
5. Consultation and education services

These required services did not provide for a total support system to replace that provided by the institution. Nor did the act specifically require the centers to take responsibility for the more disabled, more chronic psychiatrically ill. It was believed that psychiatric illnesses could be managed completely by medications and a caring community—again with no studies or research to support such ideas. To be sure, a caring community cannot be legislated, as the growing numbers of abandoned mentally ill in the streets attest.

In 1965, Congress passed Medicaid. This program discriminates against funding for the psychiatrically ill in ways that have led to further irresponsible deinstitutionalization. Medicaid in most instances does not cover care in freestanding psychiatric hospitals, either public or private; it does cover treatment in psychiatric wards of general hospitals and, under certain circumstances, nursing home costs.

These programs—Federal Aid to the Disabled (now SSI and SSDI), the Community Mental Health Centers Act, and Medicaid—offered opportunities for the states to substitute federal dollars for their own in the often lifelong care and treatment of the chronically mentally ill. All the states had to do to shift responsibility from state to federal ledgers was to transfer patients from public psychiatric hospitals, the traditional caretaker of the mentally ill, to nursing homes if the patients were elderly and to psychiatric units of general hospitals if the patients needed acute care. This massive shift of patients to nursing homes and general hospitals has undermined the support for long-term inpatient treatment. Finally, this discrimination abetted the campaign, under way since the 1950s, against the large public hospitals.

In 1966, the United States Court of Appeals for the District of Columbia ruled in *Lake v. Cameron* that a patient could not be involuntarily hospitalized if an alternative that infringes less on his or her rights to liberty (community placement) could be found. Based on the logic of *Shelton,* the decision held that before Ms. Lake could be admitted to a hospital involuntarily, one had to establish that no less restrictive alternative existed. The term "least restrictive" has become a key element in many judicial decisions and in some legislative initiatives.

The difficulty with using the least restrictive setting and deinstitutionalization is that while they sound noble in themselves, in execution they often mean simple neglect. The psychiatrically ill would have been better served had the goals of the reformers called for the greatest possible freedom from the illness and its consequences or a decent, dignified life outside hospitals with all necessary and comprehensive community services.

In 1969, the enactment of the Lanterman-Petris-Short (LPS) Act in California, passed in 1967, was a major step in the trend toward limiting involuntary commitment to dangerousness and grave disability (basically a form of dangerousness to self; Lamb and Mills 1986). Until that time, only five states had had such a limitation; within a decade almost every state had changed its code similarly (Shuman 1985). The LPS act also pioneered limits on how long a person could be hospitalized.

In the late 1960s, the federal government bolstered the antihospital trend through grant requirements that citizen boards have direction of CMHCs; local control was regarded as less suspect than state, county, or city governance. This concept, as well as direct federal subsidies to the mental health centers for a certain starting-up period, allowed the centers to remain aloof from state systems for the care of the severely mentally ill. And it created gaps in care that left no one agency—federal, state, county, city, or local—with full responsibility or accountability within any integrated, effective system for the mentally ill.

Who indeed was responsible for the mentally ill in the honeymoon period of the late 1960s that followed passage of the Community Mental Health Centers Act? As the CMHCs being built went their own ways—frequently ignoring the needs of the severely mentally ill (Torrey 1988)—no one stood up to antipsychiatry initiatives, no matter how absurd (Isaac and Armat 1990). And so, believing that the emperor of antipsychiatry had clothes, gullible, well-intentioned people thought that the mentally ill should not be treated because there was probably nothing to treat or that no matter how ill, they should be treated using milieu rather than biological therapies.

Thus, by the end of the 1960s, in the antiestablishment clime spawned by the Vietnam War, antipsychiatry themes found favor in the courts and legislatures. The psychiatrically ill were now seen as another oppressed group, like African Americans, women, or Hispanics. Furthermore, the traditional chief caretaker of the psychiatrically ill, the states, shamed by their inglorious record, declined to advocate for the seriously mentally ill. No one else—certainly few doctors, lawyers, or social workers—stepped forward.

The Seventies

In the 1970s, antitreatment and anticare trends continued, until in 1979 the families of the mentally ill shouldered their familiar burden publicly for the first time by forming the National Alliance of the Mentally Ill to press for better care for their loved ones.

In 1971, a right-to-treatment suit in Alabama, *Wyatt v. Stickney*, curiously, led to a reduction in treatment. The decision called for improved staffing and many other changes in Alabama's public mental and retardation institutions. So Alabama neatly improved staff-to-patient ratios—by decreasing the number of patients, sending them into the community or nursing homes.

A marked expansion of due process came in by a series of lawsuits, notably *Lessard v. Schmidt*. In 1972, a Wisconsin court ruled in this landmark case that the only grounds justifying involuntary commitment were dangerousness to others or to self. It also injected a spirit of criminalization in involuntary commitment by requiring that the risk of violence to self or others be demonstrated by a recent overt act plus substantial probability of recurrence. This theme became so bowdlerized in subsequent applications that as one psychiatrist put it, "You've got to grab the patient between the time [he] fires the gun and the bullet hits the victim—and just hope he's not a good shot" (Isaac and Armat 1990, p. 346).

Lessard also required a preliminary hearing within 48 hours and placed the burden of excluding less restrictive alternatives to involuntary hospitalization on the state. In addition, states were required to prove beyond a reasonable doubt, the standard of proof required in criminal proceedings, that the individual was dangerous. A less strict standard, preponderance of the evidence, usually applied in civil conflicts (Lonsdorf 1983). (In 1979, in *Addington v. Texas*, the United States Supreme Court ruled that clear and convincing evidence was the minimal sufficient standard, but a state could set the standard higher to beyond a reasonable doubt if it wanted.) *Lessard* was not binding outside Wisconsin, but it introduced techniques for blocking involuntary commitment that would be copied elsewhere. Civil commitment more and more resembled criminal proceedings (Shuman 1985).

In 1972, the Joint Commission on Accreditation of Hospitals (JCAH) (renamed the Joint Commission on Accreditation of Healthcare Organizations, or JCAHO, in 1987), an organization that had been accrediting hospitals since the 1950s, established separate standards for psychiatric hospitals. JCAH standards encouraged deinstitutionalization in two ways: 1) generally, the standards were easier to achieve when the number of patients was relatively small; and 2) specifically, the standards required treatment plans to include community placement outside the institution from the moment the patient was admitted.

In 1973, David Rosenhan's study, "On Being Sane in Insane Places," was published in the prestigious journal *Science*. Rosenhan, a disciple of Szasz, Goffman, and Laing, undertook to prove their view "that psychiatric diagnoses . . . are in the minds of the observers and are not valid summaries of characteristics displayed by the observed" (Isaac and Armat, p. 54). His study dispatched eight individuals posing as patients to a total of 12 psychiatric wards. The pseudopatients gave false histories on admission and, once admitted, immediately stopped displaying any psychopathology. Yet they were never discovered by the ward staff—despite their continuous note taking!

This study certainly raised questions about the accuracy of psychiatric evaluations and diagnoses. But it also heightened concern about treatment of the people on the wards by staff. Even though they acted as if they were "normal" after being admitted to the ward, the bogus patients were kept on the units for 7 to 52 days and at discharge were still considered to have suffered from a mental illness (Rosenhan 1973). Although the clinicians' failure to make the proper diagnosis could be attributed to false data, their dismal postadmission performance seemed to vindicate the views of Szasz and his followers.

In 1975, the United States Supreme Court ruled in *O'Connor v. Donaldson* that a psychiatrist had erred in retaining a patient, Kenneth Donaldson, in a Florida institution without treating him—although Donaldson steadfastly refused treatment for nearly his entire 14-year incarceration. After many years and much litigation, the final settlement was $20,000. The lesson for the psychiatrist working in thinly staffed public settings was that there was a simple way to avoid professional liability for inadequate treatment on the one hand and to avoid civil liability for deprivation of liberty on the other hand: avoid being responsible for the patient in the first place by discouraging admission and, if he or she were admitted, by effecting rapid discharge.

In 1975, a federal court in the District of Columbia granted hundreds of patients of St. Elizabeths Hospital a right to community placement, "the least restrictive setting," as opposed to hospitalization.

In 1979, the Massachusetts Supreme Court, relying on the state's constitution, undertook a series of decisions involving the involuntary administration of medications. In *Rogers v. Okin*, the court required the state to appoint a guardian for the patient, and the guardian's responsibilities included deciding whether to agree with a physician's decision that the patient should have antipsychotic medications administered. The court ruled that it was a conflict of interest for the physician to make the decision alone. It did allow for the prescribing under medical emergencies but defined such emergencies in policy emergency terms: "a substantial likelihood of physical harm to that patient, other patients, or to staff."

The case sparked look-alikes nationwide, although none as extreme

as in Massachusetts. The right to refuse treatment was the logical extension of the concept of those who saw psychiatric hospitalization as im-
prisonment. The patient was in the hospital for social control, not
treatment. There is evidence that the right to refuse treatment has further criminalized hospitalization, leading to a greater use of seclusion
(for psychotic, unmanageable, and untreated patients), of restraints,
and of transfer of more patients to maximum security hospitals in Massachusetts (Schultz 1982).

In addition to formalizing and hardening patient-psychiatrist conflicts, right-to-refuse judicial procedures have subtracted from resources available to the mentally ill. In California, Rappeport (1987)
reported that each treatment refusal costs the state $10,000. But in the
end, even after cumbersome and expensive court procedures, only
rarely is the patient's refusal upheld.

The right to refuse treatment pairs with another important concept—informed consent. But, obviously, in the case of the mentally ill,
because the diseased organ is the brain, it is often impossible for the
patient to give adequately informed consent without treatment. In addition, the legal basis for the informed consent has been distorted, as
Isaac and Armat (1990) explain:

> A 1914 New York Court of Appeals decision, *Schloendorff v. Society of New
> York Hospital*, is misused as a basis for affirming a mental patient's right
> to refuse treatment even after [he or she] is committed. In his opinion,
> Judge Benjamin Cardozo then wrote: "Every human being of adult years
> and *sound mind* has a right to determine what shall be done with his own
> body."
>
>   How could Judge Cardozo's words, specifically exempting the men-
> tally ill, be used as ground for giving them the same right to determine
> their treatment as normal [sic] individuals? The key has been the legal
> fiction, enshrined in state laws during the late 1960s and 1970s, that men-
> tal patients are competent. (p. 341)

Then, in 1981, the Omnibus Budget Reconciliation Act of the Reagan
administration changed federal direction and support for the psychiatrically ill by providing subsidies to the states through block grants.
Thus, the omnibus act reversed a trend toward increasing federal responsibility for the psychiatrically ill that had begun after World War
II. After more than three decades of leadership and initiatives—some
would say badly bungled ones—including providing seed money
without accountability to CMHCs, the federal government turned the
hands-on care and planning for the psychiatrically ill back to their former caretakers.

The Nineties

Today, a decade later, while it is difficult to generalize, in many states no one government agency is fully responsible for the care of the mentally ill. Splits in lines of authority across cities, counties, and states diffuse responsibility among a variety of agencies. Also, the sheer multiplicity of services the psychiatrically ill need to reside in the community, such as housing, food, education, and vocational and medical assistance, in addition to psychiatric care and social supports, further fragment responsibility for care.

Reimposing a need-for-treatment standard will require that one clearly defined agent has full responsibility for the psychiatrically ill. The present mix of federal, state, county, city, and local authorities means that no one agent is fully responsible—or accountable. It is obvious all the services needed by the severely disabled psychiatrically ill—formerly provided by the hospital—often can be provided only by the state. City or county authorities lack the ability to provide comprehensive and continuous care and treatment for this population, though as in Dane County, Wisconsin, the county mental health system can do a great deal if properly organized. Logically, the state should—once again—coordinate the myriad services—housing, food, education, vocational assistance, social support, and medical and psychiatric care—required by the psychiatrically ill.

But looming over all concerns for the mentally ill is the long shadow of antipsychiatry and an involuntary commitment criteria based on a criminal standard of dangerousness. This standard blocks care—whatever the source— for those often most in need. As Appelbaum has said, "The dangerousness standard makes no sense whatever . . . because it is not at all clear that you should be using your mental hospitals for the purpose of detaining people who are dangerous rather than treating people who need treatment" (Isaac and Armat 1990, p. 155).

In summary, the first half of the 19th century encouraged a wholly altruistic belief in the need for psychiatric treatment, called moral treatment. This phase peaked with the building of numerous state hospitals, then degenerated tragically in the second half of the 20th century. It would yield cravenly to a misinformed, even Luddite, view of mental illness as an alternative lifestyle, a matter of free will, and even a civil right. By the mid-1980s, with its victory over common sense and medical science, antipsychiatry could boast that a majority of the public—55%—did not believe there was such a thing as mental illness (Holden 1986)!

At the same time, the number of abandoned psychiatrically ill has soared. In 1986, in answer to a congressional inquiry, NIMH estimated that 104,800 schizophrenic patients were being treated in state mental hospitals (6%), 73,500 in nursing homes (5%), 225,400 in acute inpatient settings (14%), and 269,000 in outpatient settings (17%). The location of 937,000 patients (58%) was listed as unknown. Thus, NIMH could not account for the whereabouts of nearly 1 million people with schizophrenia.

Recent Developments in Involuntary Treatment

Although it is often thought that one cannot successfully treat an unwilling psychiatrically ill patient, there is considerable evidence that involuntary treatment is often effective. One substantial problem of the psychiatrically ill is that they frequently do not recognize that they are ill. When they do, their mental incapacity may make it difficult for them to cooperate. Still, when treatment is imposed, the patients' symptoms often clear, enabling them to make more rational decisions about their lives, such as deciding to continue treatment, take a job, and so on.

Because of radical changes in the perception of mental illness arising from a series of lawsuits since the late 1960s, a patient may now be committed involuntarily (e.g., because of dangerousness), yet be considered competent enough to refuse treatment. Clearly, this may transform a hospital from a place of treatment to a place of detention. Should involuntarily committed patients have the right to refuse treatment? First, let us look at some studies of committed patients.

- Gove and Fain (1977) found that 80% of 172 voluntary patients and 75% of 86 committed patients felt that they had benefited from the hospitalization.
- A follow-up study by Tomelleri and colleagues (1977) of 96 committed patients 18 months after discharge found that 20 of these patients had had 30 readmissions. Of these 30 admissions, 65% had been voluntarily.
- Kane and colleagues (1983) found that many involuntary patients had changed their minds between admission and discharge and later agreed that treatment was justified. A survey after discharge of these patients found that 64% were in compliance with treatment after discharge and—most significantly—that 93% of those in need of rehospitalization came voluntarily.
- Toews and colleagues (1980, 1981, 1984) found that 33% of a sample of committed patients felt that commitment had harmed them, whereas 46% said that it had helped them. Much larger percentages reported that they felt positive about their treating psy-

chiatrist. Only 7% felt more negative about psychiatry than they had on admission.

Incidentally, involuntary psychiatric treatment of medical and surgical patients takes place in hospitals routinely in the *parens patriae* tradition—without legal procedures—when patients, such as those suffering from Alzheimer's disease, become confused or destructive or act in bizarre ways. In studying this phenomenon at a hospital, Appelbaum and Roth (1988) found about one episode of involuntary treatment per 100 patient days. Medications and restraints were used in patients who were very disoriented or unruly.

A new form of commitment, involuntary outpatient commitment, was first used in the United States in the District of Columbia in 1972 (Band et al. 1984; Miller and Fiddleman 1984). Outpatient commitment is a court order that the patient must conform to treatment in an outpatient setting. Geller (1986) has stated some of the arguments in favor of outpatient commitment:

> To correct the "greatest failing of the modern mental health system . . . the failure of continuity of care" (Stone 1982), to desist from avoiding the care of the sickest patients, to shed feelings of impotence, and to do all this without acts of civil disobedience or moral gyrations that render him or her too exhausted to attend to patient's clinical requirements, the psychiatrist needs a sanctioned system that permits effective therapeutic intervention in community settings. One such system may be civil commitment to outpatient treatment. (p. 1262)

In a subsequent publication, Geller (1990) provided clinical guidelines for the use of involuntary outpatient treatment. His work provides specific indications for its use. Another well-stated summary of the issues around outpatient commitment appeared in a review by Mulvey and colleagues (1987):

> The most reasonable position appears to be an open recognition that there are serious threats to civil liberties posed by a policy of involuntary commitment but that little positive treatment can be done for the casualties of deinstitutionalization without accepting some element of coercion in the policy strategy. In the end, outpatient commitment is . . . a possible way to get us out of the present quandary of having to decide between the inhumaneness of institutions and the neglect involved in dumping mental patients in the community. The . . . unsuitability of our present options should push us to design a system that is sensitive to both the needs and the rights of mental patients. (p. 583)

Outpatient commitment truly has the potential to provide enforced treatment and greatly increased freedom for the patient. Liberated from psychosis, the patient becomes able to live decently in the community. In the District of Columbia in some years during the 1980s, outpatient commitment was used more than inpatient commitment. The results have been very satisfactory. For example, Zanni and de Veau (1986) found that District of Columbia patients who had been committed on an outpatient basis not only had fewer hospitalizations than previously but also briefer ones. Because noncompliance with treatment can be a reason for rehospitalization, obviously if treatment reaches the patient early enough, it can stave off a full-blown break.

A Right-to-Treatment Standard

We have reviewed the unfortunate history of the erosion of the belief in the need for involuntary commitment and treatment in the United States. We have indicated our belief in the effectiveness of involuntary treatment with both hospitalized and nonhospitalized patients. Basically, commitment based on dangerousness and the separation of commitment from competency has led to a senseless narrowing of the circumstances under which clinicians can treat and care for the psychiatrically ill involuntarily.

To reverse this direction, we would suggest that involuntary commitment reincorporate a right-to-treatment standard. We suggest using the standard formulated by Alan Stone and the APA with certain modifications. It may be recalled that Stone drafted a set of criteria in 1976 for involuntary commitment that formed the basis of the "Guidelines for Legislation on the Psychiatric Hospitalization of Adults," published by APA in 1983. The patient would be expected to meet each of the following guidelines to be eligible for involuntary commitment.

1. The person is suffering from a severe mental disorder.
2. There is a reasonable prospect that his [or her] disorder is treatable at or through the facility to which he [or she] is to be committed and such commitment would be consistent with the least restrictive alternative principle.
3. The person either refuses or is unable to consent to voluntary admission for treatment.
4. The person lacks capacity to make an informed decision concerning treatment.
5. As the result of the severe mental disorder, the person is (*a*) likely to cause harm to him[- or her]self or to suffer substantial mental or physical deterioration or (*b*) likely to cause harm to others.

The guidelines go to great lengths to protect patients' rights and allow for timely, periodic judicial reviews as well as lengthy treatment, if the patient meets these criteria.

Not surprisingly, however, we disagree with the fourth criterion, which requires that the patient be found incompetent in addition to being severely mentally ill. This separation between a diagnosis of severe mental illness justifying involuntary commitment and an intact ability to decide on treatment, in our view, has led to the root problem of current standards for commitment: it allows those already judged severely disabled enough to be involuntarily committed to have the right to refuse treatment. This amounts, in effect, to a right to remain crazy—and untreated.

Rightly, mentally ill patients were seen as being deprived of their civil rights wholesale in more primitive if not too distant times. As a rule, they forfeited their rights to vote, marry, sign contracts, or make wills after being involuntarily committed. This situation changed with the decoupling of commitment from competency (Isaac and Armat 1990), first articulated in the Senate hearings on model commitment legislation.

Based on those hearings and a rash of lawsuits regarding the right to refuse treatment, states across the country by the mid-1970s had changed their statutes to provide that hospitalized mental patients remain legally competent unless specifically judged otherwise by the court. And that bizarre separation of purely treatment—medical—decisions from civil commitment judgments has survived even in the otherwise workable APA guidelines.

In practice, what would happen if states adopted the APA's model guidelines? Two studies using the Stone criteria have been done (Appelbaum and Roth 1988; Hoge et al. 1988). The Appelbaum studies found that the competency requirement restricted the number of people qualifying for commitment. Those who conducted the study concluded, "The criterion of incompetency had, by far, the greatest effect in restricting the application of the Stone model in this group" (p. 764).

It would be helpful if an additional study used the APA guidelines themselves to deduce exactly their effect on commitment. But in the end, our concern is not the number of patients who might be committable using particular criteria but the most effective approach to caring for mentally ill patients.

On this basis, granting competency to involuntarily committed mentally ill patients to make treatment decisions is not appropriate and should not be used as a criterion in commitment guidelines. As attorney Joel Klein has suggested, if you are ill enough to be committed, then you are by definition incompetent in that situation and unable to decide on treatment (Isaac and Armat 1990). What happens to persons who are judged dangerous and competent but who refuse treatment, as frequently happens? Often, they are detained and untreated—making hospitals places of detention rather than places of treatment. And when they are not detained, they remain dangerous and untreated.

One state that has struggled successfully to find a way through the thicket of currently acceptable guidelines for involuntary commitment is Utah. In that state's code, a patient who is dangerous to self or others, who has mental illness, and who "lacks the ability to engage in a rational decision-making process regarding acceptance of medical treatment as demonstrated by evidence of an inability to weigh possible costs and benefits of treatment" is committable. In other words, Utah makes the decision that someone is incompetent (i.e., unable to decide on treatment rationally) at the time of emergency commitment. Nor do subsequent court proceedings to decide on longer-term commitment weigh the patient's competency separately. The difficulty, as usual, is that someone must still be dangerous, rather than simply ill enough, to warrant care, a standard that continues to criminalize the procedures of civil commitment. The Utah standard, in effect since 1986, was upheld in two court cases, one as high as the Federal Circuit Court of Appeals in Denver, and has remained unchallenged since.

Conclusions

In summary, involuntary treatment is frequently effective. In addition, an intermediate legal status between full hospital commitment and no treatment—involuntary outpatient commitment—allows patients whose condition is chronic to receive treatment over an extended period of time in independent, least restrictive settings in the community.

Clearly, today the mentally ill, wherever they reside, are pawns in an agenda of deinstitutionalization driven not by medical concerns but by unfounded psychiatric theories and civil rights. In many cases, remedies for their plight are divorced from true compassion and an accurate understanding of the nature of mental diseases. What has been overlooked is their right to freedom from suffering, neglect, and lack of treatment.

This nation deserves a need-for-treatment standard that will facilitate—not block—the treatment of the severely psychiatrically ill. At the same time, we urge returning responsibility for our nation's mentally ill to the states. The states, therefore, must take the lead in changing the standards for involuntary commitment and replace dangerousness-only criteria with a framework that incorporates implicit recognition of the need for treatment.

Put simply, if one is psychiatrically disabled enough to warrant involuntary commitment, one is not competent to make treatment decisions, as currently allowed in our Alice in Wonderland commitment process. Cases of mental illness requiring involuntary hospitalization, by definition, require by all standards of humane intervention a benevolent *parens patriae*—not a pretense of granting civil rights to people too ill to exercise them.

References

Addington v Texas, 441 U.S. 418 (1979), 7-7.4, 7-9.8

American Psychiatric Association: Guidelines for legislation on the psychiatric hospitalization for adults. Am J Psychiatry 140:672–679, 1983

Appelbaum PS, Roth LR: Assessing the NCSC guidelines for involuntary civil commitment from the clinician's point of view. Hosp Community Psychiatry 39:406–410, 1988

Band D, Heine A, Golfrank J, et al: Outpatient commitment: a thirteen year experience. Paper presented at the annual meeting of the American Academy of Psychiatry and the Law, Nassau, Bahamas, October 1984

Barton R: Institutional Neurosis. Bristol, England, Wright, 1959

Birnbaum M: The right to treatment. American Bar Association Journal, May 1960, pp 499–505

Caplan G: An Approach to Community Mental Health. New York, Grune & Stratton, 1961

Deutsch A: The Shame of the States. New York, Harcourt Brace, 1948

Geller JL: Rights, wrongs, and the dilemma of coercive community treatment. Am J Psychiatry 143:1259–1264, 1986

Geller JL: Clinical guidelines for the use of involuntary outpatient treatment. Hosp Community Psychiatry 41:749–755, 1990

Goffman E: Asylum: Essays on the Social Situation on Mental Patients and Other Inmates. New York, Doubleday, 1961

Gove WR, Fain T: A comparison of voluntary and committed psychiatric patients. Arch Gen Psychiatry 34:669–676, 1977

Hoge SK, Sacks G, Appelbaum P, et al: Limitations on psychiatrists discretionary civil commitment authority by the Stone and dangerousness criteria. Arch Gen Psychiatry 45:764–769, 1988

Holden C: Giving mental illness its research due. Science 232:1084–1085, 1986

Isaac RJ, Armat VC: Madness in the Streets: How Psychiatry and the Law Abandoned the Mentally Ill. New York, Free Press, 1990

Joint Commission on Mental Illness and Health: Action for Mental Health: Final Report of the Joint Commission on Mental Illness and Health, 1961. New York, Basic Books, 1961

Kane J, Quitkin F, Rifkin A, et al: Attitudinal changes of involuntary committed patients following treatment. Arch Gen Psychiatry 40:374–377, 1983

Lake v Cameron, 364 F 2d 657 (1966)

Laing RD: The Divided Self. New York, Pantheon, 1960

Lamb HR, Mills M: Needed changes in law and procedure for the chronically mentally ill. Hosp Community Psychiatry 37:475–480, 1986

Lonsdorf R: The involuntary commitment of adults: an examination of recent legal trends. Psychiatr Clin North Am 6:651–660, 1983

Miller RD, Fiddleman PB: Outpatient commitment: treatment in the least restrictive environment? Hosp Community Psychiatry 35: 1147–1151, 1984

Moynihan DP: The homeless (letter). The New York Times, March 10, 1988

Mulvey EP, Geller JL, Roth LH: The promise and peril of involuntary outpatient commitment. Am Psychol 42:571–584, 1987

O'Connor v Donaldson, 422 U.S. 563 (1975), 7-2.1, 7-4.10, 7-10.8

Rappeport J: Belegaled: mental health and the law in the United States, 1986. Can J Psychiatry 32:719–727, 1987

Rogers v Okin, 478 F. Supp. 1342 (D. Mass. 1979), 1159–1160

Rosenhan D: On being sane in insane places. Science 179:250–258, 1973

Schultz S: The Boston State Hospital case: a conflict of civil liberties and true liberalism. Am J Psychiatry 139:183–188, 1982

Shelton v Tucker 364 US 479, 81 S Ct 257, 5 L Ed 231 (1960)

Shuman D: Innovative statutory approaches to civil commitment: an overview and critique. Law, Medicine & Health Care, December 1985, pp 284–289

Solomon HC: The American Psychiatric Association in relation to American psychiatry. Am J Psychiatry 115:1–9, 1958

Szasz T: The Myth of Mental Illness. New York, Harper, 1961

Tarasoff v Regents of the University of California, 131 Cal Rptr, 551 P2d 334 (1976), vacating 118 Cal Rptr 129, 529 P2d 553 (1974)

Toews J, Prabhu V, el-Guebaly N: Commitment of the mentally ill. Can J Psychiatry 25:611–618, 1980

Toews J, el-Guebaly N, Leckie A: Patient reactions to their commitment. Can J Psychiatry 6:251–54, 1981

Toews J, el-Guebaly N, Leckie A, et al: Patient attitudes at the time of their commitment. Can J Psychiatry 29:590–595, 1984

Tomelleri C, Lakshminarayanan N, Herjanic M: Who are the "committed"? J Nerv Ment Dis 165:288–293, 1977

Torrey EF: Nowhere to Go: The Tragic Odyssey of the Homeless Mentally Ill. New York, Harper & Row, 1988

Wyatt RJ, DeRenzo EG: Scienceless to homeless (editorial). Science 234:1309, 1986

Wyatt v Stickney, 325 F Supp 781 (MD Ala 1971); enforced by 344 F Supp 373, 376, 379–385 (MD Ala 1972)

Zanni G, de Veau L: Inpatient stays before and after outpatient commitment. Hosp Community Psychiatry 37:941–942, 1986

Chapter 12

Clinical Case Management With the Homeless Mentally Ill

Felicity V. Swayze, M.S.W.

Research data and clinical experience are quickly bringing us to an understanding that the homeless mentally ill are, in fact, a particular subgroup of the chronically mentally ill. Homeless mentally ill persons present an array of service needs similar to those of other mentally ill persons being treated in the community: psychiatric care, medical care, and access to benefits and entitlements in order to ensure a reliable source of income and health insurance, substance abuse treatment, and housing. However, it is a mistake to assume that "placing" a homeless mentally ill person in housing will, in and of itself, take care of the problem. It may not even be the most desirable initial goal in intervention.

Case management is critical in delivering services to the homeless mentally ill (Belcher 1988; Gold Award 1986; Lamb and Lamb 1990). Case management services are being delivered in the shelters, in the streets, and in agencies. However, a clear conceptualization of case management for this population is needed. Where should case management services be located? Who should deliver them? What professional or paraprofessional background is most useful? How should these services be integrated into communities, into existing mental health systems, and, above all, into the social networks and shadow world of homeless mentally ill people? So far, case management for this population has been represented in traditional terms—as a linking or facilitating mechanism—rather than as a clinical intervention that in-

The author thanks Sharon Miller, M.S.W., clinical case manager, for contributing her rich clinical experience to the stories in this chapter.

corporates and manages the entire spectrum of the individual's psychosocial needs.

New approaches to case management are emerging in the community-based treatment of psychiatrically disabled individuals. Clinical case management, with its emphasis on the clinical relationship between the case manager and the patient, is proving effective in ensuring the consistency and availability of the full range of services over time to the deinstitutionalized psychiatric population (Harris and Bergman 1988). Recently, as a result of work being carried out in the homeless shelters of the nation's capital, we as clinicians are becoming convinced that clinical case management can also provide coherent and effective strategies for engaging the homeless mentally ill, treating their psychiatric illness, and placing them in stable living situations, with the result being a decrease in relapse and recidivism to the streets and shelters.

A particular conceptualization of case management underlies this work. Clinical case management encompasses a knowable set of treatment strategies and clinical skills. It is a treatment intervention in which the clinical case manager focuses simultaneously on treating the individual and the individual's environment. Treatment of the individual occurs through the development of a clinical relationship between patient and case manager. Treatment of the environment occurs as the case manager intervenes in the patient's external world to create a responsive care environment.

The Patient and the Environment: The Story of Ms. E

A clinical story will help illustrate ways in which the clinical case manager develops and carries out a plan incorporating the dual focus of treatment.

Clinical Case

Ms. E, a 40-year-old Hispanic woman, was referred to the clinical case management agency by a shelter worker. She had been living in shelters and on the streets for at least 7 years. Alienated from family, her only solid contact was a volunteer representative payee, a well-meaning man who found himself acting as case manager. In the previous year, he had moved her 12 times from shelter to shelter. Each move was precipitated by her increasing paranoia, as the intensity of interpersonal contact in the shelter became intolerable to her.

When we first met her, she was experiencing symptoms of a long-untreated mental illness. Her speech was almost unintelligible, as she mumbled and looked down at the table between us. We were inside on a dark day, but she wore sunglasses throughout our meeting. The shelter staff had arranged the interview; this first time, it was enough that she actually came and stayed for a few minutes. The agency case manager returned frequently to the shelter, always communicating the day and time to Ms. E and to the shelter worker. Soon, Ms. E came to know when the agency case manager would be at the shelter and, increasingly, came to the shelter at those times.

The case manager understood that Ms. E was beginning to become engaged with her, and decided on the next move. Working again with the shelter staff, she arranged an appointment for Ms. E with the consultant psychiatrist at the shelter. She persuaded Ms. E to see him and assured her that she would also be there. The psychiatrist made a diagnosis of schizophrenia and prescribed appropriate psychotropic medications. The case manager worked with the shelter staff around supervision of the medications. By this time, the case manager was developing a good working relationship with Ms. E and could discuss medications with her without major resistance.

Psychiatrically, Ms. E improved markedly; the sunglasses came off and she spoke more clearly. As the relationship developed and work went increasingly smoothly, the case manager began to consider residential placement. Initially, she ruled out a group home because Ms. E did not see herself as a patient and, as she well knew, these were homes for "patients." The case manager suggested an independent living arrangement in a house shared with three other agency clients.

Trouble started during the first visit, when Ms. E saw that she would be living with Ms. I, whom she had known at the shelter and whom she distinctly disliked. Ms. E started a fight in the front hallway. She then began to deteriorate psychiatrically and continued to unravel at the shelter. After some consideration, the case manager came to the conclusion that Ms. E was fearful of the demands, both practical and interpersonal, represented by the new living situation. She approached Ms. E with a new plan and a new message.

The case manager's new message to Ms. E was based on an understanding of her deficits. She told Ms. E that the agency had a group home available in which she would not have to do any cleaning, cooking, or anything. She told Ms. E that this placement was a way for her to get out of the shelter and have a place to live so she would not have to spend all day outside. The placement was made quickly and has been successful.

Goals of Clinical Case Management

Clinical case management assesses a patient's deficits at the outset and, in this way, recognizes the enormous psychic disorganization that persons with chronic mental illness experience. For the homeless mentally ill person, surviving in a transient and particularly chaotic world, the disorganization takes on global dimensions. The external world is almost a disorderly, concrete representation of the person's internal state.

The story of Ms. E indicates ways in which the clinical case manager can use the relationship with the patient as a means of accomplishing necessary tasks of case management. In this way, the case manager treats the individual and the individual's environment and works to develop a better integration between the patient's internal and external worlds. Our tale also illustrates the two important goals of clinical case management with the homeless mentally ill.

The first goal is to achieve some reduction in psychiatric symptomatology. Unlike most individuals discharged from psychiatric hospitals, the homeless mentally ill frequently are experiencing an untreated mental illness at the very moment that attempts are being made to connect them to services. Psychiatric intervention and the ability to introduce medications are necessary in order to enhance psychosocial functioning to at least some minimum level. Without these services, case managers are like Sisyphus pushing the stone up the hill; all efforts at engagement and provision of services fall back upon themselves.

It is my observation that case managers and others charged with trying to help these people frequently may have little formal training in understanding mental illness, its profoundly disabling effects, and its treatment. Clinical case management, with its comprehensive framework, empowers, expects, and trains case managers to understand major mental disorders, be familiar with medications, and advocate for and secure psychiatric services for the patient. Psychiatrists, in their turn, can learn to work with case managers who are informed in this way. A clinical case manager can provide the medicating psychiatrist with invaluable information on the current life situation and ongoing mental status of a patient; the case manager can also make observations about possible side effects of medications. Most critically (as in the case of Ms. E), the case manager, by working through the relationship with the patient in the patient's environment, can develop mechanisms for medication supervision that will promote compliance and an improved prognosis for reduction in psychiatric symptomatology.

The second goal, which is also evident in the story of Ms. E., is to identify and provide reasonable living situations so as to reduce the cycle of homelessness and inhibit psychiatric relapse and recidivism to the streets and shelters. The doors of the shelters revolve even faster than those of the mental hospitals. Working in a shelter, I see residents' charts. On the cover, the chart carries a label for each entry and discharge of a resident. It is not unusual to see rows of labels on a chart, a visual history of a life as a homeless person. Case managers in the shelter know which residents will return, and they also know that, between labels, these persons are usually staying in another shelter or living in the streets.

In the case of Ms. E, the clinical case manager had to identify or develop additional resources in order to achieve the two goals. Ms. E was a recipient of Supplemental Security Income (SSI) benefits, payable in an adjoining state to her volunteer representative payee. The case manager secured access to the benefits in order to pay housing costs in the group home and to transfer medical insurance to the local jurisdiction, as Ms. E would eventually need to be seen by the agency psychiatrist. Psychiatric care at the shelter was provided without charge by a psychiatrist from a public agency.

The case manager needed to work long and hard to gain the trust of both the representative payee and Ms. E before she could bring about the necessary change in the financial situation. And she could not move Ms. E into the group home until she had reasonable assurance that the funds would be available. Again, the clinical case manager works through the relationship with the patient in the patient's environment to bring about change.

Principles of Clinical Case Management

We have already identified goals of clinical case management as a treatment intervention for the homeless mentally ill. We also need practical and useful strategies that engage our own capabilities and the interest of the patient as we work to achieve them. First, however, let us review several principles that underlie clinical case management treatment of the chronically mentally ill. These principles also inform our work with the homeless subpopulation.

First, severe and persistent mental illness is a biopsychosocial disorder with devastating consequences. Nowhere is this more evident than in the shelters and on the streets of our towns and cities.

Second, services for the chronically mentally ill must be continuous and reflect an integrated plan. Case managers, whether in agencies or in shelters, are in a position to develop and direct this plan and must be empowered to do so. We see the importance of this step in the initial work with Ms. E.

Third, services should be centered, to the extent possible, on the patient's needs, both as expressed by the patient and as assessed by the case manager. Patients must perceive that services are voluntary and meet their perceived needs.

Fourth, services should be individualized, based on individual care and individual treatment planning. These patients are not well served by programs that rely on across-the-board programmatic expectations as determinants of success or failure. The clinical stories we present show how the creativity and flexibility of the case manager led to accomplishment of case management goals.

Fifth, services in the system must be responsive to the efforts of the clinical case manager working on behalf of the patient. The clinical case manager is at the center and must be empowered by the rest of the system to act. Clearly, this is difficult to achieve in the alternative treatment world that is emerging in the shelters and in the streets as the public mental health system is proving unable to care for these patients. The case manager must be skillful in many ways: as an advocate, a linking force, a detective. Frequently, the case manager creates leverage and gets systems response only by his or her physical presence in accompanying the patient (e.g., to Social Security offices, psychiatric clinics, drug programs, the courts, and elsewhere).

Strategies: Engagement and the Clinical Relationship

I will examine in greater detail the strategies and treatment approaches of clinical case management as they apply to work with the homeless mentally ill. Recall the dual focus of treatment, the individual and the environment; I will now look at each in turn.

Clinical case management treats the individual through the clinical relationship between patient and case manager. How does the relationship begin? How do we characterize it? How does the case manager maintain the relationship over time?

The relationship begins with the first contact with the case manager, or with any representative of the service provider whose contact with the patient may precede the connection to the case manager. The engagement phase is critical in providing a foundation for effective work with the homeless mentally ill (Cohen 1989). Engagement is a process that allows for an extended time frame, accepts the need to tolerate cyclical regression, and recognizes the possibility of initial residential instability.

The demands of the engagement phase are understood and mediated by the clinical case manager as he or she works with the patient through the relationship.

The First Interview: Indian Tribes

Again, a clinical scene provides a better understanding of the initial stage of engagement. The relationship begins with the first contact. Intake staff from the clinical case management agency usually conduct the first meeting with a shelter resident in pairs; one person conducts the interview and the other makes observations and takes notes. We arrived at this arrangement for a couple of reasons. First, there are considerations of personal safety. We know little about the individuals we see, and they may be actively psychotic and acutely symptomatic. Interviewing space may be isolated from or out of the view of others at the shelter. One person should not be expected to manage a disorganized patient and a chaotic environment simultaneously with no support.

Second, two observers are better than one. During one memorable interaction, my colleague and I found ourselves incorporated into the woman's delusional world within the first 15 minutes. Her world was peopled with Indian tribes, white-colored foods, and the son of the Indian chief, who clearly represented the young, attractive, male psychologist with whom I was doing the interview. (I was notably excluded from this primitive picture; she was married to the chief's son.) The hour was an extraordinary experience, as if we were all floating around together in a watery dream. It was not at all unpleasant, but when it was over my colleague and I certainly needed to help each other get fixed back in reality so that we could make an assessment of the patient's treatment needs and her ability to engage in services. We had made an attachment, however primitive.

When we arrive for this first meeting, we follow a certain path. First, we ask the person what he or she has been told about why we are at the shelter. The answer invariably focuses on housing. But, as I have stated earlier, this meeting is not necessarily the best time to suggest psychiatric intervention. Obviously other considerations must be brought to bear on the situation. We reply, "Yes, that is true, but you should also know that we are a mental health clinic." Here we pause and wait for the reaction. Sometimes it comes quickly, dramatically, and negatively. But more often than not, the person stays to listen. So, we continue and say, "Our clients are people who have some history of emotional or psychiatric problems"; another pause. Many reactions are possible, but we are not deterred. If the person is still in the room, we then say, "We have a psychiatrist at our clinic. We would probably ask you to agree to the possibility of seeing him [or her] occasionally. No more than once a month."

We present all this as disarmingly as possible, in a low-keyed way. We go on to say, "It is possible he might prescribe some medications. . . . Would you consider agreeing to the possibility of taking some medications?"

Now is the time to remember that we do not have to get this person to do anything. We can engage these patients only by looking for some embryonic inclination on their part to voluntary participation. Voluntary participation may mean simply sitting out a 10-minute interview and not shouting at us or fleeing when we say we will return. We go on to describe all that we can offer the person, including housing, the support of a case manager, and assistance with his or her financial needs.

In this first contact, we do not ask for decisions. We say we will be back at a regular time one afternoon each week, and we tell the person when it is. We may leave cards with our names. We let the person approach at his or her own rate. There are no institutionally determined discharge dates here.

Empowerment and trust are key elements in the initial phases of bringing homeless mentally ill individuals into psychiatric treatment and residential services. Our clinical experience leads us to put it more simply: Don't offer anything you can't deliver, and don't keep quiet about something you will have to ask for later but are reluctant to state in the beginning. We believe that if you do not address the mental illness, the psychiatric need, at the outset, you have probably dropped the ball at the beginning of the game. Many of these people seem to understand, at some level, that there is something seriously wrong in their internal world, but it is not necessary that they explicitly recognize it. Frequently, however, an empathic comment by the case manager, which does not require an answer or an action, registers somewhere in their minds, and a small connection is made. They may have the relatively rare experience of feeling understood.

Time to Engage: The Story of Ms. D

The first contact is the first step in engagement and provides a foundation for developing a relationship. However, we must allow an extended time frame for engagement. This approach reflects reality, and reality needs to be built into treatment approaches. Clinical work with the homeless mentally ill is characterized by sporadic attempts to engage and become engaged, both on the part of the case manager and the patient.

The story of Ms. D shows the difficulty some patients have in developing attachments.

Clinical Case

Ms. D is a 37-year-old woman who has been diagnosed with major depression. As her case manager describes her, "There is a real thread underneath that things are not right and are never going to be right." Ms. D has never lived independently. She was homeless for 16 months, after being sent to a shelter on Thanksgiving Day after a fight with her older sister, with whom she lived. Although she had had a year of college, she had always been a low-functioning person who was taken care of by her sister, who finally gave up. She was first identified as being mentally ill when she was psychiatrically evaluated at the shelter.

Ms. D is typical of many mentally ill homeless women. They have been sheltered in some tolerant or simply available living situation. The living situation ends, sometimes through the death of the family member who may be housing the woman, or after an altercation or an eviction. The woman ends up on the streets and in the shelter system. She is still not identified as being mentally ill.

The case manager worked with Ms. D for 5 months in the shelter, seeing her at least once a week, often more. This particular clinician is unusually effective in engaging the difficult, disaffiliated patient. But Ms. D simply did not want a relationship with her and stated it clearly. She said she did not trust anybody, that people always let her down, and that she expects always to be disappointed. Engagement moved at a snail's pace. The case manager came to understand that the only way to connect with this patient was at the concrete level of trying to give her exactly what she asked for, particularly in the living situation. Luck intervened and a subsidized efficiency apartment became available. There, Ms. D can live alone and shut herself in. The case manager is certain that without the availability of this living situation, we would not have been able to move her out of the shelter or be able to address any of her other treatment needs.

It is not enough, however, simply to house her. Without the continuing, though attenuated, efforts to establish a connection, a relationship with the case manager, Ms. D is at risk for psychiatric relapse. The case manager must use whatever relationship, whatever personal leverage she has, in order to gain Ms. D's participation in mental health treatment. Her acute and disabling depression makes it impossible for her to work. She has no social supports. She spends all her money within the first 2 weeks of receiving her monthly check; she buys clothes to make herself feel better. It was necessary not only to address mental health treatment at the outset but also to build it into the case management plan.

About 3 months after she moved into the apartment, Ms. D needed to obtain a medical signature on her application for general public assistance benefits. The case manager, thinking creatively, saw an opportunity. She told Ms. D that if she came into the agency, the psychiatrist would sign it for her. Ms. D agreed. However, she refused to take the medications that the psychiatrist wanted to prescribe. The case manager worked with the psychiatrist who, reluctantly, agreed not to insist on medications and to sign her form. He did state clearly to her, however, that she had a major depression and that she would benefit from medications. Again, there was an explicit recognition of her mental illness but no requirement that she make a verbal or behavioral acknowledgement of it. Ms. D was managing adequately in her isolated way.

Ms. D struggles against engaging with the case manager. Sometimes she will accept assistance and sometimes she won't. When she received her lump sum back-payment of benefits money, she let the case manager take her shopping for a television but not for furniture. The relationship is quite tenuous still. Describing her visits to Ms. D, the case manager said, "There are times when she is sleeping, or not there, or says she is ill. I only stay a few minutes. There are other times when it seems like she doesn't want me to leave."

Time to Regress: The Story of Ms. H

The clinical case manager, then, understands that developing the relationship with the patient and engaging the patient in services are extended processes. There may also be periods of cyclical regression during this phase.

Clinical Case

Ms. H is a young woman with a history of physical and sexual abuse within her family. When we first met her at the shelter, she exhibited an extremely paranoid and grandiose delusional system focusing on having lots of money and being married to famous people. Her anger and distrust were almost palpable as we sat together. However, an attachment to the case manager seemed to come very quickly, and Ms. H accepted residential placement within 2 months of our first contact. If housing the homeless mentally ill is a measure of success, then this was an outstanding achievement.

However, all has not gone well during the past year. Trust is still developing many months later. Ms. H is a striking young woman who carries herself with an angry pride. She comes to the agency and will sit with the case manager anywhere from 30 seconds to 30 minutes. In this way, she maintains control over the interaction and manages the degree of interpersonal closeness she can tolerate. Any attempt by the case manager to move the conversation away from concrete concerns to a more personal approach escalates Ms. H's delusions and her anxiety.

Recently, a dramatic episode resulted in a major setback in the relationship and in the engagement process. Another agency had applied for SSI benefits on behalf of Ms. H before she had accepted our agency's services. SSI ruled that she was not disabled based on the psychiatric diagnosis given to her by the SSI-appointed psychiatrist, and benefits were denied. Ms. H allowed the clinical case manager to initiate the appeals process, agreed to go to the hearing, and signed in advance so that the case manager could read the exhibits. However, when the judge asked the case manager if she disagreed with anything in the original application, the case manager stated that she disagreed with the original diagnosis. Even though Ms. H had told the case manager that she could say whatever she wanted, when she heard the new diagnosis presented by the case manager, she exploded in a rage. She screamed racial epithets at the case manager and continued to be abusive in the street as they went to the car.

This is a complicated business. At a concrete level, the case manager's purpose was well served by the patient's escalation during the appeals hearing. The judge had no difficulty making a decision in favor of awarding disability benefits. Ms. H now has a reliable source of income and medical insurance, both essential in reversing her homelessness and treating her mental illness. In terms of her relationship with the case manager, it is unlikely that Ms. H would have participated at all if she had not developed some sense that the case manager could be trusted. The case manager also believes that on yet another level, Ms. H went to that hearing because she knows she is mentally ill and is moving closer to accepting it.

But the entire process put an extraordinary demand on the relationship, on both sides. The ability of the case manager to tolerate this regression, as painful as it was to her personally, is a critical factor in the ongoing process of engaging a paranoid and angry young woman in services that will allow her to avoid homelessness and accept treatment for her mental illness.

Time to Try Again: Initial Residential Instability

The stories of Ms. D and Ms. H tell something of the difficulties that homeless mentally ill people and their case managers can experience in the engagement phase, as the relationship develops and the provision of services occurs. Recall that clinical case management not only focuses on the clinical relationship but also treats the individual's environment through the development of a responsive care environment. Nowhere is this aspect more important than in the living situation that we attempt to provide. We must recognize the possibility of initial residential instability in the engagement phase. We may not get it right the first time.

We remember Ms. E, who reverted to psychosis when presented with an independent living situation. Fortunately, the case manager did not attempt to force this move; it was doomed to failure from the start. Ms. H also experienced severe difficulties in the initial residential placement. She moved out of the shelter into an agency-leased apartment with another previously homeless woman with a mental illness. There was great friction from the start; it was a poor match interpersonally. The problem was made worse by the fact that everything in the apartment belonged to the other woman. But Ms. H refused to consider a move. Things went from bad to worse. After disappearing into the city for a few days, Ms. H turned up at the case manager's office, demanding to be moved. She accepted placement in a house that she shares with three other women in which she has two rooms of her own.

As we reflect on these stories and on the engagement process, it appears that there is a complicated interplay between the development of the relationship and the offering and provision of concrete services. In some instances—in the case of Ms. E, for example—the patient eases into accepting services only as a trusting relationship begins to develop. In other cases, such as that of Ms. D and perhaps of Ms. H, the patient will accept contact with a mental health professional only if it appears that instrumental needs, such as housing and benefits and entitlements, are met. In both situations, however, as time passes and the engagement process develops, the consistency of the relationship and psychiatric and residential stability become intertwined. The prognosis for breaking the cycle of homelessness becomes more hopeful.

Time to be Together: Aspects of the Clinical Relationship

We have looked at ways in which the clinical case manager considers the relationship with the patient and works, within the relationship, to engage the individual in the overall case management process. Let us look at this relationship more closely. How is it characterized and how does the clinical case manager work to maintain it over time? This conceptualization derives, as I have indicated before, from clinical case management approaches to working with the chronic psychiatric patient. Any modifications we make in reference to our work with the homeless mentally ill are a matter of degree rather than of substance. The difficulties we experience engaging any person with a long history of severe and persistent mental illness are particularly acute with the homeless mentally ill. Interpersonal factors, such as the extreme disaffiliation of these individuals, are reinforced by environmental factors present in the fragmented underworld of the urban homeless.

I will keep this in mind as I say a few things about the relationship between case manager and patient in the clinical case management model. First, it is a supportive, explicitly developed therapeutic relationship. In the case of the homeless mentally ill, the goals of the relationship are to enable the case manager to modify the environment with the purpose of assisting the patient in achieving some measure of psychiatric and residential stability.

This relationship operates on many levels, both instrumental and affective, as we have seen in our clinical examples. The relationship has many aspects. It is a real relationship that takes place in many different settings: in shelters, in stores, in offices, and in living situations. It is, however, a hierarchical relationship in which issues of authority are inherent. Case managers who work with homeless mentally ill persons must tread particularly carefully in this area, as any hint of coercion or control will certainly lead to the patient's fleeing.

It is also an affective relationship in which the case manager's natural tendency to like or dislike the patient may predispose the outcome to success or failure. Again, the person who has been living on the streets and in the shelters may frequently present in a variety of unappealing and even obnoxious ways. Psychiatric symptomatology is often present; personal hygiene may well be extremely poor. It is difficult for homeless chronically mentally ill individuals to engage themselves in a therapeutic relationship; it is as difficult for the case manager to want to attach.

This relationship also has major implications for case managers at an intensely personal level (Swayze 1988). As is true of traditional dynamic therapies, it is a relationship in which distortions of reality, stemming from the intrapsychic dynamics of both the patient and the case manager, can occur. Transference and countertransference reactions develop. Recall the story of Ms. H and her case manager at the SSI appeals hearing: Ms. H reacted to the case manager as if she were a hostile and persecutory figure. The case manager, in her turn, was expected to manage an extraordinary demand in the external world and at the same time control and mediate her own rage and fear.

Successful outcomes in clinical case management rely on an understanding of the engagement process and on the clinical relationship between case manager and patient. The case manager treats the individual through the relationship and must work to maintain this connection over time in the face of many demands.

Strategies: Systems Interventions

The demands on the case manager come as frequently from the external system as they do from interactions with the patient. Treatment focuses not only on the individual. The clinical case manager treats the environment, as well, through interventions in the system so as to reduce psychiatric symptomatology and develop and maintain a stable living situation. A principle of clinical case management asserts that services must be responsive as the clinical case manager works on behalf of the patient to accomplish goals and tasks.

The problems here are abundantly clear as one comes to know the obstacles that case managers experience as they try to secure services for their residents. The following tale bears out the analogy of Sisyphus and his stone.

A wildly symptomatic mentally ill woman presents herself at the shelter and is admitted. She has been there many times before. She is picked up again by a case manager there who is all too familiar with her. The case manager decides, this time around, that something different needs to happen. She sets about trying to find out something about the client.

In this situation, the case manager functions as a detective, hunting down elements of this person's life, trying to fill in the blanks. The woman tells the case manager, a low-keyed and skillful person with a nonthreatening manner, that she has recently been at the public mental hospital. The city's public mental health system tries to follow outpatients through a centralized computer system. Shelter and other staff can use this system to learn if the resident has had any connection to the hospital or to any of the community mental health centers (CMHCs). This system is quite useful for learning about the patient's history and other information, but it does not necessarily ensure continuity of treatment.

In this particular case, the case manager learned that the woman had had numerous psychiatric hospitalizations over the years, after which there had been many failed attempts to place her in housing and gain compliance with psychiatric treatment as an outpatient. She had been placed in at least three group homes in the few months prior to this shelter admission. Each time, the woman stayed no more than a month and then returned to live with her abusive husband. Once there, she deteriorated psychiatrically, whereupon her husband threw her out of the apartment, and she returned to the streets or to a shelter.

The case manager performed a systems intervention by arranging an appointment with the CMHC psychiatrist. Medications were prescribed, and the woman brought them to the case manager at the shelter, who arranged for her to take them under supervision. About a week later, the case manager consulted me in considerable distress because as far as she could see, the woman was as psychotic as ever, and there had been no apparent reduction in extremely disabling symptomatology. The woman was manic, couldn't sit still, couldn't stop talking, and couldn't focus her attention on anything. She certainly could not engage in a case management plan to find housing.

With guidance from me, the case manager picked her way through this situation. My approach is to assume nothing and question everything. I was puzzled, particularly as a serious attempt had been made to treat the psychiatric illness. I asked the case manager about the medications. How often is she to take them? Once a day. Where are they kept? In the locked closet in the shelter office. Who gives them out? The life coach on duty. Does the woman return to the shelter every night? Yes, she does. Does she go to the office and ask for her medications? The life coach says yes. How do you know? There is a log book where they list the residents who have taken their medications.

So far, so good. What are the medications? I ask. The case manager reads from the chart. Prolixin, Artane, Xanax. Makes sense to me, I think. What is the dosage, particularly of the Prolixin? I'm not sure, she says, 2 or something. You mean, 20 something, I said. No, I'm pretty sure it's 2, she said. Can you bring the bottles here? I ask. She goes out and returns with the medications. I read the label. It says Prolixin, 2.5 mg hs. I am not a medically trained person, but 10 years of working with the severely and persistently mentally ill have taught me some things. Give her aspirin, I say. It will do as much good.

The stone is on its way down the hill. The shelter has a psychiatrist, too. Perhaps she can be seen there. The case manager calls the CMHC. Problems develop later when the CMHC case manager calls to say that the treating psychiatrist does not want the shelter psychiatrist to see the patient or prescribe medications. The stone is at the bottom of the hill and the case manager is underneath it. It seems impossible to achieve the first goal of clinical case management, the reduction of psychiatric symptomatology.

Systems interventions by the clinical case manager are designed to integrate fragmented resource networks and treatment systems. This story also contains a clue to an obstacle to securing an appropriate and stable living situation for this woman. She left the group home each time that she had been there 30 days. A good detective case manager can deduce that she is probably payee for her own benefits check, which may be addressed to her at her husband's apartment. She goes to pick it up and spends it. Or maybe they spend it together: she hangs around, goes off her medications, which she has left at the group home, and the rest we know. A clinical case manager, committed to a coherent and responsible plan for this woman, would work toward securing a representative payee for the benefits. The financial resources would then be secure, the group home could be paid, the woman's need to return to her husband's apartment would be reduced, her medication compliance might improve, and her psychiatric symptomatology could be reduced.

Conclusions

Clinical case management is a clinical intervention that is effective in treating chronically mentally ill individuals in community settings.

With modifications in goals and emphasis, as I have described in this chapter, clinical case management can also provide a coherent framework for engaging homeless mentally ill people and bringing them into psychiatric care and stable living situations. However, a few recommendations and a caveat must be registered here if these approaches are to be useful.

First, this work cannot be done without the psychopharmacological and diagnostic expertise of the psychiatrist. Psychiatrists need to be available wherever we are trying to engage the homeless mentally ill. They must be willing to prescribe and medicate aggressively. Obviously, this approach is not without risk. It also takes time for which there is extremely little financial reward. It is not difficult to understand why physicians want to stay away from this work. However, for those who are willing to make a commitment, the clinical case manager can be a valuable partner in treatment.

Second, clinical case managers who are doing this work should be mental health professionals with expertise in chronic mental illness and its interplay with the special problems of homelessness. Training and good clinical supervision must be available for ongoing learning and support.

Third, systems organization and funding mechanisms must be developed to further integration of services and communications among those who deal with the homeless mentally ill. Some significant initiatives are already under way. For example, Social Security outreach workers have begun visiting homeless shelter sites to assist individuals in applying for benefits and entitlements. Hospitals, emergency rooms, shelters, mobile outreach teams, and agencies must find flexible ways to share information. The clinical case manager, working as a detective, can provide a valuable linking function in fragmented service networks.

I would like to close with a caveat, or perhaps what is actually a recommendation for more clinical explorations. This chapter is based on work with homeless mentally ill individuals whom we find in shelters. Although most of them have spent time on the streets, they tend not to be hard-core urban "street people," those who live on heating grates, under freeways, and in the parks and alleys of our cities. Clinical case management will undoubtedly need further modifications to reach and treat this particular subgroup.

The story of Ms. M represents our modest beginning. She was taken to a shelter by a compassionate and concerned office worker who had attempted to befriend her. Ms. M had lived under a blanket on a busy downtown street corner for 5 years. She said she wanted nothing. Wiser heads prevailed, and she was taken into the emergency psychiatric unit and referred to our agency's crisis house. Since then, she has become eligible for and is receiving benefits and is living comfortably in a group home. She is quiet and not demanding. Her psychiatric symptomatology is alleviated, and she is settled into a reasonable and stable living situation.

References

Belcher J: Defining the service needs of homeless mentally ill persons. Hosp Community Psychiatry 39:1203–1205, 1988

Cohen MB: Social work practice with homeless mentally ill people: engaging the client. Social Work 34:505–508, 1989

Gold Award: a network of services for the homeless chronic mentally ill: Skid Row Mental Health Service, Los Angeles County Department of Mental Health. Hosp Community Psychiatry 37:1148–1151, 1986

Harris M, Bergman HC: Clinical case management for the chronically mentally ill: a conceptual analysis. New Dir Ment Health Serv 40:5–13, 1988

Lamb HR, Lamb DM: Factors contributing to homelessness among the chronically and severely mentally ill. Hosp Community Psychiatry 41:301–305, 1990

Swayze F: I want to go to the circus: personal perspectives on case management. New Dir Ment Health Serv 40:79–86, 1988

Chapter 13

Homelessness and Dual Diagnosis

Kenneth Minkoff, M.D.
Robert E. Drake, M.D., Ph.D.

Psychiatry's awareness of the problem of substance use disorder among people with severe mental illness—often referred to as dual diagnosis—has grown rapidly over the past 10 years. Numerous clinical studies have documented a high prevalence (approximately 50%) of substance abuse or dependence among people who have severe mental illness (Alterman 1985; Drake and Wallach 1989; Pepper et al. 1981; Safer 1987; Schwartz and Goldfinger 1981). The Epidemiologic Catchment Area (ECA) studies also found a marked co-occurrence of severe psychiatric disorders and substance use disorders among people living in the community (Regier et al. 1990).

During the same period, the problem of people who are mentally ill and homeless has also drawn increasing attention (Lamb 1984). Although studies of homelessness have generally avoided the issue of multiple diagnoses (Arce and Vergare 1984), we now recognize that people dually diagnosed with severe mental illness and substance use disorder constitute a particularly vulnerable subset of approximately 10% to 20% of homeless people (Drake et al., in press, b; Tessler and Dennis 1989).

Both the dually diagnosed population and the homeless population are characterized by extreme diversity. The heterogeneity of dual diagnosis includes variations in type and severity of mental illness, type and severity of substance use disorder, phase of treatment, level of severity, extent of disability, and level of motivation for treatment of each disorder (Lehman et al. 1989; Minkoff, in press). The homeless population varies in terms of demographics, pathways to homelessness, presence of mental illness or substance abuse, and length of homelessness.

The heterogeneity of the population with homelessness and dual diagnosis (HDD) is even more complex. Though many homeless people have multiple impairments (Institute of Medicine 1988), individuals with HDD constitute a subgroup defined by three major problems—homelessness, severe psychiatric disorder, and substance use disorder. We will argue here that for this particular subgroup, homelessness operates metaphorically as a third diagnosis; all of the difficulties that attend dual diagnosis are amplified by a third set of complicating factors related to homelessness.

In the 7 years since the publication of the first American Psychiatric Association task force report on the homeless mentally ill (Lamb 1984), our knowledge of dual diagnosis among homeless people has grown considerably. In this chapter, we will review current thinking regarding HDD in several domains: epidemiology, barriers to care, philosophical issues related to treatment, emerging clinical models, phases of treatment, and research issues.

Epidemiology

Approximately one-third of the homeless suffer from severe and disabling mental illnesses (Morrissey and Dennis 1986; Morrisey and Levine 1987; Tessler and Dennis 1989); 30% to 40% have alcohol problems (Fischer and Breakey 1987; Koegel and Burnam 1987; Wright et al. 1987); and 10% to 20% have problems with other drugs (Milburn 1989). Approximately 10% to 20% of the people who are homeless are dually diagnosed with severe mental illness and alcohol and/or other drug problems (Tessler and Dennis 1989), which suggests that 30% to 60% of people who are homeless and mentally ill have coexisting substance abuse or dependence.

In a recent review of research on homelessness, Fischer (1990) identified 10 studies that differentiated between individuals with a single diagnosis of alcohol, drug, or mental health problems and those with dual or multiple diagnoses. The rate of mental disorder plus alcohol use disorder ranged from 3.6% to 26% in seven studies; the rate of mental disorder plus drug use disorder ranged from 1.7% to 2.5% in three studies; and three studies reported a co-occurrence of mental disorders and alcohol and/or drug use disorders ranging from 8% to 31.1%. In a similar review, Tessler and Dennis (1989) reviewed studies of homelessness funded by the National Institute of Mental Health (NIMH). Mental disorder plus substance abuse (alcohol and/or drug use disorder) ranged from 8% to 22% in the five studies that reported comorbidity. In four of the five studies, nearly half of the subjects with mental disorders also had substance use disorders. Even with the lack of standardization in reporting categories, assessment methods, and sampling, both reviews support a 10% to 20% rate of dual diagnosis for the homeless.

Few epidemiologic studies have examined the relationship between dual diagnosis and homelessness. Koegel and Burnam (1988) found that the rate of schizophrenia was nine times as high in homeless alcoholic subjects compared to non-homeless alcoholic subjects in the Los Angeles ECA study. Similarly, bipolar disorder was seven times as prevalent in homeless alcoholic subjects as in non-homeless alcoholic subjects. Koegel and Burnam (1987) also found that a majority of persons with HDD began alcoholic drinking years before they became homeless; for some others, the combination of homelessness and mental illness may have led to substance abuse.

Clinical studies indicate that dually diagnosed patients are strongly predisposed to homelessness because their substance abuse and treatment noncompliance lead to disruptive behaviors, loss of social supports, and housing instability (Belcher 1989; Benda and Dattalo 1988; Drake and Wallach 1989; Drake et al. 1989a, 1989b, 1991). For example, Belcher (1989) found that 36% of mentally ill patients discharged from a state hospital became homeless within 6 months of discharge and that the use of alcohol and other drugs strongly predicted homelessness. Interviews with families and third parties confirm the view that dual diagnosis predisposes individuals to homelessness (Lamb and Lamb 1990).

Not surprisingly, the HDD population has been found to have greater difficulties and to require more services than other subgroups of homeless people (Fischer 1990). They are more likely to be in pain and to exhibit psychological distress and deterioration, to trade sexual favors for food and money, to be estranged from their families, and to become incarcerated (Koegel and Burnam 1987). Fischer and Breakey (1991) found that people with HDD were more likely to experience harsh living conditions, such as living on the streets rather than in shelters. Further, Fischer's review (1990) indicated that people with HDD were more likely to be unemployed or disabled and to have longer periods of homelessness than other subgroups.

Barriers to Care

The high prevalence and increasing visibility of HDD persons, with their extensive service needs, have challenged clinicians, programs, and systems of care. Bachrach (1987) described the dually diagnosed population as "system misfits" who do not readily conform to expected client roles within the addiction system or the mental health system. Homeless people are also excluded from traditional care systems and experience great difficulty in obtaining services (Bachrach 1984). Specific barriers to care for people who are homeless and mentally ill are described in other chapters in this book. We will discuss specific barriers to obtaining care that are related to dual diagnosis, how these difficulties are amplified by homelessness, and possible strategies for developing programs and care systems to serve the HDD population.

Barriers Related to Dual Diagnosis

Barriers to care for dually diagnosed people arise primarily from the separation between the addiction system and the mental health system. Programs designed to treat mentally ill people are not prepared to address coexisting substance abuse; programs designed to treat addiction are not prepared to address mental illness. Dual diagnosis is therefore underdiagnosed in both systems (Helzer and Pryzbeck 1988). Clients with dual disorders who seek services within either system are often denied access or prematurely discharged (Galanter et al. 1988). Moreover, the mental health and substance abuse systems have different, sometimes conflicting philosophies and a history of poor cooperation (Ridgely et al. 1987). The net result is that dually diagnosed people are frequently bounced back and forth between systems and programs that cannot help them effectively.

Intersystem barriers are reinforced at every level of the care system: governmental agencies, funding resources, institutions, programs, and clinicians. On the federal level, the Alcohol, Drug Abuse, and Mental Health Administration (ADAMHA) is organized into three separate institutions (NIMH, the National Institute on Alcohol Abuse and Alcoholism, and the National Institute on Drug Abuse). A similar separation of administrative authority for mental health and substance abuse services exists in 21 of the 55 U.S. states and territories, and few states have a single authority to develop, coordinate, and fund integrated dual-diagnosis services (Ridgely et al. 1990).

Third-party insurance carriers, as well as Medicare and Medicaid, may not reimburse adequately for complicated dual-diagnosis cases, thereby excluding such patients from eligibility for treatment (Ridgely et al. 1990). Similarly, prospective payment systems and diagnosis-related groups (DRGs) encourage shorter hospital stays, which may be less effective for complex cases (Scherl et al. 1988). Determinations of eligibility for disability or hospitalization benefits may also fail to take the severity of comorbidity into account.

Efforts to integrate mental health and substance abuse programs and care systems at state and local levels are further complicated by differences in training and philosophy. For example, addiction clinicians and mental health clinicians often disagree over which diagnosis should be considered primary. They also may disagree about the benefits of psychotropic medications, the roles of various caregivers, the importance of abstinence as a condition of treatment, the usefulness of allowing clients to deteriorate until they are motivated to seek treatment, and the value of confrontational techniques (Ridgely et al. 1986, 1987).

To overcome the barriers just described, several authors (Lehman et al. 1989; Ridgely et al. 1987; Sciacca 1987) recommend the development of dual-diagnosis programs that combine mental health and substance abuse treatments in one setting (often termed integrated, or hybrid, programs) or that provide a high level of coordination between mental health and substance abuse providers in separate systems (termed parallel treatment). Clinical techniques and program models that combine treatments in an integrated or parallel fashion are rapidly developing (Bartels and Thomas, in press; Drake et al., in press, a; Evans and Sullivan 1990; Minkoff 1989; Osher and Kofoed 1989; Ridgely, in press; Ridgely et al. 1987; Sciacca, in press; Teague et al. 1990), and some of them specifically target HDD populations (Kline et al., in press; Pepper and McLaughlin, in press).

Barriers Related to Homelessness and Dual Diagnosis

Problems of combining addiction and mental health treatments are magnified considerably by the addition of the homelessness service system. Instead of one set of intersystem boundary problems, there are now three: homelessness plus mental illness, homelessness plus addiction, and addiction plus mental illness. The homelessness service system consists of those agencies that are specifically concerned with the provision of housing (temporary or permanent) to all homeless individuals and families. On the federal level, this system includes the Department of Housing and Urban Development and other components of Health and Human Services outside ADAMHA; on the state and local level, the homelessness system consists of networks of service providers, missions, outreach agencies, and housing providers, as well as local social service and welfare agencies.

Attempts to provide integrated services or to coordinate parallel services among all three systems can be extraordinarily difficult. HDD individuals encounter more than double jeopardy because the extent of their difficulties makes them easy to exclude (Drake et al., in press, b). For example, housing programs for mentally ill people often exclude substance abusers; those for clients who abuse substances often exclude severely mentally ill persons; and programs for dually diagnosed individuals may exclude people who are homeless. Overcoming these barriers clearly requires an enormous amount of intraservice integration or interservice coordination.

Philosophical Issues

Although a variety of program models have been successful for dually diagnosed patients, the field remains divided by important controversies. Minkoff (in press) has identified several issues related to dual diagnosis that must be addressed in order to incorporate specific program models into a comprehensive and continuous care system. Similar issues are also critical for HDD services.

Primary Versus Secondary Distinction

A frequent tension between the homelessness service system and the addiction and mental health systems involves the prioritization of needs. Advocates for the homeless point out that homelessness is defined by the lack of a home and is neither a mental health nor a social service problem per se (Baxter and Hopper 1984). They argue that the need for housing, therefore, takes precedence over the need for treatment. By contrast, clinicians in the field of mental health and addiction sometimes argue that the provision of housing without provision of treatment is ineffective and even may enable the addictive behaviors to continue. Thus, for example, current housing programs for homeless substance abusers often require abstinence (Argeriou and McCarty 1990).

This tension extends to the issue of permanent versus transitional housing. Some assert that homeless people need stable housing, not crisis or transitional housing (Baxter and Hopper 1984; Blanch and Carling 1988; Carling 1990); others emphasize that transitional housing may facilitate control of symptoms, engagement in treatment, and placement in more permanent housing (Kline et al., in press; National Resource Center 1990).

To the extent that these tensions represent disagreements over clinical effectiveness rather than ideological beliefs, they may be partially resolved by offering a comprehensive, continuous, and integrated care system (Minkoff, in press) and by conceptualizing the provision of basic services as an initial phase in the process of engaging people in treatment (Drake et al., in press, b). In addition, these tensions may be framed as important hypotheses related to the organization, delivery, and financing of limited resources that require careful services research (Drake et al., in press, b).

Care Versus Confrontation

In the community support system model (Stroul 1989), case management emphasizes active outreach and provision of services to psychiatrically disabled individuals according to their needs. If the client refuses help, the case manager attempts to minimize the negative consequences (to the client) of this refusal. Traditional 12-step addiction treatment programs, by contrast, emphasize the client's responsibility and motivation. To achieve sobriety, clients must develop motivation for recovery through being confronted—in a caring way—with the negative consequences of their addiction; help is therefore based on what clients are willing to ask for. If an addicted person refuses help, clinicians are encouraged to detach and to allow the person to bear the responsibility for whatever negative consequences ensue. In other words, mental health treatment stresses the caregiver's responsibility, whereas addiction treatment emphasizes the client's choice.

The homelessness service system overlaps both of the other systems with regard to this issue. On the one hand, advocates for homeless people, like mental health clinicians, emphasize the active provision of basic needs such as those for food, clothing, and shelter (Hopper 1989). On the other hand, like addiction clinicians, homelessness providers emphasize that clients should be engaged in programs according to what they want rather than what professionals want to do for them. Homeless people, even those who are dually diagnosed, often want help with food, clothing, shelter, and money rather than treatment (Drake et al., in press, b; Mulkern and Bradley 1986).

To bring this issue into sharper focus, let us consider the following common clinical situation. A dually diagnosed individual living in a mental health community residence is actively drinking. His behavior when intoxicated is disruptive to the residential program, but he refuses treatment for alcoholism. Repeated efforts to contract for sobriety have been unsuccessful. Should the client be terminated from the residence, even though he would become homeless? Addiction treatment philosophy would tend to say that he should be offered treatment for alcoholism and discharged if he refuses. Discharge to a shelter would be seen as a necessary consequence to stimulate motivation for addiction treatment. Mental health clinicians and homelessness advocates might view the prevention of homelessness as a higher priority and recommend that the client be kept in the residence until hospitalization or another residence could be arranged. Neither approach is always effective.

Pragmatically, a treatment system should balance care, support, and the provision of services with empathic confrontation so that people can take as much responsibility as possible for their own rehabilitation and recovery. Moreover, because people with HDD vary among themselves and over time in their levels of disability, competence, and motivation, the service system should offer a range of programs and interventions that combine care and detachment in differing proportions for different clients.

Abstinence Orientation (Wet, Damp, or Dry?)

A common dilemma in designing inpatient, outpatient, or residential programs for dually diagnosed clients is whether to mandate abstinence as a precondition of treatment or to encourage abstinence as a goal. Although traditional 12-step addiction programs view mandatory abstinence as necessary for credibility and effectiveness, requiring abstinence at the outset often prevents the engagement of dually diagnosed people in treatment (Teague et al. 1990). Consequently, many dual-diagnosis programs offer abstinence as a goal, and clients are encouraged to progress toward that goal gradually, through incremental reduction in the amount and frequency of substance use.

In HDD programs, even setting abstinence as a goal may prevent some people from receiving basic services (Hopper 1989). Shelters that allow drinking within (often termed "wet" shelters) or outside (termed "damp" shelters) may at least provide a modicum of stability so that the process of engagement in treatment can begin (Blankertz and White 1990; Kline et al., in press). Similarly, establishing group homes (Blankertz and White 1990) and single-room-occupancy (SRO) hotels (Coalition of Voluntary Mental Health, Mental Retardation, and Alcoholism Agencies 1989) with minimal demands for abstinence has been proposed. These programs, of course, will be unable to serve clients who require and request a completely abstinent environment in order to initiate or maintain sobriety (Minkoff, in press; Teague et al. 1990).

A continuum of housing in which policy toward abstinence corresponds to the client's stage of treatment may be optimal (Kline et al., in press). Thus, a comprehensive HDD care system might include a combination of "wet," "damp," and "dry" programs, each with clear guidelines that define its respective roles.

Deinstitutionalization Ideology
Versus Rehabilitation Ideology

The treatment of chronically mentally ill people has been dominated for several decades by the ideology of deinstitutionalization (Minkoff 1987), in which success is defined by the reduction in state hospital census and the maintenance of clients in the least restrictive settings in the community. Policies related to this ideology continue to reduce the availability of long-term hospitalization in most states. Meanwhile, critics of deinstitutionalization and those who study homelessness point out that overly optimistic predictions of the clinical benefits of community care have contributed to homelessness by underestimating the needs of many chronically mentally ill persons for long-term care and ongoing structure (Group for the Advancement of Psychiatry 1982; Lamb 1984; Lipton and Sabatini 1984).

In recent years, an ideology that emphasizes rehabilitation and long-term outcome has begun to supplant the ideology of deinstitutionalization (Group for the Advancement of Psychiatry 1992; Harding et al. 1987; Minkoff 1987). The ideology of rehabilitation in mental illness is similar to the ideology of recovery in 12-step addiction treatment (Minkoff 1989). Both emphasize mastery, rather than cure, of chronic illness; both emphasize the long-term goal of maximizing stability and/or sobriety, functional level, and quality of life; and both de-emphasize the locus of care.

Though advocates of deinstitutionalization favor limiting inpatient care, a rehabilitation-oriented approach suggests that long-term outcome rather than short-term avoidance of the hospital should be the primary goal. Certain individuals with HDD may require the judicious use of highly structured treatment and living settings, and may sometimes need lengthy hospitalization, to stabilize both disorders simultaneously (Bachrach 1984; Drake and Adler 1984; Lamb 1984; Lipton and Sabatini 1984). In other words, some clients may require intensive short-term help in highly restrictive settings in order to attain successful long-term outcomes. Research is needed to match clients with settings, approaches, and lengths of treatment. At this point, whether or not lengthy hospitalization can facilitate rehabilitation and improve long-term outcomes remains a question for empirical research.

Integrated Versus Parallel Treatments

Concurrent treatments of substance use disorder and major mental illness can occur in either integrated or parallel programs. Kline and colleagues (in press) analyze the comparative benefits of integrated and parallel approaches to treatment for an HDD population. The benefits of integrated programs include the provision of simultaneous treatment of homelessness, mental illness, and substance abuse under one supervisory umbrella, with a unified case management perspective, by specifically trained clinicians. This model puts the burden of resolving philosophical and other differences on the caregivers rather than on the clients. The major limitation of the integrated treatment model is the difficulty of developing sufficient numbers and variations of hybrid programs to accommodate the size and heterogeneity of the HDD population.

Parallel treatment permits utilization of existing treatment resources (with some modification, consultation, and staff training) in all three care systems, and allows for clients to progress through the care system with more flexibility. Parallel treatment also encourages participation in widely available and free addiction treatment programs (such as Alcoholics Anonymous or Narcotics Anonymous), which are sometimes more acceptable to clients than programs in the mental health system (Minkoff, in press). Significant limitations of parallel treatment are the burden placed on both clients and case managers to maintain continuity and integration through multiple episodes of treatment in diverse programs in distinct systems of care, as well as the difficulty of finding suitable providers for HDD clients.

Minkoff (in press) argues that a comprehensive care system for dually diagnosed clients should include both types of programs. By extension, a comprehensive system for individuals with HDD might balance the development of integrated programs with the pragmatic use of generic shelters, crisis housing services, and other existing programs for homeless mentally ill or homeless substance-abusing people. A prerequisite for the success of integrated and parallel services for homeless dually diagnosed people may be the development of a unified conceptual framework that provides a common language and philosophy for assessment, treatment, and program development.

A Conceptual Framework

Minkoff (1989, in press) describes an integrated conceptual framework for treating co-occurring severe mental illness and substance dependence. His conceptualization includes the following key elements:

1. Both long-term psychotic disorders and substance dependence are viewed as examples of chronic illness with many common characteristics (biologic etiology, heritability, chronicity, incurability, treatability, potential for relapse and deterioration, denial, associated shame and guilt), despite distinctive differences in symptomatology.
2. Both illnesses fit into a disease and rehabilitation model with goals of stabilizing acute symptoms and engaging the client in a long-term program of maintenance, rehabilitation, and recovery.
3. Each disorder is considered primary. People with dual disorders should receive specific treatments for both concurrently.

4. Both disorders have phases of treatment that may be regarded as parallel. Minkoff (1989) identified four phases of treatment: acute stabilization, engagement in treatment, prolonged stabilization/maintenance, and rehabilitation/recovery. Osher and Kofoed (1989) also described four phases of substance abuse treatment for dually diagnosed clients—engagement, persuasion, active treatment, and relapse prevention—that are compatible with Minkoff's formulation.

5. Because progress in rehabilitation depends on the individual's readiness or motivation, which often differs for the two disorders, the pace of treatment for each disorder may vary and be relatively independent. Thus, some clients may be engaged in active treatment to maintain stabilization of psychosis while still refusing treatment for substance abuse; others may be actively sober in addiction treatment yet deny the need for psychotropic medication for mental illness.

This conceptual framework can be extended to clients with HDD by defining homelessness as a third major problem, analogous to another diagnosis in terms of complications and treatment complexity. Though not an illness per se, homelessness is a potentially chronic and deteriorating condition with varying levels of severity and characteristic patterns of disability that must be addressed as a primary problem in its own right (Hopper 1989). The goals of the intervention are 1) to stabilize the acute manifestations of homelessness through the provision of basic necessities such as food, clothing, and shelter, and 2) thereafter to encourage the homeless person to participate in a long-term program to acquire and maintain stable housing arrangements.

Homelessness can also be regarded as having phases of rehabilitation that parallel those of addiction and mental illness: acute stabilization (shelter), engagement, active treatment (crisis housing or short-term hospitalization), prolonged stabilization/maintenance (transitional supported residential program or halfway house), and rehabilitation/recovery (permanent supported residence or independent living). Although progress in the recovery from homelessness is often affected by and interacts with progress in the treatment of coexisting psychiatric and substance use disorders, it may proceed independently, depending on the individual's readiness and motivation for the intervention and the level of disability associated with each condition. Some people with HDD, for example, may proceed from acute stabilization to a stable independent residence with the help of a payee, even while refusing continued treatment of either mental illness or substance abuse. Others with HDD may become sober and/or stabilized on anti-

psychotic medication in a shelter before progressing to more permanent housing. Nonetheless, addressing homelessness through the provision of adequate housing usually facilitates the successful treatment
of coexisting psychiatric and substance use disorders (Kline et al. 1987;
Lipton et al. 1988; Teague et al. 1990; Wittman 1989).

A Model System of Care

Specific programs for HDD should be designed in accordance with the
specific goals of the conceptual framework described above within a
comprehensive care system. The ideal care system would include program elements that meet the needs of clients in each phase of rehabilitation for each disorder, address various levels of severity and
disability in each phase, and correspond to clients' levels of readiness
for treatment of each disorder. An ideal care system would provide for
continuity as well as for comprehensiveness of care through the different phases of treatment (Bachrach 1986). Some HDD programs might
be extensions of existing generic programs within the addiction, mental health, or homelessness service system; others might be integrated
programs that address two or three major problems simultaneously
(Minkoff, in press). The ideal care system would necessarily include
intensive case management, phase-specific treatments, and collaboration with families (Drake et al., in press, a).

Intensive, Integrated Case Management

People with HDD typically experience multiple crises and episodes of
acute stabilization in different care systems before they engage in treatment, achieve stability, and pursue rehabilitation and recovery. Intensive case management can promote this process. In the intensive case
management model, teams of clinicians with small caseloads engage
clients through assertive crisis intervention, outreach, and practical assistance and support them through the phases of rehabilitation for
each disorder (Drake et al., in press, a). Because dually diagnosed clients are difficult to engage regardless of their housing status, many
programs, such as the New Hampshire continuous treatment team
model, regard intensive case management as the central treatment vehicle (Drake et al. 1990b). Clients with HDD typically require even
greater intensity of effort by case managers during the engagement
process (Kline et al., in press).

Models of intensive case management for people with dual disorders emphasize the importance of integrating or linking the addiction
and the mental health treatments. Although some dual-diagnosis case

management programs are created entirely within the mental health system (Harris and Bergman 1987), most such programs arise through statewide collaborations between mental health and substance abuse authorities (Drake et al. 1990b; Illinois Department of Mental Health and Developmental Disabilities 1990; Teague et al. 1990).

Phase-Specific Treatment

Appropriate programs for HDD should vary according to the phase of treatment of each disorder. An ideal care system would include programs to address each phase of each disorder.

Acute stabilization of psychiatric disorders frequently occurs in an acute psychiatric inpatient unit and sometimes in outpatient or day hospital settings. To treat people with coexisting substance use disorders, the psychiatric inpatient unit must have the capacity to provide detoxification, to identify substance abuse and dependence, to initiate engagement and education regarding substance abuse, and to link clients to programs in the community that can continue the process of engagement and stabilization for both substance use disorders and psychiatric disorders (Minkoff, in press).

Within the addiction system, acute stabilization is usually provided in detoxification programs. Generic detoxification programs are potentially appropriate for dually diagnosed clients who are not psychotic, those whose psychotic symptoms are stabilized by medications, and those who are not disruptive and threatening. Such programs must be able to provide maintenance (nonaddictive) medications, protocols for assessment of coexisting psychiatric disorders, availability of psychiatric consultation, and appropriate referral linkages for both disorders (Minkoff, in press). Specialized detoxification programs have been developed in some settings for clients who have behavioral disorders or are self-destructive when they are intoxicated.

For homeless individuals, shelters and drop-in centers are the most common settings for acute stabilization of homelessness. For those with HDD, hospitals and detoxification centers may also serve this function. Because dually diagnosed people who are homeless tend to be more difficult to engage in treatment than those who are domiciled, extended outreach efforts—in shelters or on the streets—are often necessary prior to hospitalization or detoxification. Although shelters may provide an opportunity for stabilization, screening, and assessment, they often fail to offer the basic security and supports that would facilitate engagement (Dockett 1989; Drake et al., in press, b; Martin 1989). Although some people with HDD will accept psychotropic medications and become more stable while residing in the shelter, many others require a more protected setting; and those with the most severe psychiatric disabilities may need involuntary commitment and/or extended hospitalization.

Engagement in treatment among people with HDD can occur in a variety of programs. A setting that provides acute stabilization of the most pressing problem often serves as the entry point. Because people with HDD typically are not ready for treatment of all three problems simultaneously, engagement occurs sequentially and incrementally. Maximizing opportunities in a care system for a person to receive treatment for any one problem will therefore increase the likelihood that engagement and stabilization related to concurrent problems will eventually take place.

Engagement in HDD treatment (voluntarily or involuntarily) often begins in an acute psychiatric inpatient unit. Following acute stabilization of psychotic symptoms and possibly detoxification, clients receive education regarding mental illness and are discharged to outpatient and/or residential programs. The most severely disabled individuals may require prolonged hospitalization before they are able to engage in outpatient treatment (Group for the Advancement of Psychiatry 1982; Lamb 1984). Because psychiatric units often fail to address substance abuse, integrated addiction and mental health units are a critical resource, particularly if severe mental illness precludes an individual's access to programs in the addiction system (Minkoff 1989). These integrated units can also address diagnostic dilemmas (Lehman et al. 1989). When integrated programs are not available, concurrent parallel treatment in collaborative units can also work (Ridgely et al. 1990).

Even when integrated inpatient programs are available, dually diagnosed clients often are not ready to address their substance use disorders during the index hospitalization. Therefore, they must be referred to outpatient and residential programs in the mental health system, and these programs must engage them in substance abuse treatment as well as in mental health treatment. Several such models have been described (Bartels and Thomas, in press; Hellerstein and Meehan 1987; Kofoed and Keys 1988; Kofoed et al. 1986; Osher and Kofoed 1989; Sciacca, in press) and in NIMH-sponsored reviews and demonstration projects (Bartels and Thomas, in press; Drake et al. 1990b, in press, a; National Institute of Mental Health 1989; Ridgely et al. 1987, in press; Teague et al. 1990), including some that specifically addressed HDD clients (Kline et al., in press). These programs include several common features:

- Abstinence is initially a goal, not a requirement.
- Clients with substance abuse and dependence problems are treated together.

- Peer-oriented group models, ranging from purely educational groups to interactive, behavioral, and skill-building groups, are fundamental.
- Clients learn to develop substitute activities and relationships to reinforce an abstinent lifestyle.
- Clients whose substance dependence is disruptive in outpatient mental health settings may be referred for formal addiction treatment in more controlled settings.
- Families are involved whenever possible.

People with HDD often enter programs such as these through the homelessness service system. They may be engaged while in shelters, drop-in centers, day programs, soup kitchens, or other gathering places for people who are homeless, rather than in hospitals, through intensive case management or other outreach programs (Harris and Bergman 1987). Examples of well-described programs include the Salvation Army Clitheroe Center Shelter in Anchorage, Alaska (Dexter 1990), the Phoenix Club Drop-In Center in Somerville, Massachusetts (Wittman and Madden 1988), and Community Connections, Inc., in Washington, DC (Kline et al. in press).

To engage clients in addressing homelessness, inpatient hospitalization (or, less commonly, stabilization in a community-based case management program) may stabilize both substance abuse and mental illness sufficiently to permit a transition to permanent housing. However, many people with HDD are unable or unwilling to adhere initially to the level of expectations regarding either structure or control of substance use that is required for participation in some housing programs. Premature placements not only fail to prevent relapse into homelessness or institutionalization but also reinforce the person's sense of demoralization.

An ideal housing system would be maximally flexible during this phase of treatment (Drake et al., in press, b; Kline et al., in press). Engagement in housing may be more likely to take place in residences that have a high tolerance for both substance abuse and psychotic behavior. "Wet" or "damp" housing programs, though controversial, may reduce the morbidity of continued homelessness and permit further engagement, stabilization of mental illness and addiction, and transition to permanent housing (Blankertz and White 1990; Coalition of Voluntary Mental Health, Mental Retardation and Alcoholism Agencies 1989; Hopper 1989).

Finally, a significant portion of people with HDD will engage in treatment through the addiction system during the rehabilitation phase of inpatient treatment for substance dependence. Programs that mandate commitment to abstinence as a condition of participation are often suitable for clients who are stabilized on medications without severe residual psychiatric disability. To accommodate dually diagnosed clients, addiction programs often need to expand their psychopharmacologic and psychodiagnostic capabilities through consultation and training. Some clients with HDD can make the transition into halfway houses in the addiction system, and subsequently into independent living, particularly if intensive case management is available to help maintain linkages with mental health treatment services.

Ongoing stabilization and rehabilitation for people with HDD may occur in a range of outpatient, day treatment, and residential settings. The most severely ill and least compliant clients may require long-term residential treatment and self-contained day programming, sometimes in mental hospitals; those with illnesses of moderate severity typically may live successfully in supervised residences or in the care of family members and participate in ongoing day programming; and those with the least severe illnesses often live independently and participate in outpatient treatments (Minkoff, in press).

Ongoing stabilization and rehabilitation of clients with HDD may require an integrated continuum of residential services, some based in the addiction system and some in the mental health system. For example, extended support to maintain sobriety is available within the addiction system in most states through a network of halfway houses (stays of 3 to 12 months), therapeutic communities (stays of 12 to 24 months), and sober houses (long-term stays), all of which mandate abstinence (Minkoff, in press). These settings are appropriate for motivated clients who are otherwise capable of independent living, use reasonable social skills, and have stable psychiatric disorders. Dually diagnosed clients must be permitted to self-administer stable regimens of nonaddictive psychotropic medications (Minkoff, in press) and must be linked to both outpatient psychiatric and addiction treatments.

For people with more severe psychiatric disabilities, halfway houses in the mental health system can be modified by adding substance abuse treatment programs either within the residence or as part of affiliated day programs. Residential dual-diagnosis programs are less tolerant of substance use on premises than are so-called wet residences, but often they do not require total abstinence. Clients with HDD living in crisis housing or in residences with low expectations might graduate to such dual-diagnosis residential programs once their psychiatric disorders are stable and they have agreed to limit substance use and follow program rules.

Each program must define the level of substance-related problem behavior that it cannot tolerate (e.g., obvious intoxication, belligerence, selling or using drugs on premises, etc.) and develop a clear set of policies that determine the behavioral consequences for violations (Sciacca, in press). These limits are not punitive but rather provide protection from drugs and alcohol, safety for other program participants, and leverage to encourage offending clients to accept more intensive addiction treatment. Consequences are valid only if they can be enforced, and provision must be made in the care system for clients who are suspended or discharged due to persistent problematic substance use. Although "wet" crisis housing is available in some locations (Blankertz and White 1990), in most systems state hospitals may need to be available for severely psychiatrically disabled, actively addicted, and unmotivated clients who otherwise might become homeless.

For dually diagnosed clients who are psychiatrically disabled but committed to abstinence, residences that provide integrated psychiatric care and addiction treatment in a substance-free environment are essential. Transitional living communities (Hannigan and White 1990) have been developed in New York City by integrating addiction treatment into psychiatric halfway houses. Another New York City residential program for HDD has been developed by integrating psychiatric treatment into an addiction therapeutic community (Pepper and McLaughlin, in press). Community Connections, in Washington, DC, uses highly supervised apartments staffed by housing personnel with addiction treatment backgrounds who keep drug dealers out (Kline et al., in press). New Hampshire has instituted a series of long-term psychiatric residences that facilitate integrated treatment during a transition from residential care to day programming and then to treatment in the community (Bartels and Thomas, in press).

Ultimately, many clients with HDD can make the transition to independent living arrangements by relying on outpatient psychiatric and addiction services. Active treatment as well as relapse prevention can be effective as long as the individual's living setting provides safety and relative freedom from the constant drug purveyance and usage that affect some neighborhoods (Teague et al. 1990). For clients with HDD to live in areas that are strongly affected by alcohol and other drug use, it may be necessary to provide active protection (Drake et al., in press, b).

Given an appropriate independent living situation, clients can participate in integrated outpatient programs in either the mental health or the substance abuse system. For example, in New Hampshire's mental health system, dually diagnosed clients move from persuasion groups (for those who have not yet acknowledged a substance abuse problem) to active treatment groups (for those who are learning skills to control or eliminate substance use) and finally to relapse prevention groups, for those who have achieved abstinence (Drake et al., in press, a; Noordsy and Fox, in press). In addition, 12-step programs in the addiction system, particularly those such as "double trouble" groups that are designed for people with dual diagnoses, may be appropriate for active treatment or relapse prevention (Kofoed et al. 1986; Ridgely et al. 1987). Clients with HDD may need special preparation to select suitable groups and to learn how to use them (Kline et al. in press; Minkoff 1989, in press; Ridgley et al. 1987).

Family Involvement

Families of homeless people, including those with HDD, are often overlooked. Families frequently do not have the supports or skills necessary to deal with either severe mental illness or addiction, and the excessive family burden that attends dual disorders may precipitate homelessness (Lamb and Lamb 1990). Research in New Hampshire indicates that the majority of clients with HDD maintain regular contacts with their families and that the families provide a great deal of support, treatment, and financial assistance (Clark et al., unpublished data, 1991). Clinical programs often have the explicit goal of engaging families as collaborators in the treatment process (Drake et al., in press, a; Kline et al., in press). Sciacca (in press) has developed a staff-supported, peer-oriented support and recovery program for families of mentally ill chemical-abusing (MICA) clients called MICA-Non. Early intervention with families who are caring for their dually diagnosed relatives, especially efforts to help families set limits and use respite housing and hospitalizations rather than extrude their relatives, may actually prevent homelessness in this population.

Current Research Issues

Drake and colleagues (in press, b) have identified several research issues related to HDD that require further study. For example, reliable and valid assessments of the dually diagnosed homeless population are critical, yet standardized instruments have not been validated in this population (Lovell and Shern 1990). Research should examine the assessment of severe mental illness (Susser and Struening 1990), substance abuse (Drake et al. 1990a), and other key dimensions of attitudes, behavior, and environments. One key variable to assess is living preference—the client's attitudes toward comparative living environments (Drake and Wallach 1979, 1988, in press). Validity can then be increased by aggregating observations over time and situation, by collecting information from collaterals, and by modifying standard instruments so that they assess behaviors that are relevant for this population (Drake et al., 1990a).

In some areas, qualitative approaches may be appropriate. Koegel (in press) argues persuasively for ethnographic research—longitudinal studies to assess the homeless person's behaviors, attitudes, and beliefs in the homeless living situation. For example, intensive participant observation with a few homeless individuals over time might counterbalance current reliance on cross-sectional self-report data and allow us to learn more about how homeless people actually survive and make decisions regarding living situations, treatment participation, and substance abuse. Schwab and colleagues (Schwab 1990; Schwab et al., in press), for example, used participant observation to clarify the significance of lost children in the lives of many people with HDD.

Numerous coping efforts, support systems, and societal protections must fail before people become homeless. Dual diagnosis interacts in a complex way in this longitudinal process (Benda and Datallo 1988; Lamb and Lamb 1990). However, few longitudinal data regarding HDD are available. High-risk populations such as people with dual disorders should be followed longitudinally to clarify patterns of homelessness as well as the risk factors and protective factors that are associated with developing and recovering from homeless episodes. Complex sociocultural processes like homelessness may be more amenable to intervention at early stages. For example, working closely with families, delaying discharges, or providing specific types of housing for people with dual disorders may be more effective than trying to engage these individuals on the streets. Those on the streets should not be ignored, but strategies for preventing homelessness may be more clinically effective and cost-effective and should be explored vigorously.

Current studies of services for homeless dually diagnosed people focus on models of integrating alcohol, drug, and mental health treatments with models of providing temporary and permanent housing (National Institute of Mental Health 1989, 1990; Teague et al. 1990). Critical issues include which type of service models to offer, when and how to link clients to these services, and how the services themselves should be integrated. Housing is critical but difficult to study (Goldman and Newman 1990; Wittman 1989). Research is needed in several areas: the usefulness of transitional versus permanent housing, group versus independent settings, and congregate versus scattered site alternatives; when and how to institute "wet," "damp," and "dry" housing; and how to use Section 8 vouchers most effectively. Current ideologies and hypotheses should be tested with designs that are scientifically rigorous and sensitive to costs.

Nearly all dual-diagnosis programs and homelessness programs recommend intensive case management, yet few studies address how case management should be organized, staffed, and performed. Many current models prescribe cross-training of clinicians and integrated treatment (Drake et al., in press, a). Researchers are currently investigating the role of nonprofessionals who share some key background experiences with the clients (National Institute of Mental Health 1990).

Conclusions

People with HDD have three complicated sets of problems that require a continuous and comprehensive care system—one that integrates or coordinates interventions in the mental health system, the addiction system, and the homelessness service system. Psychiatric disorders, addictive disorders, and homelessness should each be regarded as primary, but interactive, problems. Specific program models should address the many combinations of severity, disability, phase of treatment, and readiness for treatment that are related to each condition. The unified conceptual framework for people with HDD presented here emphasizes a broad continuity of services in all care systems— ranging from "wet" housing to long-term, hospital-based, dual-diagnosis programs—to enable clinicians and program planners to understand the role of current programs and to develop needed programs to fill gaps. Services research related to these hypotheses, theoretical concepts, and programmatic elements is of critical importance.

References

Alterman AI: Substance abuse in psychiatric patients, in Substance Abuse and Psychopathology. Edited by Alterman AL. New York, Plenum, 1985

Arce AA, Vergare MJ: Identifying and characterizing the mentally ill among the homeless, in The Homeless Mentally Ill: A Task Force Report of the American Psychiatric Association. Edited by Lamb HR. Washington, DC, American Psychiatric Association, 1984

Argeriou M, McCarty D: Treating alcoholism and drug abuse among homeless men and women: nine community demonstration grants. Alcoholism Treatment Quarterly 7:1–164, 1990

Bachrach LL: The homeless mentally ill and mental health services: an analytical review of the literature, in The Homeless Mentally Ill: A Task Force Report of the American Psychiatric Association. Edited by Lamb HR. Washington, DC, American Psychiatric Association, 1984

Bachrach LL: The challenge of service planning for chronic mental patients. Community Ment Health J 22:170–174, 1986

Bachrach LL: The context of care for the chronic mental patient with substance abuse. Psychiatr Q 58:3–14, 1987

Bartels SJ, Thomas W: Lessons from a pilot treatment program for people with dual diagnosis of severe mental illness and substance use disorder. Psychosocial Rehabilitation Journal (in press)

Baxter E, Hopper K: Shelter and housing for the homeless mentally ill, in The Homeless Mentally Ill: A Task Force Report of the American Psychiatric Association. Edited by Lamb HR. Washington, DC, American Psychiatric Press, 1984

Belcher JR: On becoming homeless: a study of chronically mentally ill persons. Journal of Community Psychology 17:173–185, 1989

Benda BB, Dattalo P: Homelessness: consequence of a crisis or a long-term process? Hosp Community Psychiatry 39:884–886, 1988

Blanch AK, Carling PJ: Normal housing with specialized supports: a psychiatric rehabilitation approach to living in the community. Rehabilitation Psychology 33:47–55, 1988

Blankertz L, White KK: Implementation of rehabilitation program for dually diagnosed homeless. Alcoholism Treatment Quarterly 7:149–164, 1990

Carling PJ: Major mental illness, housing, and supports: the promise of community integration. Am Psychol 45:969–975, 1990

Coalition of Voluntary Mental Health, Mental Retardation and Alcoholism Agencies: Low demand residence discussion paper. New York, Coalition of Voluntary Mental Health, Mental Retardation and Alcoholism Agencies, 1989

Dexter RA: Treating homeless and mentally ill substance abusers in Alaska. Alcoholism Treatment Quarterly 7:25–30, 1990

Dockett KH: Street homeless people in the District of Columbia: characteristics and service needs. Washington, DC, Agriculture Experimental Station, 1989

Drake RE, Adler DA: Shelter is not enough: clinical work with the homeless mentally ill, in The Homeless Mentally Ill: A Task Force Report of the American Psychiatric Association. Washington, DC, American Psychiatric Association, 1984

Drake RE, Wallach MA: Will mental patients stay in the community? A social psychological perspective. J Consult Clin Psychol 47:285–294, 1979

Drake RE, Wallach MA: Mental patients' attitudes toward hospitalization: a neglected aspect of hospital tenure. Am J Psychiatry 145:29–34, 1988

Drake RE, Wallach MA: Substance abuse among the chronic mentally ill. Hosp Community Psychiatry 40:1041–1046, 1989

Drake RE, Wallach MA: Patients who are attracted to the mental hospital: correlates of living preference. Community Mental Health Journal (in press)

Drake RE, Osher FC, Wallach MA: Alcohol use and abuse in schizophrenia: a prospective community study. J Nerv Ment Dis 177:408–414, 1989a

Drake RE, Wallach MA, Hoffman JS: Housing instability and homelessness among aftercare patients of an urban state hospital. Hosp Community Psychiatry 40:46–51, 1989b

Drake RE, Osher FC, Noordsy DL, et al: Diagnosis of alcohol use disorders in schizophrenia. Schizophr Bull 16:57–67, 1990a

Drake RE, Teague GB, Warren RS: New Hampshire's dual–diagnosis program for people with severe mental illness and substance use disorders. Addiction Recovery 10:35–39, 1990b

Drake RE, Wallach MA, Teague GB, et al: Housing instability and homelessness among rural schizophrenic patients. Am J Psychiatry 148:330–336, 1991

Drake RE, Antosca L, Noordsy DL, et al: Specialized services for the dually diagnosed, in Dual Diagnosis of Major Mental Illness and Substance Use Disorder. Edited by Minkoff K, Drake RE. San Francisco, CA, Jossey-Bass (in press, a)

Drake RE, Osher FC, Wallach MA: Homelessness and dual diagnosis. Am Psychol (in press, b)

Evans K, Sullivan JM: Dual Diagnosis: Counseling the Mentally Ill Substance Abuser. New York, Guilford, 1990

Fischer PJ: Alcohol and Drug Abuse and Mental Health Problems Among Homeless Persons: A Review of the Literature, 1980–1990. Rockville, MD, National Institute of Alcohol Abuse and Alcoholism and National Institute of Mental Health, 1990

Fischer PJ, Breakey WJ: Profile of the Baltimore homeless with alcohol problems. Alcohol Health Research World 11:36–37, 1987

Fischer PJ, Breakey WJ: Correlates of homelessness in a Baltimore dual diagnosed population. Paper presented at the annual meeting of the American Psychiatric Association, New Orleans, LA, May 1991

Galanter M, Castaneda R, Ferman J: Substance abuse among general psychiatric patients: place of presentation, diagnosis, and treatment. Am J Drug Alcohol Abuse 14:211–235, 1988

Group for the Advancement of Psychiatry: The Positive Aspects of Long-Term Treatment in the State Mental Hospital. New York, Brunner/Mazel, 1982

Group for the Advancement of Psychiatry: Beyond Symptom Suppression: Improving Long-Term Outcomes of Schizophrenia (GAP Report No 134). Washington, DC, American Psychiatric Press, 1992

Goldman HH, Newman S: Financing and reimbursement issues, in Homelessness and Mental Illness: Toward the Next Generation of Research Studies. Edited by Morrisey JP, Dennis DL. Washington, DC, U.S. Department of Health and Human Services, 1990, pp 95–104

Hannigan T, White A: Housing hard-to-place mentally ill women—350 Lafayette Transitional Living Community. Status report of programs of Columbia University Services. New York, Columbia University, 1990

Harding CM, Brooks GW, Ashikaga T, et al: The Vermont longitudinal study of persons with severe mental illness, II: long-term outcome of subjects who retrospectively met DSM-III criteria for schizophrenia. Am J Psychiatry 144:727–735, 1987

Harris M, Bergman H: Case management with the chronically mentally ill: a clinical perspective. Am J Orthopsychiatry 57:296–302, 1987

Hellerstein DJ, Meehan B: Outpatient group therapy for schizophrenic substance abusers. Am J Psychiatry 144:1337–1339, 1987

Helzer JD, Pryzbeck TR: The co-occurrence of alcoholism with other psychiatric disorders in the general population and its impact on treatment. J Stud Alcohol 49:219–224, 1988

Hopper K: Deviance and dwelling space: Notes on the resettlement of homeless persons with alcohol and drug problems. Contemporary Drug Problems 16:391–414, 1989

Illinois Department of Mental Health and Developmental Disabilities: Task Force Report for the Mentally Ill Substance Abuser. Springfield, IL, Illinois Department of Mental Health and Developmental Disabilities, 1990

Institute of Medicine: Homelessness, Health, and Human Needs. Washington, DC, National Academy Press, 1988

Kline MV, Bacon J, Chinkin M, et al: The client tracking system: a tool for studying the homeless. Alcohol Health Research World 11:66–67, 1987

Kline J, Bebout R, Harris M, et al: Models of treatment for dually diagnosed homeless adults, in Dual Diagnosis of Major Mental Illness and Substance Use Disorder. Edited by Minkoff K, Drake RE. San Francisco, CA, Jossey-Bass (in press)

Koegel P: Understanding homelessness: an ethnographic approach, in Homelessness: A Prevention-Oriented Approach. Edited by Jahiel R. Baltimore, MD, Johns Hopkins University Press (in press)

Koegel P, Burnam MA: The Epidemiology of Alcohol Abuse and Dependence Among the Homeless: Findings From the Inner City of Los Angeles. Rockville, MD, National Institute of Alcohol Abuse and Alcoholism, 1987

Koegel P, Burnam MA: Alcoholism among homeless adults in the inner city of Los Angeles. Arch Gen Psychiatry 45:1011–1018, 1988

Kofoed L, Keys A: Using group therapy to persuade dual-diagnosis patients to seek treatment. Hosp Community Psychiatry 39:209–1211, 1988

Kofoed L, Kania I, Walsh T, et al: Outpatient treatment of patients with substance abuse and co-existing psychiatric disorders. Am J Psychiatry 143:867–872, 1986

Lamb HR (ed): The Homeless Mentally Ill: A Task Force Report of the American Psychiatric Association. Washington, DC, American Psychiatric Association, 1984

Lamb HR, Lamb DM: Factors contributing to homelessness among the chronically and severely mentally ill. Hosp Community Psychiatry 41:301–305, 1990

Lehman AF, Myers P, Corty E: Assessment and classification of patients with psychiatric and substance abuse syndromes. Hosp Community Psychiatry 40:1019–1025, 1989

Lipton FR, Sabatini A: Constructing support systems for homeless chronic patients, in The Homeless Mentally Ill. Edited by Lamb HR. Washington, DC, American Psychiatric Association, 1984

Lipton FR, Nutt S, Sabatini A: Housing the homeless mentally ill: a longitudinal study of a treatment approach. Hosp Community Psychiatry 39:40–45, 1988

Lovell A, Shern D: Assessing mental health status among adults who are homeless, in Homelessness and Mental Illness: Toward the Next Generation of Research Studies. Edited by Morrisey JP, Dennis DL. Washington, DC, U.S. Department of Health and Human Services, 1990, pp 69–77

Martin MA: Report to the New York City Transit Authority, 1989

Milburn N: Drug abuse among the homeless, in Homeless in the United States, Vol 2. Edited by Momeni J. Westport, CT, Greenwood Press, 1989

Minkoff K: Beyond deinstitutionalization: a new ideology for the postinstitutional era. Hosp Community Psychiatry 38:945–950, 1987

Minkoff K: An integrated treatment model for dual diagnosis of psychosis and addiction. Hosp Community Psychiatry 40:1031–1036, 1989

Minkoff K: Components of a comprehensive integrated care system for mentally ill patients with substance disorders, in Dual Diagnosis of Major Mental Illness and Substance Use Disorder. Edited by Minkoff K, Drake RE. San Francisco, CA, Jossey-Bass (in press)

Morrissey JP, Dennis DL: NIMH-Funded Research Concerning Homeless Mentally Ill Persons: Implications for Policy and Practice. Washington, DC, U.S. Department of Health and Human Services 1986

Morrisey JP, Levine IS: Researchers discuss latest findings, examine needs of homeless mentally ill persons. Hosp Community Psychiatry 38:811–812, 1987

Mulkern V, Bradley VJ: Service utilization and service preferences of homeless persons. Psychosocial Rehabilitation Journal 10:23–29, 1986

National Institute of Mental Health: Currently Funded Research Grants on Services on Persons With Mental Disorders That Co-occur With Alcohol and/or Drug Abuse Disorders. Rockville, MD, Biometric and Clinical Applications Branch, Division of Biometry and Applied Sciences, National Institute of Mental Health, 1989

National Institute of Mental Health: Mental Health Services Research. Rockville, MD, Division of Applied and Services Research, National Institute of Mental Health, 1990

National Resource Center on Homelessness and Mental Illness: Working With Dually Diagnosed Homeless Persons: An Overview. Delmar, NY, Policy Research Associates 1990

Noordsy DL, Fox L: Group intervention techniques for people with dual disorders. Psychosocial Rehabilitation Journal (in press)

Osher FC, Kofoed LL: Treatment of patients with psychiatric and psychoactive substance abuse disorders. Hosp Community Psychiatry 40:1025–1030, 1989

Pepper B, McLaughlin P: Modifying the therapeutic community for the mentally ill substance abuser, in Dual Diagnosis of Major Mental Illness and Substance Use Disorder. Edited by Minkoff K, Drake RE. San Francisco, CA, Jossey-Bass (in press)

Pepper B, Kirshner MC, Ryglewicz H: The young adult chronic patient: overview of a population. Hosp Community Psychiatry 32:463–469, 1981

Regier DA, Farmer ME, Rae DS, et al: Comorbidity of mental disorders with alcohol and other drug abuse. JAMA 264:2511–2518, 1990

Ridgely MS: Creating integrated programs for severely mentally ill persons with substance disorders, in Dual Diagnosis of Major Mental Illness and Substance Use Disorder. Edited by Minkoff K, Drake RE. San Francisco, CA, Jossey-Bass (in press)

Ridgely MS, Goldman HH, Talbott JA: Chronic Mentally Ill Young Adults With Substance Abuse Problems: A Review of the Literature and Creation of a Research Agenda. Baltimore, MD, Mental Health Policy Studies, University of Maryland School of Medicine, 1986

Ridgely MS, Osher FC, Talbott JA: Chronic Mentally Ill Young Adults With Substance Abuse Problems: Treatment and Training Issues. Rockville, MD, Alcohol, Drug Abuse, and Mental Health Administration, 1987

Ridgely MS, Goldman HH, Willenbring M: Barriers to the care of persons with dual diagnoses: organizational and financing issues. Schizophr Bull 16:123–132, 1990

Safer DJ: Substance abuse by young adult chronic patients. Hosp Community Psychiatry 38:511–514, 1987

Scherl DJ, English JT, Sharfstein SS (eds): Prospective Payment and Psychiatric Care. Washington, DC, American Psychiatric Association, 1988

Schwab B: An ethnographic approach to evaluating case management. Paper presented at the First Annual Case Management Conference, Cincinnati, OH, September 14, 1990

Schwab B, Clark RE, Drake RE: An ethnographic note on clients as parents. Psychosocial Rehabilitation Journal (in press)

Schwartz SR, Goldfinger SM: The new chronic patient: clinical characteristics of an emerging subgroup. Hosp Community Psychiatry 32:470–474, 1981

Sciacca K: New initiatives in the treatment of the chronic patient with alcohol/substance use problems. T.I.E.-Lines 4:3, 1987

Sciacca K: An integrated treatment approach for severely mentally ill individuals with substance dependence, in Dual Diagnosis of Major Mental Illness and Substance Use Disorder. Edited by Minkoff K, Drake RE. San Francisco, CA, Jossey-Bass (in press)

Stroul BA: Community support systems for persons with long-term mental illness: a conceptual framework. Psychosocial Rehabilitation Journal 12:9–26, 1989

Susser ES, Struening EL: Diagnosis and screening for psychotic disorders in a study of the homeless. Schizophr Bull 16:133–145, 1990

Teague GB, Schwab B, Drake RE: Evaluation of Services for Young Adults With Severe Mental Illness and Substance Use Disorders. Arlington, VA, National Association of State Mental Health Program Directors, 1990

Tessler RC, Dennis DL: A Synthesis of NIMH-Funded Research Concerning Persons Who Are Homeless and Mentally Ill. Rockville, MD, NIMH Division of Education and Service System Liaison, 1989

Wittman FD: Housing models for alcohol programs serving homeless people. Contemporary Drug Problems 16:483–504, 1989

Wittman F, Madden P: Alcohol Recovery Programs for Homeless People. Rockville, MD, National Institute for Alcohol Abuse and Alcoholism, 1988

Wright JD, Knight JW, Weber-Burdin E, et al: Ailments and alcohol: health status among the drinking homeless. Alcohol Health Research World 11:22–27, 1987

Chapter 14

Medical Concerns of Homeless Persons

Philip W. Brickner, M.D.

The homeless bear the largest burden of untreated illness in the United States. Although the diversity of this population is well recognized, certain generalizations can be allowed.

Homeless persons live in poverty, and thus can be understood as a segment of the poor in our country. Arguably, the health care of the poor and of the homeless are the same subject, and in considering such matters as health insurance for these populations, grouping them together is a useful approach. In regard to clinical disorders, however, as I shall discuss below, the homeless suffer to an extraordinary degree beyond others who are impoverished. They are at risk. On the streets, in shelters, there is danger; and danger can be random, as a news item from *The New York Times* (1989) revealed.

WILD PAVING ROLLER CRUSHES SLEEPING MAN IN NEW JERSEY
    Bordentown Township, N.J., Sept 13 (AP) — A homeless man was reported in critical condition today after a paving roller ran over him while he was sleeping.
    The victim, 44 years old, was at the Cooper Medical Center in Camden with a crushed chest, internal injuries, broken legs and a broken hip, the police said.
    The accident occurred about 3:20 A.M. Tuesday at a truck stop near Exit 7 on the New Jersey Turnpike. Authorities are searching for the person who started the paving roller, which moved across a parking lot into a wooded area where [he] was sleeping.
    "All we know is that somebody started the machine and let it go," a police dispatcher said.

The homeless are also courageous. Without courage, in these situations, survival is unlikely: and a sense of humor helps, as illustrated by the story of RR, a 48-year-old alcoholic African American man with a past history of schizophrenia.

> RR lived in a room at the Keller Hotel in Manhattan, where a Health Care for the Homeless Program team met him. This grim single-room-occupancy (SRO) hotel is dirty and foreboding. Its stairwells are intermittently lit by 20-watt bulbs. The residents tend to remain locked in their 8- by-11-foot rooms, afraid of drug-addicted predators. The manager observes the entrance from behind wire, protected by two German shepherds.
>
> RR, in contrast, managed to obtain some white paint and redecorated his room. He found a scrap of rug for the floor. He kept an Alaskan husky, impeccably groomed and well trained, as a pet and for protection. He had crocheted a motto which he had framed and hung on the wall. It read "Cubicle Sweet Cubicle."

By generalizing about homeless persons, clinicians run the risk of stereotyping. It is essential, however, if services for the homeless are to prove workable, that each person be recognized, appreciated, and valued as an individual human being. If homeless persons are not regarded as individuals, they will respond with alienation, anger, and suspicion and will not develop the confidence essential for health care to take place.

Outreach

The broad experience of programs that provide health care for the homeless over the last decade shows that bringing teams of physicians, nurses, and social workers into the places that homeless persons congregate can be effective in bridging mistrust (Breakey et al. 1989; Brickner et al. 1986, Gelberg and Linn 1989; Reuler 1989). Establishment of clinics at shelters, in church basements, and at food lines and drop-in centers is workable; sending homeless persons to busy emergency rooms or hospital outpatient departments fails.

However, merely setting up an examining room at the shelter is not sufficient. Outreach is required. Reaching out to the homeless with the purpose of encouraging them to attend the shelter clinic engages staff members in what is largely a new discipline but one that incorporates tasks and qualities familiar to health workers; educating patients one to one, reassuring them, empathizing with them, keeping promises, and fulfilling expectations. Regarding the outreach team, the psychiatrist Barry Blackwell and colleagues (1990) point out that its members are chosen for attributes that lessen social distance from clients, and they use strategies of relationship building and power sharing designed to create trust. Team members function as case finders, case managers, and advocates, dealing with multiple problems, meeting basic needs, and providing linkages between the clients and disparate parts of the human resource system. (p. 190)

Formerly homeless men and women have proven to be effective outreach workers. They often can engender trust with far more validity than the professional staff.

In addition to employing outreach staff, these clinic settings require the following:

- Physicians, nurses and social workers, present on a consistent basis, able to offer continuity of care in an honest, nonjudgmental manner, with sensitivity training for staff;
- A hospital prepared to back up the program with a full range of services, including inpatient beds, emergency room, subspecialty clinics, laboratory, X-ray facilities, and pharmacy;
- Care given regardless of ability to pay; and
- Availability of transportation for accessing services.

Attention to these points is especially indicated for the homeless, a population characterized by high indices of mental illness and extraordinary need for reassurance. The consequences of the deinstitutionalization movement are considered elsewhere (Chapter 2), but the absence of asylum for homeless persons, and the protection, nourishment, and shelter that the word asylum implies, is a devastating indictment of the ideologues who pursued the goal of deinstitutionalization without following through to assure development of alternative, concrete services. They made an unholy alliance with government officials, who abandoned these disabled persons to the streets. The fate of Ella Hartley, reported by *The New York Times*, illustrates this tragedy.

WOMAN IN RULING ON MENTALLY ILL DROWNS
Huntington, W. Va., Nov. 30 (AP) — A woman whose court case gave West Virginia's psychiatric patients freedom to live with as few restrictions as possible drowned after wandering off during a visit to a doctor, the authorities say.

Ella Hartley, 53 years old, died on Tuesday. She was last seen alive at a boat dock on the Ohio River where she told bystanders she was going for a swim, said Capt. Paul Price.

The court decision resulted from a lawsuit filed on Ms. Hartley's behalf by the Appalachian Research and Defense Fund, a public advocacy group. The suit sought more freedom for mentally ill people able to care for themselves.

In what became known as the Hartley decision, the Kanawha County Circuit Court ruled in 1982 that mentally ill people should be kept in "the least restrictive environment possible."

After the decision, the mental patient population at Huntington State Hospital fell from 1,500 to 90.

State health officials refused to discuss Ms. Hartley's case.

Clinical Concerns

The clinical disorders of homeless persons are those of all human beings. The factors that distinguish the health status of the homeless from those who are housed, and magnify their risks, are in large part external: exposure to extremes of heat and cold, dampness, burns, crowding in shelters, assault, vehicular accidents, and unremitting anxiety about where to find the next meal and a safe place to lie down. In part, the medical problems of homeless persons are the consequences of alcoholism, substance abuse, and mental illness.

The several characteristic conditions discussed here represent the panoply of disease that afflicts these persons. Many of the data derive from the national Health Care for the Homeless Program sponsored by the Robert Wood Johnson Foundation and Pew Charitable Trusts, a 19-city project spanning the years 1984 through 1989, and from other service efforts, some spanning several decades (Bassuk 1984; Breakey et al 1989: Lamm and Reyes 1985: Lindsey 1989; Neibacher 1990; Ropers et al. 1985; Somers et al. 1990; Wright 1990; Wright and Weber 1987: Wright et al. 1987; Wytham Hall 1989). In all, information about more than 200,000 individuals and family members seen at shelter clinics is available.

Transmissible Conditions: Infections and Infestations

For those living in shelters, or for families crowded into small hotel rooms, the spread of viral and bacterial respiratory diseases, scabies, and lice is routine. Beyond the fact that such conditions are transmitted through close personal contact, infectibility of homeless persons is enhanced by the likelihood of poor underlying health status, malnourishment, and the detrimental effects of depression and anxiety. The impact on homeless children is perhaps most striking. In 1988 the health status of 101 children placed with mother and siblings in two New York City SRO hotels was compared with that of 72 children living in the same neighborhood in public housing. Over a 6-month period, rates of otitis and sinusitis were more than 30% higher among the children living in the hotel. Their rates of gastroenteritis were more than 100% higher and of skin infections more than 300% higher (Lee et al. 1990).

There is a striking parallel between the situation in large congregate shelters in our major cities today and the condition of slaves in the South before the Civil War.

> The state of slave health depended not only on disease immunities and susceptibilities but also on living and working conditions.
>
> Most slaves on plantations or farms lived in a well-defined area known as the quarters. Here was a setting ideal for the spread of disease. At the slave quarters, sneezing, coughing, or contact with improperly washed eating utensils and personal belongings promoted transmission of disease-causing microorganisms among family members. Poor ventilation, lack of sufficient windows for sunshine, and damp earthen floors added to the problem by aiding the growth of fungus and bacteria on food, clothing, floors, and utensils, and the development of worm and insect larvae. (Savitt 1988, p. 133)

Trauma

A life on the streets is not safe, and the risks in large congregate shelters are not appreciably less. Homeless persons are subject to danger from vehicular accidents, from burns resulting from fires set in dangerous circumstances in an attempt to stay warm, and from assault. In the inner city, any individual perceived as weak is at risk of attack; thus, the elderly homeless and women and children are in double jeopardy. James Wright analyzed the presenting complaint of 63,079 adults seen in 17 cities supported by Johnson-Pew grants in 1985–1987. Trauma was the reason for seeking help in 25% of cases. Lacerations and wounds were noted more frequently, followed by sprains, bruises, and fractures (Wright and Weber 1987).

The impact of trauma is well shown by a specific example.

> A 46-year-old homeless male diabetic suffered multiple rib fractures when a garbage truck emptied into its compactor the dumpster in which he was asleep. A 35-year-old homeless female alcoholic sustained a skull fracture when she was beaten and raped by four men in a deserted building where she was sleeping. (Kelly 1985, p. 87)

Peripheral Vascular Disease

Homeless persons often cannot lie down at night. Local housing regulations bar drop-in centers from installing cots, and those seeking shelter sit on chairs until dawn. Others remain on park benches because they fear indoor shelters. Many feel that safety requires walking all night long, or standing, rather than sleeping and becoming a victim while lying helpless. As a consequence, fluids pool in the lower legs, by force of gravity. In time, edema compresses the microcirculation of the skin. Inflammation and cellulitis ensue, leading to overt infection, skin breakdown, and ulceration.

Treatment of this problem in homeless persons is challenging, as the following example demonstrates.

> A shelter staff member observed a homeless woman with hugely swollen legs swathed in dirty bandages. On examination, the woman's skin was found to be inflamed and her feet swollen. The worker urged and pleaded with the woman to go to the local hospital emergency room (ER) for treatment. She finally agreed, took the bus token that was offered, and in due time arrived at the ER. There she waited 5 hours to be seen because, in fairness, she was not truly an emergency case. When at last she was examined by a physician, she was told to go home, elevate her legs for a week, and have somebody help her soak them in wet, warm dressings for several hours each day. He gave her a prescription for an antibiotic and made an appointment for her to return to the clinic in a week.

What is the reality of this case? The woman has no home, no bed to lie in for a week, no way to soak her legs, nobody to help her do so, no money with which to purchase the antibiotic, and no assured way to return to the clinic. It is likely that by the time she managed to return to the shelter she would have missed the lineup for the evening meal and a cot for the night. Such instances demonstrate the need for development of shelter-based clinics and respite care areas (Goetcheus and Gleason 1990).

The Health of Homeless Children

About 15% of homeless persons are children (Wright and Weber 1987), defined as newborns through age 18. These years are a vast span of time, encompassing the physical and emotional developments characteristic of both early and adolescent life.

Most of the younger children in shelters and hotels are identified as family members. Usually, the word family means a woman (often pregnant) with one or more children. Young children living in these environments are in danger. In addition to experiencing marked increases in rates of respiratory illness compared to housed children, they suffer from high indices of failure to thrive, physical injury, abuse, chronic diseases such as iron deficiency anemia and asthma, congenital disorders, and inadequacy of immunizations. They are at risk from predators in their buildings, as well.

The older children often play the role of adult, creating a hazardous ambiguity in which neither child nor adult has full responsibility or authority. The case of CW, a 15-year-old girl with a 3-month-old infant, is a good example.

> CW has been homeless since she left her mother's house after an argument shortly after the baby's birth. She was placed in a shelter for teenagers with children after spending 2 weeks on the streets. On initial admission examination at the shelter the infant, JW, was noted to have thrush and monilial diaper rash. He also failed to gain weight.
>
> CW was instructed to give medications every 8 hours and to feed JW at least 3 ounces every 8 hours with ready-to-feed formula. She was also instructed to keep a record of his feeding and medication times. When seen for follow-up 3 days later, JW showed no improvement. On further investigation, it was found that CW was too embarrassed to acknowledge that she could not tell time or count (Lee et al. 1990).

Tuberculosis

Human beings faced with poverty, overcrowding, minority status, alcohol abuse, and poor nutrition have long been understood to be at increased risk of developing pulmonary tuberculosis (TB) (Abeles and Feibes 1970; Barry et al 1986: Friedman et al. 1987; LaForce et al. 1973; Patel 1985; Stead et al. 1990; Teller 1988; "Tuberculosis in minorities" 1987; Wehrle and Top 1981). These factors aptly depict the status of many homeless persons, and perhaps it should not be surprising that the incidence of TB is high in this population. TB is, in fact, so strikingly prevalent among the homeless that it has influenced significantly the trend for the United States population as a whole.

The incidence of TB declined progressively each year from 1900 through 1984, and in 1985 the United States Centers for Disease Control announced that our country was nearing its goal of reducing the incidence to eight new cases of TB per 100,000 population (MMWR 1985). In that year, however, the almost century-long favorable trend reversed, and in 1989 new cases reached the level of 9.46 per 100,000 ("Summary of notifiable disease, 1989" 1990c). This phenomenon is particularly striking in New York City. In 1989, the total number of cases was 2,545, whereas in the first 10 months of 1990 more than 3,000 had already been diagnosed ("Cases of specified notifiable diseases, 46th week" 1990a).

A continuing 10-year study of men seen at a clinic in a large New York City shelter has shown that 42.8% had a positive skin test, indicating they were infected with TB, and that 6% had active disease (McAdam et al. 1990a). The study revealed that increasing age of the men and African American or Hispanic minority status were independent risk factors for development of tuberculous infection or disease. Especially striking was that length of time in the shelter was positively associated with both infection and disease, and that those who were intravenous drug users (IVDUs) had a risk of active disease more than three times that of non-IVDUs.

This last point has led to the recognition that TB, intravenous drug use, and human immunodeficiency virus (HIV) are inextricably related. The most recent findings of the study suggest strongly that almost every person with active TB tested positive for HIV (McAdam et al. 1990a; Torres et al. 1990).

The situation is similar in other cities in which homeless persons live closely together in dormitories. Small outbreaks of active TB have been identified in Seattle and Boston shelters, in the latter instance leading to grave concern that antibiotic-resistant bacteria would seriously compromise the success of TB treatment. In these instances, aggressive action by local public health authorities and shelter staff to identify cases through screening, and to place patients under treatment promptly, halted the epidemics (L. L. Scharer, unpublished data, 1991; see also McAdam et al. 1990b; Nardell et al. 1986).

HIV Disease

HIV infection among the homeless in the United States is difficult to quantify or characterize, largely because this transient population lacks adequate access to standard health care. The fear and fatalism commonly associated with HIV disease and AIDS, in combination with the alienation of many homeless persons, also contribute to statistical uncertainty. However, staff members who work with the homeless in larger cities note a growing numbers of patients with the infection. Transmission through sexual activity and sharing of needles and syringes ("the works") certainly takes place in shelters, and for IVDUs it is feasible to make an educated guess about the numbers infected.

For instance, through the investigative work of Don Des Jarlais, it is known that about 60% of IVDUs in New York City are HIV positive (Des Jarlais et al. 1989; Spira et al. 1984). Data derived from the national Health Care for the Homeless Program show that about 13% of homeless men use heroin or cocaine or both (Wright and Weber 1987). A reasonable estimate is that about 7,800 of the 60,000 homeless men in New York are HIV positive.

The nature of HIV disease in the homeless is perhaps better illustrated by the following case history, obtained by James Kennedy, medical director of Covenant House of New York, an organization that offers shelter and services for runaway youths (Kennedy et al. 1990).

Madeline arrived at Covenant House in November 1987 following the death of her mother from a crack-induced stroke. Her father had been in jail for the last 2 years. She did not complete the 8th grade because of a pregnancy and marijuana use. She had never had a job. She used crack daily for 8 months before coming to Covenant House. Her first child has AIDS and is still in a hospital: her second pregnancy ended with a miscarriage in the fourth month. She had had a total of three male sex partners. The father of her first child was neither an intravenous drug addict nor gay. He did have two other girlfriends who were intravenous drug addicts. The father of her second child (and this pregnancy) denied IV drug use and homosexuality, but he was raped at the age of 8 (with anal penetration) by a male baby sitter.

She's been arrested and is on probation for "child abandonment." She told the nurse who interviewed her that "She felt good about herself," and was looking forward to being an executive secretary. . . . She and her boyfriend tested HIV antibody positive. She lost custody of the baby when it tested positive for cocaine. The baby stayed in the hospital when it tested positive for HIV antibody, and she was discharged to the street where she lived until 1989 when she again presented to the shelter . . . pregnant for the fourth time. She had made three firm decisions: she would stop using crack, she would have an abortion, and she would not tell her current boyfriend she was infected by the AIDS virus. She stuck to all three. Her two surviving children have AIDS and remain in the custody of child welfare agencies.

Conclusion

The health concerns of many homeless persons can be resolved by improving their access to help. It is an elementary point that for care to be given staff and patients must meet. Many of the homeless do not seek care at the establishment. Barriers of poverty, anger, fear, confusion, and depression exist. For some, treatment of disease is a lower priority than obtaining food, a bed for the night, or substances of abuse. Lack of funds for transportation to a clinic or hospital is also a concern; and, in frankness, many health care institutions do not welcome the homeless.

Yet it is in everybody's interest that effective health care for homeless persons be arranged. The care of patients with diabetes mellitus is illustrative. Diabetes exists in 5% of the United States population but is of substantially higher prevalence in African Americans and Hispanics ("Regional variation in diabetes mellitus prevalence, United States,

1988 and 1989" 1990), minorities overrepresented among the homeless. Diabetes is properly treated by a medical diet and the use of oral hypoglycemics or insulin injections.

In reality, however, no medical diet is available in shelters, and if pills are required, money for their purchase is unlikely to be at hand (Martinez-Weber 1987). Insulin, to maintain potency, must be stored safely and at a steady temperature. Syringes and alcohol swabs to cleanse the injection site must be purchased, but in the homeless person's unsafe environment they are subject to theft for their street value. Even if homeless diabetics escape early death from hyperglycemia and diabetic coma, they risk the long-term vascular effects of coronary artery disease, stroke, chronic renal disease or blindness, leaving them helpless and expensive wards of the state.

There is a better way. If we intend to give effective health care to the homeless we must go where they are: food lines and soup kitchens, drop-in centers, SRO hotels, shelters, the parks, river banks, under viaducts, and on the streets. We must reach out to them and wherever feasible give direct, hands-on primary care services on the spot. Many programs that provide health care for the homeless have worked out systems to obtain benefits for the homeless, provide proper food, purchase and store medications safely, and give basic health education.

Perhaps the most significant lesson learned through these programs is that for the effort to be effective, staff members must feel genuine respect for their patients, keep promises, be present consistently at the site of care, and work persistently to build trust, motivation, and self-esteem among the homeless.

References

Abeles H, Feibes B: The large city prison: a reservoir of tuberculosis. Am Rev Respir Dis 101:706–709, 1970

Barry MA, Wall R, Shirley L, et al: Tuberculosis screening in Boston's homeless shelters. Public Health Rep 101:487–494, 1986

Bassuk E: The homeless problem. Sci Am 215:40–45, 1984

Blackwell B, Breakey W, Hammersley D, et al: Psychiatric and mental health services, in Under the Safety Net: The Health and Social Welfare of the Homeless in the United States. Edited by Brickner PW, Scharer LK, Conanan BA, et al. New York, WW Norton, 1990, pp 184–203

Breakey WR, Fischer PJ, Kramer M, et al: Health and mental health problems of homeless men and women in Baltimore. JAMA 262: 1352–1357, 1989

Brickner PW, Scanlan BC, Conanan B, et al: Homeless persons and health care. Ann Intern Med 104:405–409, 1986

Cases of specified notifiable diseases, 46th week. MMWR 39:837, 1990

Des Jarlais DC, Friedman SR, Novick DM, et al: HIV-1 infection among intravenous drug users in Manhattan, New York City, from 1977 through 1987. JAMA 261:1008–1012, 1989

Friedman LN, Sullivan GM, Bevilaqua RP, et al: Tuberculosis screening in alcoholics and drug addicts. Am Rev Respir Dis 136:1188–1192, 1987

Gelberg L, Linn LS: Assessing the physical health of homeless adults. JAMA 262:1973–1979, 1989

Goetcheus J, Gleason MA, Sarson D, et al: Convalescence: for those without a home, in Under the Safety Net: The Health and Social Welfare of the Homeless in the United States. Edited by Brickner PW, Scharer LK, Conanan BA, et al. New York, WW Norton, 1990, pp 169–183

Kelly JT: Trauma: with the example of San Francisco's shelter program, in Health Care of Homeless People. Edited by Brickner PW, Scharer LK, Conanan B, et al. New York, Springer, 1985, pp 77–91

Kennedy JT, Petrone J, Deisher RW, et al: Health care for familyless, runaway street kids, in Under the Safety Net: The Health and Social Welfare of the Homeless in the United States. Edited by Brickner PW, Scharer LK, Conanan BA, et al. New York, WW Norton, 1990, pp 82–117

LaForce FM, Huber GL, Fahey JM: The focality of urban tuberculosis. Am Rev Respir Dis 108:553–558, 1973

Lamm D, Reyes L (eds): Health Care for the Homeless: A 40-City Review. Washington, DC, United States Conference of Mayors, 1985

Lee MA, Haught K, Redlener I, et al: Health care for children in homeless families, in Under the Safety Net: The Health and Social Welfare of the Homeless in the United States. Edited by Brickner PW, Scharer LK, Conanan BA, et al. New York, WW Norton, 1990, pp 119–138

Lindsey AM: Health care for the homeless. Nurs Outlook 37:78–81, 1989

Martinez-Weber C: The homeless person with diabetes: a diagnostic and therapeutic challenge. Postgrad Med 81:289–298, 1987

McAdam JM, Brickner PW, Scharer LL, et al: The spectrum of tuberculosis in a New York City men's shelter clinic (1982–1988). Chest 97:798–805, 1990a

McAdam JM, Brickner PW, Scharer LL, et al: Tuberculosis in the homeless: a national perspective, in Under the Safety Net: The Health and Social Welfare of the Homeless in the United States. Edited by Brickner PW, Scharer LK, Conanan BA, et al. New York, WW Norton, 1990b, pp 234–249

Nardell E, McInnis B, Thomas B, et al: Exogenous reinfection with tuberculosis in a shelter for the homeless. N Engl J Med 315:1570–1575, 1986

Neibacher S: A public–private partnership in health care for the homeless, in Under the Safety Net: The Health and Social Welfare of the Homeless in the United States. Edited by Brickner PW, Scharer LK, Conanan BA, et al. New York, WW Norton, 1990, pp 340–353

Patel KR: Pulmonary tuberculosis in residents of lodging houses, night shelters, and common hostels in Glasgow: a five-year prospective survey. Br J Dis Chest 79:60–66, 1985

Regional variation in diabetes mellitus prevalence, United States, 1988 and 1989. MMWR 39:806–812, 1990

Reuler JB: Health care for the homeless in a national health program. Am J Public Health 79:1033–1035, 1989

Ropers R, Robertson M, Boyer R: The Homeless of Los Angeles County: An Empirical Evaluation (Basic Research Project, Document No 4). Los Angeles, CA, University of California at Los Angeles, 1985

Savitt TL: Slave health, in Disease and Distinctiveness in the American South. Edited by Savitt TL, Young JH. Knoxville, TN, University of Tennessee Press, 1988

Somers S, Rimel R, Shmavonian N, et al: Creation and evolution of a national health care for the homeless program, in Under the Safety Net: The Health and Social Welfare of the Homeless in the United States. Edited by Brickner PW, Scharer LK, Conanan BA, et al. New York, WW Norton, 1990, pp 56–66

Spira TJ, Des Jarlais DC, Marmor M, et al: Prevalence of antibody to lymphadenopathy-associated virus among drug-detoxification patients in New York (letter). N Engl J Med 311:467–468, 1984

Stead WW, Senner JW, Reddick WT, et al: Racial differences in susceptibility to infection by Mycobacterium tuberculosis. N Engl J Med 322:422–427, 1990

Summary of notifiable disease, 1989. MMWR 38:54, 1990c

Teller ME: The Tuberculosis Movement. New York, Greenwood Press, 1988, pp 101–102

Torres RA, Mani S, Altholz J, et al: Human immunodeficiency virus infection among homeless men in a New York City shelter. Arch Intern Med 150:2030–2036, 1990

Tuberculosis in minorities. MMWR 36:77–80, 1987

Wehrle PF, Top Sr FH (eds) Communicable and Infectious Diseases. St. Louis, MO, CV Mosby, 1981, p 671

Wild paving roller crushes sleeping man in New Jersey. New York Times, September 13, 1989

Woman in ruling on mentally ill drowns. New York Times, November 30, 1990, p A12

Wright JD: The health of homeless people: evidence from the national health care for the homeless program, in Under the Safety Net: The Health and Social Welfare of the Homeless in the United States. Edited by Brickner PW, Scharer LK, Conanan BA, et al. New York, WW Norton, 1990, pp 15–31

Wright JD, Weber E: Homelessness and Health. Washington, DC, McGraw-Hill, 1987

Wright JD, Rossi PH, Knight JW, et al: Homelessness and health: effects of lifestyle on physical well-being among homeless people in New York City, in Research in Social Problems and Public Policy, Vol 4. Edited by Lewis M, Miller J. Greenwich, CT, JAI Press, 1987

Wytham Hall: Annual Report, 1989 (117 Sutherland Avenue, Maida Vale, London W9 2QJ, England)

Chapter 15

Day Treatment in a Shelter: A Setting for Assessment and Treatment

Frederic I. Kass, M.D.
David A. Kahn, M.D.
Alan Felix, M.D.

Assessment, treatment, and formulation of a sound plan for residential placement should be performed in a setting that the patient already perceives as helpful and noncoercive. The on-site day treatment program is an ideal vehicle for this purpose. A number of authors have described related impressions. Gounis and Susser (1990) elaborate on the importance of understanding how men enrolled in a shelter's day treatment program perceive their own needs and the difficulties of applying traditional treatment goals in this population. Morrissey and colleagues (1986) emphasize that recruiting homeless men to a shelter with comprehensive, on-site mental health services requires that professionals accept a "reinterpretation" of traditional resources, such as acknowledging the patient's view that a mental health clinic may have greater significance as a source of subway tokens than as a treatment program.

Preliminary evidence suggests that on-site mental health services in residences or shelters have positive impacts. Lipton and colleagues (1988) found that homeless mentally ill men placed in a residence with integrated treatment services similar to those found in a day program fared better on a variety of outcome measures than control subjects placed in residences without such services. Caton and colleagues (1990) found that after completing our own program, men were able to live more successfully in community housing, utilized mental health aftercare, and engaged in less criminal behavior.

What is novel in all of these programs, reversing traditional models, is the extent to which full evaluation and treatment sometimes fol-

The authors thank Karen Ferrara, M.A., for her comments.

low—by weeks or months—initial engagement of patients. At our day treatment program, our approach is to create a flexible, individualized environment in which both evaluation and engagement are continuing processes that may alternate as the chief focus of care.

The purpose of this chapter is twofold. First, we will describe how the program, actually located in a shelter, facilitates the engagement, assessment, treatment, and placement in appropriate residential settings of homeless mentally ill persons. We then discuss in some detail the crucial task of comprehensive psychiatric assessment, which must precede individualized and rational planning.

Initial Contact: Referral and Outreach

The day treatment program at Columbia Presbyterian Medical Center (Caton et al. 1990) is located in a large armory that serves as a nightly shelter for up to 850 men. The program area comprises several secure rooms that are well separated from the large, open floor where the men sleep. Sixty to 70 men are enrolled at any time, for an average stay of 6 months. To summarize the demographic characteristics of the men, the median age is 32, 94% are single, 87% are unemployed, 78% are minority (African American or Hispanic), 63% are high school graduates, 19% are military veterans, and 44% have been in prison. Eighty percent have had at least one prior psychiatric hospitalization, primarily for a psychotic disorder, and 63% meet criteria for substance abuse.

We try to enroll every man who is referred or asks for help; given estimates that about 25% of shelter residents have mental illness (Susser et al. 1989), it is clear that we reach only a minority of those in need. All shelter residents are seen by case workers to assist with concrete needs. The case workers may refer patients to the program, but because they are not trained in mental health, they may miss individuals who do not display overtly bizarre behavior. Men who desire help and have heard of the program may also refer themselves. A further source of referrals is the psychiatric emergency room of Presbyterian Hospital, located across the street from the shelter. Men from the shelter may present themselves there or be brought by the shelter staff. The emergency room, in effect, serves as a safety net for those initially not identified by shelter case workers.

It has become clear to us, however, that many men either are never referred to our program or do not follow through. Thus we have developed outreach methods, similar to those described by others (Cohen et al. 1984). Nonuniformed, streetwise security guards from the program receive on-site training in outreach techniques. They share ethnic, linguistic, and socioeconomic backgrounds with many of the homeless men, factors that create rapport and make them effective outreach workers. Case workers and psychiatrists, together with the guards, have formed two outreach teams, one based in the shelter and the other on the street. The two teams collaborate and share some staff in order to provide continuity of care to the sometimes overlapping clientele and to facilitate the goal of relocating the men from the street to the shelter and then to a community residence.

The teams seek out men who were referred for treatment and did not show up, or who appear obviously disturbed by virtue of bizarre behavior or self-neglect. This task may also be undertaken by higher-functioning patients in the program, who are often our most effective outreach workers. These shelter residents are often better able than professional staff to reach out to their mentally disturbed peers, gain their trust, and recruit them into the program.

Engagement

Initial engagement is accomplished by meeting the men on their own terms and addressing what they perceive as their most pressing needs. The program literally offers a safe haven from the violence of the shelter and initially emphasizes concrete needs such as food and clothing. During their first visit to the program, prior to formal enrollment, men enter a low demand prescreening phase of 1 to 2 weeks, although for those men who are well-motivated we proceed with active treatment planning. For others, the only expectation is daily attendance. In exchange, we offer services and comfort, including cigarettes and coffee for those who attend the morning community meeting.

We ask questions only to learn what each man wants, such as help obtaining benefits or housing. Many of the men fear involuntary treatment. We will offer medication to a man who is obviously psychotic but do not force it or make it a condition for participation in the program. On the contrary, we appear as advocates for empowerment (e.g., by emphasizing rights to refuse treatment).

During the prescreening period, each of the eight or so staff members of the shelter program interacts informally with the prospective patient. This interaction facilitates an unobtrusive first assessment of social skills and psychopathology. Decisions to offer enrollment are made by consensus at a weekly staff meeting. Only men with severe antisocial behavior that would endanger other program members are excluded. Each newly accepted man is congratulated by the staff and offered the option to enroll. A staff member is then assigned as case manager, although all staff will continue to work actively with the patient to allow the patient to form numerous independent relationships.

Assessment

Underlying Philosophy

Although the homeless mentally ill share many clinical characteristics, they do not form a monolithic group. Individuals vary widely in terms of specific biological, psychological, and social strengths and weaknesses. The goal of comprehensive psychiatric assessment is to identify the characteristics of an individual that may serve as a foundation for focused treatment planning. The assessment techniques described in this chapter were developed in the day treatment program we operate for residents of a large men's shelter. The shelter has been described in detail elsewhere (Caton et al. 1990). Assessment also occurs on the street and in the emergency room, but we will not discuss those locations here. Mobile outreach work on streets and in other public places is covered in Chapter 10.

As a preamble to our discussion of assessment, we first want to emphasize our overall philosophy in working with this population. We agree with a now widely recognized view, articulated by Susser and colleagues (1990), among others, that by and large, traditional outpatient techniques of intake evaluation such as scheduling office visits and obtaining complete histories in the first few interviews are not useful. Instead, the pace of evaluation must move slowly and piecemeal, often over months, beginning with informal and unconventional contacts.

MacKinnon and Yudofsky (1986) have pointed out that all psychiatric assessments have two components that are at once interdependent yet conflicting: developing an open, empathic relationship that will form the basis for treatment and obtaining the information needed to formulate a diagnosis and treatment plan. The conflict arises even in the most highly functional patients because of natural mechanisms of resistance against revealing oneself to a stranger until trust has developed. Balancing the tasks of developing trust and gathering accurate information about history and symptoms, thus, is a core skill for the clinician. Nowhere is this skill more demanded than in work with the homeless mentally ill, where both trust and information are hard to come by.

Clinical Assessments

Specialized clinical assessments are performed by a psychiatrist, internist, social worker, nurse, vocational and recreational counselors, and nonprofessionals who work as case managers and administrators. Although preliminary evaluations are completed within a few weeks of official enrollment, it is not unusual for the staff to require months to complete their detective work, particularly fully eliciting delusions, understanding substance abuse patterns, corroborating past history, and reaching family members.

We document all assessments in a standard medical chart utilizing forms that meet requirements of the mental health agencies that routinely audit the program us for quality assurance. We attempt to complete a basic assessment within a few weeks of enrolling a new patient, knowing that it may take months to flesh out a skeletal initial understanding.

The psychiatrist seeks standard historical and mental status information to make a DSM-III-R multiaxial diagnosis (American Psychiatric Association 1987). Interview techniques are often modified to accommodate our patients' fear of coercion. The psychiatrist states that a reason for the interviews is to gain information in order eventually to obtain housing for the individual; the emphasis is not necessarily on treatment. Although most of the men are able to sit for one or two hour-long interviews, some can be seen for no more than a few minutes at a time. The psychiatrist continually reassures the client that he will not be subjected to forced hospitalization or medication. Empathy, sympathy, encouragement, humor, and informality are essential tools.

The social worker attempts to locate cooperative family members to provide further history. We always seek access to clients' prior hospital records, as well as other possible sources of information, such as outpatient medical contacts, the Department of Veterans Affairs, and parole officers. With diligence, family members or prior records or both are located for the majority of men. They are extremely useful for corroboration of clinical impressions.

Substance abuse history is obtained by the nurse and psychiatrist. Many men openly describe their drug use; toxicology is occasionally screened when specifically indicated for diagnostic purposes. Much later in treatment, routine toxicology is obtained as a housing requirement. The nurse also evaluates hygiene, dental condition, and general health knowledge and attitudes especially about risks of human immunodeficiency virus (HIV).

With men who have a history of chronic psychosis, we often feel unable to make a specific diagnosis. For example, it is difficult to diagnose schizophrenia subtypes or to distinguish between bipolar and schizoaffective disorders or among schizotypal personality, dysthymic disorder, and residual schizophrenia in this population. The difficulties arise from many factors: the frequency of drug-induced psychosis; the men's reluctance to report all symptoms and their inability to articulate symptoms; and the inadequate sources of past history. Based on their collaboration with diagnostic research teams (Caton et al. 1988), our clinicians know that subtle or extremely paranoid delusions may be concealed from researchers only to be revealed very slowly to program staff members.

Furthermore, some individuals have been exposed to extreme trauma as children, such as witnessing the murder of one parent by the other. The emotional blunting and suspiciousness they demonstrate may meet criteria for schizophrenia although, we feel, the disorder is not truly present. Depressive disorders are difficult to distinguish from demoralization or apathy, and we prescribe antidepressants cautiously. Mood symptoms may fluctuate with prospects for housing. Withdrawal may dramatically improve with involvement in the treatment program. The presence of cognitive impairment, which appears commonly, raises questions of mental retardation, organic illness, or severe cultural deprivation.

Each patient receives a medical assessment consisting of a physical examination, ECG, blood work, chest X ray, tuberculin test by purified protein derivative (PPD), and optional HIV test (chosen by 25%). The assessment is performed by a moonlighting resident from the department of medicine at our hospital. The residents are self-selected for this job and are well motivated. Although one might expect to encounter many medical problems that could alter mental status, we have not found this to be the case on routine evaluations. The most common problems are mild anemia, inactive tuberculosis, early syphilis, gonorrhea, lice, venous stasis, and cellulitis.

We do not have systematic data on the prevalence of HIV infection in our program but so far are aware of only a few known cases of active disease. Because medical illness and substance abuse are covered in other chapters of this book, we will not address them further here.

Together, the social worker and case manager begin to assess the social resources that may be available to the homeless individual. They assist the men to obtain appropriate entitlements and make every effort to find family and friends (and are successful with surprising frequency). Occasionally, family and friends serve as an eventual source of housing, but of equal importance, they may help counter feelings of demoralization and rejection that perpetuate homelessness. Reawakened ties to family and community may be a decisive factor in persuading the homeless individual to agree to drug counseling or psychiatric treatment.

We conduct several assessments pertaining to social skills in addition to the informal evaluations made by all staff members. Vocational personnel initially evaluate work and school backgrounds; schooling in our patients ranges from seventh grade through college. Basic work skills, such as ability to concentrate, read, do math, follow a schedule, and perform simple errands, are examined. Arrangements for literacy or high school equivalency classes are made when appropriate. Prevocational and rehabilitative services are offered, including several shelter-run work programs such as a can recycling business. A recreational assessment evaluates ability to participate in activities ranging from simple checker games to more complex group activities, such as drama and creative arts workshops, community meetings, and housing or job planning groups. The activities provide role modeling and positive reinforcement for improved emotional expression, social and communication skills, and daily living skills such as money management and hygiene.

We must emphasize the tentative nature of the conclusions of the initial assessment, especially conclusions regarding prognosis. Grunberg and Eagle (1990) have hypothesized that the desperate circumstances of prolonged shelter life leads to "shelterization," a syndrome characterized by decreased interpersonal responsiveness, neglect of personal hygiene, increased passivity, and increased dependency on others. For some individuals, these behaviors may be an adaptive way to foster feelings of mastery. Individuals may even develop bizarre, psychotic-like behavior as a conscious mechanism to ensure safety. Such shelter-acquired behaviors may mimic aspects of mental illness, such as the negative symptom cluster of schizophrenia (Kay et al. 1987).

Therefore, we regard with caution many of the initial assessments we make, as we see each man during a particularly difficult time in his life. A phenomenological assessment alone is not an adequate guide to prognosis, if the phenomena are the result of residing in a shelter.

Neuropsychiatric Assessment

Some of our patients appear to the clinical staff to be cognitively impaired or at least lacking in basic language, literacy, and planning skills. We are not surprised, given both the association of schizophrenia with cognitive dysfunction and the potential for conditions associated with homelessness to cause neurological impairment, such as head trauma, malnutrition, and abuse of alcohol and drugs (Kass and Silver 1990). Checklist surveys may have underestimated the prevalence of cognitive impairment among the homeless at only 3% to 8% (Farr et al. 1986; Fischer et al. 1986; Koegel et al. 1988). In addition, it seems probable that routine medical screenings may miss more subtle evidence of neurological impairment.

To explore these possibilities we recently undertook a detailed study utilizing formal neuropsychological test batteries and structured neurological and medical examinations (Kass et al., in press). Over a 2-month period in 1989 we evaluated all 14 men enrolled in the shelter program who met DSM-III-R criteria for chronic schizophrenia and were willing to be assessed. Thirteen were able to complete the study. Their mean age was 31.6 years. Eleven were African American and two were Hispanic, comparable to the general population of the shelter. Most had abused multiple substances in the past, but all had negative urine toxicologies the day each was studied. Nine were receiving neuroleptic medication.

A neurologist performed a thorough medical and neurological examination using a standardized format, and a large battery of blood work was obtained. A neuropsychologist administered standardized tests including the Wechsler Adult Intelligence Scale-Revised, using the abbreviation of Satz and Mogel; the Wide Range Achievement Test, Revised; the Gray Oral Reading Test; the Wechsler Memory Scale-Revised; the Neimark Memorization Strategies Test; the Boston Naming Test; the Controlled Oral Word Association; the Token Test; the Trail Making Test; and the Modified Wisconsin Card Sorting Test. The total evaluation took 6 hours. In keeping with our previous experiences, we provided meals, cash payments, and considerable encouragement.

Eight subjects showed some neurological abnormality, which was only partially attributable to neuroleptics. There were high rates of neurological soft signs, and two patients had previously unnoticed gait difficulties, one of whom was discovered to have sarcoidosis of the central nervous system. Another subject was discovered to have active AIDS. Both had been suspected of having severe illness during the program's intake assessment; their work-ups were accelerated following our research findings. Thus, careful medical and neurological screening resulted in two new diagnoses of life-threatening illness.

We found that the neuropsychological tests were well tolerated by the men, despite taking up 3 hours of their time. Rather than becoming frustrated by difficulties, the men appreciated the attention they received. The neuropsychologist made a number of modifications in her usual procedures. Because many of the men had very short attention spans, she gave breaks as often as every 5 minutes. She shortened tests and simplified directions whenever possible. To maintain interest, she alternated tasks whenever possible.

The Satz and Mogel abbreviation of the Wechsler IQ test omits every other question, but the 90 minutes still required was a great effort for many of the men. The Trail Making Test, which requires holding several instructions simultaneously in memory, proved very difficult.

Tests with complicated instructions are perhaps best avoided in this population, in favor of those that measure simple output, such as verbal fluency tests.

Many tests are clearly affected by cultural background and measure experience as much as innate skill. For example, tests of reading aloud would be more difficult for someone who had been taught in very crowded classrooms and had been given minimal individual practice at this task. Selecting the father's motivation from a multiple-choice list based on a story in which a father gives a present to his child would be difficult for someone not raised in an intact, functional family.

With these caveats, we felt the test results accurately reflected current conditions of the men, although they left unanswered questions of etiology. The mean full scale IQ was 77.7, and the range was anywhere from normal to mildly retarded. Achievement tests revealed marked illiteracy and poor arithmetic skills in almost all of the men. Although a number of them could read single words, virtually none understood written sentences. Memory and learning skills ranged more widely, with one-half to two-thirds showing impairment on various tests and others functioning in the average range. Verbal output skills tended to be a stronger area for most men. Tests of following verbal commands, however, showed impairment in all men as instructions became more complex.

We have not formally explored the value of the tests, but based on individual score distributions we feel it is likely that at least some men, those with higher intelligence but lower skills, could be taught and measurably helped in key areas of literacy. The assessments also highlight the importance of providing the men with structured assistance, given their difficulty in comprehending complex instructions, at least at this phase in their lives. For example, we would expect that successful transition to independent housing would require continued concrete support in managing work, daily tasks, and entitlements.

Case Histories

To illustrate some of our points, we will present two cases. Both illustrate clearly the great amounts of time and effort required to fully understand the lives and the psychopathology of homeless individuals and the flexibility required by professional staff to design treatment programs. Both men received neuropsychological testing after they had been in the shelter for some time (the first in our research program and the second while hospitalized), and we show how the new information helped us define each man's strengths and limitations.

Clinical Case 1

Mr. A was an intelligent, literate, 34-year-old single African American man in the throes of a severe psychosis when he first entered the psychiatric day program at the Presbyterian Hospital men's shelter in July 1986. He came to the program because he was recognized by some of the staff who had known him at his previous shelter. Mr. A did not feel he had a mental illness, but he was willing to talk with the staff whom he knew. One, the program social worker, knew Mr. A to be paranoid, but considered this to be an "underlying aspect of his personality."

Mr. A had never been hospitalized or medicated when he entered the day program. He had dropped out of college, where he was a philosophy major, in his junior year. He was using cocaine at the time. Mr. A became homeless when he and his girlfriend split up in 1985. Shortly after entering a shelter, Mr. A enlisted in the army, but he was discharged during basic training because of delusions that the government was monitoring him. In fact, he revealed that he entered the army to build himself up so he could improve his fight against the American government. In addition, Mr. A acknowledged that he heard conversations when he was alone. He also held delusions that he was given an "indirect spinal tap" in high school that "gave my life force to a white guy."

Despite being markedly psychotic, Mr. A was able to speak clearly and logically for extensive lengths of time. Furthermore, he usually denied hallucinating and kept his delusions to himself. In fact, he was so adept at covering over his psychosis that the program psychiatrist assessed him as a "charming, cheerful, alert, unemployed, undomiciled man with a calm, friendly, boyish attitude, without evidence of any Axis I disorder." Our psychiatrist at that time worked part-time and did not obtain any of the client's history from the program social worker. Family members were not contacted. Mr. A was enrolled, but medication was not considered. He became an active participant in the day program but became increasingly outwardly psychotic, talking to himself, screaming out windows, and becoming filthy and lice infested.

In July 1987, a full-time psychiatrist joined the day program staff and had the opportunity to observe and speak with Mr. A daily. The psychiatrist had the benefit of the staff's past knowledge of the patient and he spoke extensively with Mr. A's sister. The sister revealed that Mr. A became psychotic during his junior year of college. A family doctor and the school recommended that he be hospitalized, but he refused, and the family let him be. They attributed his symptoms to cocaine use.

The program psychiatrist revised Mr. A's psychiatric diagnosis as chronic paranoid schizophrenia and cocaine abuse, in remission. Low doses of perphenazine, then haloperidol, were initiated several months after Mr. A developed a trusting relationship with the day program staff.

Realizing that Mr. A had strong language skills and an interest in writing, the program director appointed him to be keeper of the minutes of the daily community meeting. This appealed to Mr. A and enhanced his self-esteem. In fact, Mr. A had the highest IQ (verbal IQ, 106; Performance IQ, 98; and full-scale IQ, 102) of the 13 schizophrenic patients who were tested. However, Mr. A had more neurological soft signs than any of his fellow patients, and his reading comprehension was in the lowest percentile.

Unfortunately, taking medication did not appeal to Mr. A and he became expert at "cheeking meds." Thus, he remained psychotic even as he became increasingly attached to the program. Even though the program psychiatrist knew Mr. A was not taking his medication most days, he confronted him about his behavior very gently, recognizing that not taking medication met Mr. A's need to deny his illness. Thus, the need for medication was considered from the patient's perspective.

When the program director left in the summer of 1989, Mr. A left too. He began to sleep in parks in his old neighborhood and to visit his sister frequently. This disturbed her and she feared that her brother would spread disease to her or hurt her young children. The sister called the day program and a family meeting was held.

The problem was approached from a psychoeducational perspective. Mr. A and his family agreed that if Mr. A took medication daily, applied for Supplemental Security Income, and obtained housing, he would be a welcomed visitor at the home of any family member. Mr. A followed through on each of these conditions and was accepted into a new residential care center for adults, where he has lived for the past 6 months.

Clinical Case 2

Mr. B, a 32-year-old, tall, husky, black man from Trinidad, entered a shelter after leaving a state hospital against medical advice. His shelter case worker referred him to the day program with the assessment, "Client loses meal ticket frequently." On initial evaluation, Mr. B appeared paranoid and agitated, and he reported having shot a drug dealer in the leg after the dealer stole some marijuana from him when the patient was 19 years old. He admitted to having been arrested and serving 4 years in prison, but he denied that he was ever hospitalized. A check with the state office of mental health revealed an extensive state hospitalization history over the previous 10 years. Because of his poor language skills, the patient was able to provide little in the way of history. His speech had marked poverty of content, and he took minutes to form a sentence and then repeated it several times. He could not provide the phone number or address of a relative or friend.

Soon after his arrival Mr. B revealed his AWOL status. The psychiatrist contacted the state hospital and learned that because Mr. B had been a voluntary patient, he was discharged after he went AWOL. He had been on fluphenazine, clonazepam, and benztropine. He had not undergone an organic workup except for a basic physical, chest X ray, ECG, and blood tests, which were unremarkable. His diagnosis was chronic schizophrenia and probable mental retardation.

Initially, Mr. B made the day program staff uncomfortable. His size and history were intimidating. Furthermore, he refused to take any medications. On the encouraging side, Mr. B did appear to be in control of his behavior, he was able to understand and follow program rules, and he seemed to want to be a part of the program. His main interest was in playing table tennis, and the staff, including the director and psychiatrist, played with him often. In addition, the director held a meeting with Mr. B every morning and brought him a muffin to eat with the coffee the program supplied. A patient, nonconfrontational approach was taken, using humor as a means of creating a desirable, supportive milieu.

For 2 years, Mr. B was followed in the day program on no medication. He did not become acutely psychotic, violent, or agitated during that time. His language difficulties, along with poverty of content and some looseness of associations, persisted. A functional assessment revealed marked deficits in self-care skills, self-direction, social functioning, and ability to concentrate on tasks.

It became clear that Mr. B was more likely to be a victim of shelter violence and crime than a perpetrator of them. He was frequently threatened, his money was stolen, and he was physically assaulted. He responded to these conditions by either moving briefly to another shelter or demonstrating suicidal behavior (threatening to jump from a balcony onto the floor where the shelter residents sleep). He had one hospitalization because of his suicidal behavior and was placed on neuroleptics again, but he promptly refused them as soon as he was discharged back to the shelter.

Mr. B's treatment in the program focused on improving his self-care skills and socialization. Despite some improvement, he remained severely limited in his ability to function with any independence. Even so, an overly optimistic intensive case manager from an agency outside the day program arranged for him to be placed in a community residence. After approximately 1 month there, Mr. B was hospitalized due to bizarre and threatening behavior. He barricaded himself in his room, broke off a metal towel rack that he appeared to be keeping for self-defense, and took the underwear of a female resident, cutting holes in the crotch. He was again medicated with neuroleptics and returned to the shelter day program.

Mr. B returned to his previous level of adaptive functioning in the program and, after a brief period, was placed in a low-demand, shelter-based transitional living community. He fared somewhat better there than in the community residence but again required brief hospitalization when he became agitated while discussing with his case manager the possibility of taking an HIV test. He was kept on 50 mg of chlorpromazine. Neuropsychological testing revealed a verbal IQ of 64, a performance IQ of 68, and a full-scale IQ of 64. He demonstrated global impairment but had especial difficulty with abstract thinking and was markedly distractible. No evidence of thought disorder or psychotic features were found.

On review of the case, the program staff felt that the patient's "well-documented history of behavioral problems, typified by impulsivity and agitation would appear to reflect poor neurobehavioral (neurologically based) control, rather than primary psychiatric disorder." Using these reported findings from the neuropsychological testing, the staff revised the DSM-III-R diagnosis to organic personality disorder and mild mental retardation in addition to a probable chronic psychotic process.

Mr. B returned to the transitional living community but eventually chose to return to the shelter day program where he settled comfortably into his old routines. Our staff has concluded that the familiar, low-demand, relatively tolerant atmosphere of the shelter is the best setting they can arrange for this patient at the present time. However, we will continue to search for a more permanent residence with these characteristics.

The possibility that Mr. B was infected with HIV, which had been considered by the transitional living community staff, has become a greater concern due to the presence of weight loss, lymphadenopathy, and anal warts, the latter indicating that he takes part in high-risk sexual behavior. Whether HIV infection is playing a role in his organicity remains to be seen. Ongoing attempts will be made to obtain informed consent for HIV testing and to provide AIDS education to the extent the patient can tolerate. In addition, the general condition of his health will be regularly monitored by the program nurse and physicians.

Conclusions

Thorough psychiatric assessment of homeless mentally ill individuals make it possible for programs to provide psychosocial interventions, including placement in appropriate residential settings and somatic treatments, targeted to the individual. Assessment of many individuals require modification of traditional methods. A caretaking, relatively unpressured setting such as a day program is a preferable alternative for conducting such assessments compared with more structured settings such as standard hospital-based clinics and emergency rooms, which may be experienced as coercive. Availability of staff who share a cultural affinity with patients is helpful. Developing the trust of homeless individuals over time yields greater cooperation and validity of information. It also may result in eventual participation of reluctant family members in treatment.

The optimal basic assessment of the sheltered homeless person is a multidisciplinary team evaluation, performed in the day program milieu. Formal neuropsychiatric work-up may be valuable as well. In all situations, clinicians must avoid premature conclusions about prognosis based on a "cross-sectional" diagnosis made during the initial presentation. That is particularly true for individuals who have been homeless for a long time and have been subjected to severe social and physical environmental stress. Treatment and assessment evolve hand in hand over time. The caring and concern shown in a comprehensive evaluation becomes an important influence on the outcome of treatment.

References

American Psychiatric Association: Diagnostic and Statistical Manual of Mental Disorders, 3rd Edition, Revised. Washington, DC, American Psychiatric Association, 1987

Caton CLM, Wyatt RG, Grunberg J, et al: An evaluation of a mental health program for homeless men. Am J Psychiatry 147:286–289, 1990

Cohen NL, Putnam JF, Sullivan AM: The mentally ill homeless: isolation and adaptation. Hosp Community Psychiatry 35:922–924, 1984

Farr RK, Koegel P, Burnam A: A Study of Homelessness and Mental Illness in the Skid Row Area of Los Angeles. Los Angeles, CA, Los Angeles County Department of Mental Health, March 1986

Fischer PJ, Shapiro S, Breakey WR, et al: Mental health and social characteristics of the homeless. Am J Public Health 76:519, 1986

Gounis K, Susser E: Shelterization and its implications for mental health services, in Psychiatry Takes to the Streets. Edited by Cohen NL. New York, Guilford, 1990, pp 231–255

Grunberg J, Eagle PF: Shelterization: how the homeless adapt to shelter living. Hosp Community Psychiatry 41:521–525, 1990

Kass F, Silver JM: Neuropsychiatry and the homeless (editorial). Journal of Neuropsychiatry and Clinical Neurosciences 2:15–19, 1990

Kay SR, Fiszbein A, Opler LA: The Positive and Negative Syndrome Scale (PANSS) for schizophrenia. Schizophr Bull 13:261–275, 1987

Koegel P, Burnam MA, Farr RK: The prevalance of specific disorders among homeless individuals in the inner city of Los Angeles. Arch Gen Psychiatry 45:1085–1092, 1988

Lipton FR, Nutt S, Sabatini A: Housing the homeless mentally ill: a longitudinal study of a treatment approach. Hosp Community Psychiatry 39:40–45, 1988

MacKinnon RA, Yudofsky SC: The Psychiatric Evaluation in Clinical Practice. Philadelphia, PA, JB Lippincott, 1986

Morrissey JP, Gounis K, Barrow S, et al: Organizational barriers to serving the mentally ill homeless, in Treating the Homeless: Urban Psychiatry's Challenge. Edited by Jones BE. Washington, DC, American Psychiatric Press, 1986, pp 93–109

Susser E, Struening E, Conover S: Psychiatric problems in homeless men: lifetime psychosis, substance abuse, and current distress in new arrivals at New York City shelter. Arch Gen Psychiatry 46:845–850, 1989

Susser E, Goldfinger SM, White A: Some clinical approaches to the homeless mentally ill. Community Ment Health J 26:463–480, 1990

Chapter 16

Challenge and Opportunity: Rehabilitating the Homeless Mentally Ill

Jerome V. Vaccaro, M.D.
Robert P. Liberman, M.D.
Sally Friedlob, L.C.S.W., O.T.R.
Susan Dempsay, B.A.

A multidimensional, interactive model of mental illness that considers stress, vulnerability, and protective factors can guide the field of psychiatric rehabilitation for homeless mentally ill individuals. According to this model, symptoms and their associated social disabilities are the result of stressors impinging upon a person's enduring psychobiological vulnerability. The noxious effects of stress superimposed on vulnerability can be modulated by protective factors, from either among the personal resources of the individual (e.g., social competence) or the individual's social environment (e.g., supportive and tolerant family members and responsive community treatment services; Liberman et al. 1989). This conceptualization has stimulated new methods of psychiatric rehabilitation that train skills or provide social prostheses for patients.

The field of psychiatric rehabilitation has emerged as an organizing force in the comprehensive community care of individuals with psychiatric disorders. Over the past decade, a coherent body of interventions, rooted in sound theoretical principles, has developed that has shown its efficacy in reducing relapse and disability among individuals with mental illness (Farkas and Anthony 1989; Liberman 1988, 1991). The aim of psychiatric rehabilitation is to improve the long-term adaptive capabilities of individuals with psychiatric disabilities for living, learning, working, socializing, and adjusting to life circumstances as normally as possible (Anthony and Liberman 1986).

When the population is the homeless mentally ill, a number of issues having to do with accessibility and acceptability of rehabilitation services must be addressed. For example, because of the mobility and low

279

frustration tolerance of homeless persons, services need to be accessible immediately, without waiting periods. It is critical to address homeless persons' immediate needs for shelter, food, and clothing as elements in the initial engagement process. Without these essentials, homeless individuals will find it difficult, if not impossible, to successfully participate in rehabilitation efforts. For instance, because many homeless mentally ill individuals desire and accept appropriate housing options, and because having a stable residence is a prerequisite for the long-term learning inherent in psychiatric rehabilitation, incorporating rehabilitation services with housing can facilitate positive outcomes.

The rehabilitation process may be separated into six overlapping stages: engagement, functional assessment and goal setting, prevocational skill training, work adjustment, job seeking and acquisition, and sustained employment. The individual's rehabilitation goals may include a job in work environments that are traditionally viewed as mainstream employment settings or other adaptive roles, such as part-time worker, transitional employee, supported employee, volunteer, or psychosocial club member.

In this chapter, we will review these six stages of rehabilitation and then suggest ways these components of rehabilitation might be incorporated into community programs. This will be accomplished partly by describing a modified clubhouse program for the homeless mentally ill with which we are associated called Step up on Second. Step up on Second is located in an area of Los Angeles that has a high concentration of homeless individuals, and it caters to the special needs of those who are both seriously mentally ill and homeless. Most members of the program also carry a second diagnosis of substance abuse or dependence. The program is available to members 7 days a week during most daytime hours.

While they are beyond the scope of this chapter, it should be understood that a reliable, symptom-based diagnosis, administration of appropriate types and judicious dosages of psychotropic drugs, and monitoring of symptoms and warning signs of relapse all must be interwoven with a comprehensive rehabilitation program. In fact, control of florid symptoms with medication may be a prerequisite of rehabilitation, as severe thought disorder or symptom-evoked deviances may be incompatible with the sustained and sometimes arduous learning process implicit in rehabilitation modalities.

It is axiomatic that rehabilitation must proceed from the adaptive capacities, aspirations, and goals of each individual. Epidemiological and ethnographic surveys have identified the special assets, problems, and needs of the homeless mentally ill (Koegel and Burnam 1988; Koegel et al. 1988); in particular, homeless mentally ill individuals have many coping skills that can serve as starting points for treatment and rehabilitation. Survival skills that have been honed on urban streets can become building blocks for performing social and vocational roles and for overcoming the comorbidity of substance abuse with serious mental disorders.

Engagement

It is widely recognized that the formation and maintenance of the therapeutic alliance is critical to the success of treatment and rehabilitation. That is especially true, yet often more difficult to achieve, for the homeless mentally ill individual. Too often, these individuals, whose adaptive skills are daily put to the test under the most extreme of circumstances, are asked to adapt to services that are not designed with their special needs in mind. The following case vignette illustrates the importance of engaging homeless mentally ill individuals in a way that addresses the needs they see as most important to their survival in the community.

> Stan is a 28-year-old man who was first diagnosed as having schizophrenia at the age of 22. He had a deteriorating clinical course and had become progressively more socially isolated, delusional, and hallucinatory. He was evicted from his family home when his parents and siblings could no longer tolerate his poor self-care and florid psychotic symptoms. Before evicting him, his parents took him to the local community mental health center for treatment. He resisted going to the clinic for services and was seen several times before he finally said that he saw no value to the services he was receiving and refused to return to the clinic.
>
> Once he left his family, Stan lived on the local beaches while remaining in a psychotic state. He was physically assaulted many times. His family was very concerned about him and repeatedly sought help for him at the community mental health center. They were given many appointments for Stan, but he refused to go to the clinic, saying the clinicians did not understand him and could not address his needs.
>
> Finally, the center began a new program to work with homeless and other patients who were difficult to engage in an effort to make services more user-friendly. The treatment team was staffed by a psychiatrist and several master's-level social workers who worked with their patients in the community. The psychiatrist and social worker began their work with Stan by speaking with his family, as he was too isolated and paranoid to interact directly with them. They began by bringing him food. Gradually, they were able to speak with him, and he told them that the two most critical things he needed were to reestablish relations with his family and to get safe room and board. He also was able to articulate the steps that led him to attain these goals, as depicted in Table 16–1.

This approach differed from earlier efforts in several ways. Stan was met in his own environment, which allowed him to have more of a sense of comfort and control. In addition, he himself identified his most pressing needs, and he eventually came to consider solutions to these life problems rather than having a treatment plan offered to him by clinicians. Thus, great care was devoted to enhancing Stan's sense of empowerment. Eventually Stan was able to trust and then engage with treatment staff at the center.

Functional Assessment and Goal Setting

Often, clinicians are hesitant to engage their patients in discussions about their goals because of concerns that patients either will have unrealistic goals or be unable to articulate meaningful ones. Thus, this critical component of treatment and rehabilitation planning is ignored to spare the patient the demoralizing process of unveiling his or her inability to plan for the future. Indeed, once homeless mentally ill individuals are confronted with the enormity of their problems, they may feel overwhelmed and seek to avoid addressing their difficulties unless they see some relationship between smaller, attainable steps and their larger problems.

Thus, the goal setting process must begin with an open, supportive discussion of the social and occupational roles in which the individual wishes to engage, relationships the individual wants to establish or improve, and other goals. Assessing the patient's adaptive functioning in family, work, and other social roles as well as pinpointing community resources and skills that will have to be mobilized for achieving goals are intrinsic to this stage in the rehabilitation process. With the stage set in this manner, homeless individuals are freer to explore their desires and set realistic steps to attain these goals.

One common problem in setting goals lies in the difficulty many

Table 16–1.   Rehabilitation goal setting by Stan

Goal	Step
Improve family relations	Control behaviors that my family finds weird, such as talking to myself and staying in my room all day
	Take better care of myself—shower regularly, wear cleaner clothes
	Get help from someone to learn to talk with my family without fighting
Get safe room and board	Get money
	Look for a cheap, safe place to live and talk with the person who has the place

patients have differentiating between goals and solutions. The following case vignette illustrates this point.

Keith is a 25-year-old man who was diagnosed as suffering from schizophrenia after a 3-year decline in functioning. He had attended college and needed about 20 credits to receive a degree in engineering when he became floridly psychotic. The cognitive disorganization and psychotic thinking he experienced during his last 2 years in college prevented him from completing his education. His family places great value on education and upward mobility: his father is a physician, his mother is an educator, and his siblings are all in graduate or medical schools. Thus, Keith felt extremely demoralized after dropping out of college. He perceived his homelessness and inability to meet his basic needs as further evidence of his inadequacy.

Because of his low self-opinion, the therapist had difficulty engaging Keith in the goal setting process. He did, however, begin to address his goals by telling his therapist that he wanted to immediately reenroll in college and complete his engineering degree during the next semester, which was to begin in 2 weeks.

The therapist explored the reasons why Keith had identified this lofty goal, and learned that his family had been most supportive and had helped him provide for his basic needs while he was enrolled in school. In addition, Keith had been at his happiest during these years and fondly remembered the days when he "had a life and aspirations," as he put it. The therapist helped Keith see that his real goals were to feel valued by his family and meet his basic needs for shelter and food, and that reenrolling in college was his proposed method of attaining these goals. What ensued was a lively dialogue in which Keith articulated more attainable goals for his rehabilitation. As a first step, after getting his psychotic symptoms under control, he enrolled in an automotive school. His family was pleased that he again aspired to some vocational goals and helped support him while he applied for public assistance and admission to the mechanics' school.

The therapist in this situation helped Keith distinguish between his underlying goal of being viewed as a successful and productive family member and of returning to school in a sudden, ill-considered manner. With this task accomplished, Keith was able to plan the steps in his rehabilitation more sensibly and establish attainable objectives leading to the achievement of his goals.

Prevocational Skills Training

Once the patient is successfully engaged in goal setting and a therapeutic alliance is established, the process of training the individual in specific types of prevocational instrumental and affiliative skills begins. Table 16–2 depicts a representative sample of such social and independent living skills. For example, an individual whose basic grooming and self-care skills and conversational abilities are impaired might begin rehabilitation by learning these skills. These areas of social and independent living skills may be considered basic building blocks necessary to achieve stability of functioning before beginning vocational rehabilitation. These and other skills can then be applied and generalized in occupational settings, all but assuring success in vocational roles. The next case report illustrates how self-care skills may be generalized to a vocational setting.

> Bob is a middle-aged man who was first diagnosed as having schizophrenia in his early twenties. When he was first seen by his rehabilitation counselor, he was living in a homeless shelter and had not been in stable housing for the past 4 years. In his evaluation interviews, he was poorly groomed and had poor conversational skills. He told the counselor that he wanted to find a place to live that was safe and secure, to improve his relationship with his family, and eventually to begin to return to some form of "low-stress work, where I don't have to talk to too many people," as he put it. He had never worked at a full-time job, but had volunteered at community agencies in the past.
>
> He successfully applied to have his public welfare benefits reinstated and found housing, with the assistance of his case manager, in a single-room-occupancy hotel. As part of the plan he developed with his rehabilitation counselor, Bob enrolled in a social skills training program where he took classes in grooming and self-care, basic conversational, and medication management skills. As the next step in his rehabilitation, Bob volunteered at a local library, where he filed books and worked at the photocopy machine. His work schedule was gradually increased to suit

Table 16–2.   Examples of instrumental and affiliative skills

Type of skill	Specific skill
Instrumental	Purchasing goods in a store
	Asking for directions for a bus trip
	Reporting side effects of a medication and asking for relief from a physician
	Inquiring about rental housing
	Talking with a social worker about Social Security benefits
Affiliative	Greeting a friend
	Going to a movie with a friend
	Exchanging comments with an acquaintance about sports, the weather, or an illness
	Asking a spouse how he or she feels

his needs: he started by working 1 to 2 hours once per week and now works 3 or 4 hours per day, 4 days per week.

Once he started work at the library, Bob and his rehabilitation counselor discussed ways in which he could apply his newly learned conversational skills at work. Bob practiced transferring the skills during role play and homework exercises. As a result, Bob made several new friends and was regarded as a pleasant and competent worker.

Bob began his rehabilitation by gaining basic instrumental skills in classes specifically designed for individuals with chronic mental illnesses. The social skills training programs were developed, validated, packaged, and disseminated in modular form by the UCLA Clinical Research Center for Schizophrenia and Psychiatric Rehabilitation (Eckman et al. 1990; Liberman and Eckman 1989). Once Bob had learned these social and independent living skills, his counselor worked with him to apply them in a variety of work and social settings.

Work Adjustment and Job Training

Once the patient has learned basic social skills, the process of adjusting to work and gaining job-specific skills may begin. Opportunities to adjust to the work environment may be provided in special settings for individuals with psychiatric impairments or in programs designed for the general population. A major aim of this stage of rehabilitation is to provide "work-hardening" experiences in a supportive environment offering psychiatric consultation and liaison. Such programs usually include a combination of classroom or laboratory learning and practical exposure to job tasks.

For example, the rehabilitation service of the Brentwood Veterans Administration (VA) Medical Center offers training in janitorial, office machine repair, and horticulture skills. The curricula in these programs include didactic experiences whose nature is very practical as well as on-the-job training opportunities. In this way, trainees acquire knowledge necessary to perform work-related tasks and apply this knowledge in order to obtain requisite skills and attitudes. The story of Lee, a 35-year-old man who was diagnosed as schizophrenic while he was in the military, illustrates the importance of providing a range of options to tailor services to meet individual needs.

After discharge from the military, Lee spent over 9 years living in board-and-care homes. At the age of 29, he became addicted to crack cocaine. As a result of the financial strain created by his addiction and his increased aggressiveness while under the influence of cocaine, he was evicted from the board-and-care facility in which he lived. For the next 5

years, he lived on the streets of Los Angeles, frequently being rehospitalized after becoming psychotic following binges of cocaine use. During
one of his hospitalizations, he was referred to a new board-and-care facility and was enrolled in a drug-abuse relapse prevention program. He
was also referred to the psychiatric rehabilitation service at the VA hospital and enrolled in its social skills training classes.

Lee took classes in medication self-management, symptom self-management, recreation and leisure, and basic conversation skills. He expressed the desire to get some form of work and said he would like to
learn janitorial skills. He was enrolled in the 6-week janitorial training
program run by the rehabilitation service. He did very well in the content
portion of the program, but the trainer assessed that he was not yet ready
to work, mainly because of slow performance. Lee and his counselor decided that he would become a member of the service's shared job crew,
in which several patients share one full-time job. He is very satisfied with
this arrangement and feels great pride in his achievements.

Lee began his involvement with the rehabilitation program while his
basic needs for shelter and financial security were addressed. The sense
of self-worth he experienced from learning basic social and coping
skills led him to venture further along in his rehabilitation to the point
that he requested referral to a work-skill training program.

Even after acquiring basic social and coping skills and studying job-
specific skills, many individuals who have been unemployed for long
periods of time require some form of sheltered, transitional, or supported work experience to develop or regain work stamina and adjust
to the demands of a work routine. In these sometimes protracted experiences, they can learn appropriate workplace behavior and apply
newly acquired social skills in a safe and secure work setting. Finally,
this stage of rehabilitation provides a new opportunity for individuals
to reexamine their goals and either redirect their efforts or make mid-
course corrections.

Job Seeking and Placement

The penultimate step in the rehabilitation process is perhaps the most
critical. At this point, the individual has decided to pursue a particular
course of action, whether it be as a full- or part-time worker in the competitive market, a volunteer in a community agency, or a member of a
psychosocial program's work crew. Then it is time to plot a course and
endeavor to secure this position. Often, patients lack the skills to conduct a job search, such as completing applications, interviewing, and
conducting negotiations about job expectations and compensation.
Homeless mentally ill individuals usually need to account for large

gaps in their work histories.

Finally, they often lack basic resources for sustaining a job search such as a place to get mail, make telephone calls, and fill out applications. These services may be provided through job finding clubs, a prototype of which has been developed at the Brentwood VA Hospital in conjunction with the UCLA Clinical Research Center for Schizophrenia and Psychiatric Rehabilitation (Jacobs 1991; Jacobs et al. 1984). The benefits of job-finding clubs are demonstrated by the case of Jack.

> Jack is a 32-year-old man with bipolar affective disorder with onset when he was 25. Since becoming ill, Jack had been intermittently homeless and had worked at a variety of jobs for brief periods. He had found that he had special aptitude in the area of office machine repair. His social and independent living skills were at a high level; thus, he did not require training in these domains. Once his basic needs for shelter and financial support were met, he enrolled in a course of study in office machine repair that resulted in certification. He and his counselor agreed that he lacked many of the skills necessary to establish and sustain a successful job search, and he was referred to the job finding club.
>
> Once a member of the club, Jack received instruction and guided practice in seeking out potential employers, filling out job applications, and interviewing for work. He was also given a mailing address and access to a telephone. After several setbacks in applying for jobs, he was granted an interview with a small typewriter repair firm. He performed well at the interview and was eventually hired.

Often, homeless mentally ill individuals who successfully traverse the rehabilitative process and secure competitive employment experience difficulties in maintaining that employment. Applying skills learned in the prevocational phase, showing poor generalization of problem-solving abilities to the work setting, experiencing changes in the nature of their jobs, and requiring hospitalization are among the difficulties that adversely affect sustained employment for these individuals.

In order for people who are homeless and mentally ill to remain in the work force, ongoing support in the form of on-the-job counseling and coaching is required. Job coaches boost patients' abilities to generalize previously learned skills, successfully negotiate with employers, and integrate themselves into the work force (Bond 1991). This approach reflects a trend toward "place-train" techniques, in which patients' skills are shaped while on the job, and away from the previous emphasis on "train-place" methods. Joe, described next, benefited markedly from this approach.

Joe is a 28-year-old man diagnosed as schizophrenic. After spending time in a work training program he successfully secured a job in a printing shop. He enjoyed the job very much, and as a result of his good performance he was given additional work responsibilities and greater visibility in the shop's customer service section. Although flattered at the promotion, he was stressed by the change because he felt he would be unable to successfully interact with customers. He attempted to communicate his misgivings to his employer, but his boss responded by giving Joe a pep talk reassuring him he could perform adequately in this new role.

Joe called Ron, his job coach, who came to the work site to speak with Joe. They discussed the problem at some length and decided that Joe would go to his employer and suggest that he begin a staged increase in responsibility, wherein he would first take on work duties in the copying section. Once he performed adequately in this role, he and the employer would reevaluate the situation to determine whether he would then move into the customer service section. Joe successfully negotiated this compromise with his employer and eventually assumed the new responsibilities.

Putting It All Together

From the foregoing discussion it should be clear that the organization of the elements of rehabilitation services for the homeless mentally ill is as critical as the elements themselves. For example, emphasis must be placed on the entry point for services so that they are user- or consumer-friendly and have minimal or no waiting periods. Further, services should initially be of low intensity to allow for adequate engagement and then increase in intensity leading up to the development and implementation of a comprehensive rehabilitation plan. For these reasons, the clubhouse approach as articulated by Beard and colleagues (1982) is a sensible and feasible way to accomplish these goals. Step up on Second, the rehabilitation program for the homeless mentally ill described below, incorporates these principles.

Step Up is a daytime program that has an evening component for individuals with dual diagnoses of major psychiatric and drug dependence disorders. It is informed by clubhouse theories and principles and learning and behavior theories and offers social skills training and case management. Its stated purpose is to assist members as they struggle to gain self-confidence, relearn lost skills, utilize mental health and drug abuse treatment services, prepare for entry into the job market, and escape from homelessness.

The program is open 7 days a week and provides comprehensive services through educational classes, recreational programming, prevocational training, vocational opportunities, social activities, access to psychiatric care, and referrals to community resources. No time limits are placed on services; members are allowed to remain with the program indefinitely, through periods of stable housing, homelessness, symptom remission, or relapse. An open-door policy is maintained by employing broad, inclusive criteria for admission. Recovering members are given priority for jobs within the program, so that some members have moved from vocational training through supported employment, work team supervisor, and full-time agency staff. The agency, in fact, was founded and is directed by a family member of a young man with schizophrenia.

One of the most important interventions at Step Up is teaching assertiveness skills to the members through the assertion training group. Learning such skills empowers homeless mentally ill individuals with experiences of mastery, self-control, and success in attaining personal goals, thereby making a dent in environments where they have felt rejected, helpless, and hopeless. Achieving the goals that they set in the assertion training group also reconnects them in constructive ways to mainstream society in such areas as housing, food services, social welfare agencies, medical and psychiatric agencies, and family ties. The name assertion training was chosen because it connoted bold, confident, and normative behavior.

The assertion training group addresses four levels of responses that are the focus and goals of the program. The levels are depicted in Figure 16–1. At the bottom of the inverted pyramid are accurate and reality-based perceptions and discriminations of social situations that surround the homeless mentally ill individual's efforts to achieve his or her personal goals. These are also termed receiving skills using an information processing model of social competence.

The second level focuses on teaching the group member how to make appropriate decisions for action, taking into account his or her range of alternatives and the social norms that govern the consequences of behavior. These problem-solving skills are also termed processing skills. The third level encompasses verbal and nonverbal skills, also called sending skills, that an individual must employ appropriately in social interaction once a realistic option is chosen for achieving a goal. The fourth level, namely, a more assertive style and quality of life, grows out of successes in the use of effective receiving, processing, and sending skills (Liberman et al. 1989).

For the homeless members of the Step Up psychosocial rehabilitation center, life on the streets is generally unpredictable; thus, learning how to size up situations, how to generate alternatives and weigh their likelihood of success, and how to realistically appraise the response tendencies of others are the keys to effective problem solving, as the story of Bill illustrates.

> Bill was able to find a part-time janitorial job at a garage. One day, his boss's unreasonable criticism triggered angry feelings in Bill. Even though Bill appropriately used verbal and nonverbal sending skills to express his anger, he was promptly fired. What was lacking in his assertive response was ability at the second level of assertiveness—namely, anticipating the consequences of standing up to his boss after such a short time on the job.

A frequent pitfall for participants in the assertion training group is to select interpersonal goals that are too global and, often, beyond their

---

Figure 16–1.   Levels of responses and outcomes as Goals for Assertion Training Group.

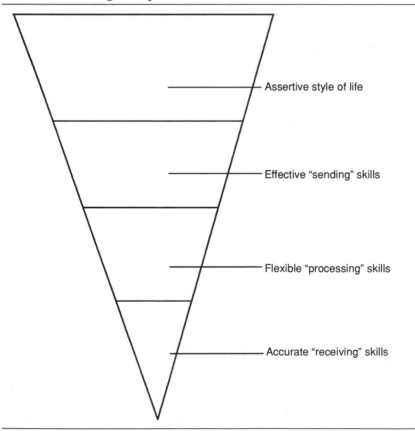

control to influence. For example, asking someone on a date, obtaining Section 8 housing, ensuring that a Social Security check arrives on time, or avoiding being accosted by police are not usually possible to achieve in a predictable fashion. The leader of the group, a psychiatric social worker who is the third author of this chapter, expends a great deal of time helping members to reformulate their goals into more attainable forms. Thus, using self-disclosure with a friend to successfully maintain a conversation, or getting a Housing and Urban Development official to assist in filling out Section 8 application forms, are proximal to the longer-term goals and more likely to be achieved. Sam's experience illustrates the usefulness of reformulating goals.

> Sam was helped in modifying his goal of being invited to his grandparents for dinner to expressing a desire for a visit and letting them know how much he enjoys his grandmother's cooking. Sam had been raised by his grandparents and felt close to them; however, as his mental illness progressed, he caused them much suffering by stealing money from them and insulting them. Finally, they terminated all contact with him. At a later point in his involvement in the assertion training group, Sam was able to modify his goal of "having my grandparents accept me" to "calling them and letting them know I've entered a rehabilitation program and would like to tell them about my progress." Sam realized that his grandparents might continue to reject him and that he might choke up when communicating with them; nonetheless, he felt the potential for reestablishing contact with his grandparents was worth the risk of being rejected.

Weighing the relative risks and benefits of using assertiveness learned in the group is another facet of the group work. The probability of rejection has to be anticipated, and members must be coached to understand that their efforts increase the likelihood of reaching goals but do not guarantee success. Members must also be counseled to expect to feel anxiety, which is also a consequence of breaking new ground in relationships by using assertiveness. In the following case, Georgia's decision not to behave assertively reflected an understanding of the risks and benefits of confronting others.

> A transsexual, Georgia slept in a public shelter while saving money to rent her own room. She was frightened and lonely. Her goal in the assertion training group was to become more firm with the only two people who had befriended her but who constantly borrowed money from her without returning it. She was able to practice appropriate refusal skills in the group but did not employ them with her friends because she considered the risk of alienating her limited social network was too great.

Setting interpersonal goals in the context of a benefit-risk assessment of the consequences of assertiveness often leads members to find compromise solutions. One set of compromises involves giving to others in order to get from them in return. Through repeated goal setting and application of skills in real life, participants become aware of the values of benevolent self-interest and social responsibility in achieving a higher level of community adaptation, as the following cases illustrate.

> Joe, a Vietnam War veteran, always shared cigarettes with his buddies in combat—a common currency of cohesion in his military unit that was instrumental for survival. On the streets, Joe had difficulty saying no to peers who requested cigarettes, even when his generosity left none for himself. Ted, another group member, said to Joe, "You should be able to say no to any moocher with no exceptions, period!" Joe, however, decided on a goal of sharing up to four cigarettes a day and saving the rest for himself. Ted could understand the compromise position that Joe staked out for himself.

> After a lengthy wait, George finally obtained an apartment through the Section 8 housing program. He complained to the group that his apartment was adjacent to the noisy laundry room and he couldn't concentrate or sleep. He set a goal to ask the apartment manager for a different apartment but offered to repaint the apartment because he knew that the manager was reluctant to reassign apartments because of the cost and effort of redecorating them.

> Jean and Randy wanted to participate in a demonstration organized by the Los Angeles Mental Health Association to advocate against cuts in the county mental health budget. Their goal in the assertion training group was to practice expressing themselves positively as mental health consumers with citizens they might encounter at the Civic Center.

Group members often present issues that reflect the stigma and rejection they experience as homeless persons from the community at large. While distressing and at times overwhelming, these experiences can charge group members to heightened levels of participation, as in the cases of Craig and Jerry.

> Craig, who had been sleeping outdoors and consequently was unkempt, felt embarrassed when he entered a local mini-market with money to buy coffee and a roll for his breakfast. His embarrassment lurched to feelings of degradation when he was sternly told by the clerk to leave the market, even before he could make his purchase. His immediate response was humiliation, choking up to the point of muteness and then meekly leaving the market. The other group members were outraged and empathic-

ally helped Craig articulate a response for future situations that would enable him to maintain his self-respect.

Jerry, another disheveled and homeless member of Step Up who had participated in the session with Craig, reported during the following week that he had encountered a similar situation in a grocery store while buying cigarettes. Having vicariously learned in the previous session how to assert his rights as a paying customer, he utilized his assertion skills with the clerk. When she responded by pointing to a sign that said "We Reserve the Right to Refuse Service to Anyone," he asked to see the manager and succeeded in using his newly learned assertiveness skills.

The assertion training group is the most popular activity offered at Step Up. Attendance ranges between 10 and 20 participants at the weekly sessions, almost all of whom come prepared and motivated to present their problems and formulate their goals. Monitoring the effectiveness of the training has indicated that between 50% to 75% of the goals set in the group are actualized in real-life situations. Gaining personal effectiveness through expressing feelings and fulfilling needs has been a key element in the struggle for daily survival and for improved quality of life among homeless mentally ill individuals.

Future Prospects

The neurobiological, sociocultural, and behavioral determinants of homeless mentally ill individuals require a multifaceted approach to rehabilitation that must integrate pharmacological with innovative and empathic psychosocial interventions. There is no place for unidimensional treatment and rehabilitation strategies, nor for single modalities that in the past have been trumpeted as remedies for the misery of severe mental illness.

For psychiatry to maintain its leadership in solving the problems of the homeless mentally ill, psychiatrists must enlarge the scope of their responsibilities to become politicians, social networkers, and team leaders. Clinical services to the homeless mentally ill must be provided in all biopsychosocial dimensions. That means clinical roles for psychiatrists must extend beyond traditional diagnosis and pharmacotherapy to encompass functional assessments, goal setting, skills training, vocational rehabilitation, development of housing and other psychosocial resources, and supervision of case management. Although the varied needs of the homeless mentally ill must be met by individualized approaches, psychiatrists cannot undertake the treatment and rehabilitation effort as solitary practitioners. They must forge partnerships with families, social agencies, housing authorities, and the criminal justice system, each with the active direction and participation of the patient in the clinical biopsychosocial decision-making process.

Stigma still rears its ugly head within the profession, as hard-to-serve homeless mentally ill individuals are avoided by practitioners who stubbornly cling to "do what I tell you" attitudes. Optimum delivery of rehabilitative services to the homeless mentally ill is not compatible with a one-size-fits-all approach to psychiatric care. With community linkages and networking, the differentiated needs of the homeless mentally ill can be met by collaboration with patients in setting goals, interventions tailored for symptom control, illness education, self-management, health promotion, nutrition, fitness, family involvement, housing, and vocational rehabilitation.

The essential strategies and elements for effective rehabilitation of the homeless mentally ill include:

- A spectrum of accessible, continuous, and consumer-friendly service options to meet the varied and individualized needs, assets, interests, and deficits of the homeless;
- Flexible levels of intervention requiring increases in the amount, form, and degree of outreach services provided, depending on the individual's present needs and circumstances;
- Encouragement of active participation in the rehabilitation process by the patient and his support network, including teaching patients and their significant others to set realistic goals and advocate for the resources required for progress;
- Availability of long-term, reliable, and mutually respectful therapeutic relationships that permit stepwise progress toward independent functioning; and
- Administrative and programmatic support for comprehensive, continuous, and coordinated services.

The special challenges, barriers, and obstacles posed by mental health systems, social agencies, consumers, and practitioners in providing services to the homeless mentally ill can spur creativity in the design of new treatment and rehabilitative interventions. Two examples of creative designs for rehabilitation service delivery for the homeless mentally ill are presented here to stimulate innovative thinking and planning.

To attract and engage the homeless mentally ill in the lengthy and effective process of rehabilitation, a "shopping mall" of needed and valued services could be constructed in a large commercial space or warehouse. A number of programs, several of which are described in the literature, use this type of approach in offering comprehensive services to the homeless mentally ill. The mall would include various "shops" or "stalls" in which the browsing, window-shopping, homeless mentally ill person might find:

- Dental hygiene services, staffed by students;
- Medical drop-in services, similar to the growing number of storefront Urgent Care centers located in the community;
- Hair salon and barbershop, staffed by students;
- Showers;
- Lounge for resting or napping;
- Laundromat;
- Nutritious fast foods;
- Clothing boutique comprising donated items;
- "Real estate" bureau listing shelters, low-cost housing, residential treatment facilities, and even secure places on the streets and parks around town that could be safe havens for homeless individuals;
- Entertainment center with video arcades and other stimulating and enjoyable activities; and
- Telephone services for calling relatives, agencies, and friends.

The shopping mall could also include outreach workers who could approach the homeless mentally ill in their natural locales and "market" the mall's services with flyers, with personable advertising, and even with judicious use of food and other tangible reinforcers that could gradually influence the sampling and participation of even reluctant individuals. This approach was used in a storefront setting with hard-to-reach juvenile delinquents and resulted in marked reductions in recidivism (Schwitzgebel 1966).

Involving homeless mentally ill individuals in a longitudinal process through which they can take on more of the responsibility of managing their own illnesses, symptoms, discomfort, or stress could be another promising avenue for rehabilitation. Already, data suggest that chronically disabled schizophrenic individuals can learn to self-manage their medication and symptoms (Eckman et al. 1990; Wirshing et al. 1990) with the help of a rehabilitation technology that employs video-assisted training modules. Just as people who have diabetes learn to monitor their own blood and urine sugar and people with hypertension are taught to take their blood pressures, the homeless mentally ill could be engaged in a learning process aimed at helping them identify their warning signs of relapse and work collaboratively with their physicians and other caregivers in titrating their medications.

The availability of antipsychotic medication that can be administered intermittently at the minimal effective dose may also provide a means of engaging otherwise resistant persons with schizophrenia and bipolar disorder in time-limited "experiments" to accept medication while evaluating its effects on symptoms and functioning. Homeless mentally ill persons should be taught the knowledge and skills necessary to manage the benefits and side effects of their medication. Such education would make possible a true partnership between patient and clinician in managing pharmacotherapy that could yield improved compliance and reduced relapses.

Through these and similar efforts, we may begin to alleviate the suffering caused by homelessness and begin to rehabilitate individuals who are both homeless and mentally ill. However, these goals will be accomplished only if we are able to change our clinical practice and our systems of care to address needs in a continuous, comprehensive manner that attend to the many and diverse needs of the homeless mentally ill.

References

Anthony WA, Liberman RP: The practice of psychiatric rehabilitation: historical, conceptual, and research base. Schizophr Bull 12:542–559, 1986

Beard JH, Propst RN, Malamud TJ: The Fountainhouse model of psychiatric rehabilitation. Psychosocial Rehabilitation Journal 5:47–53, 1982

Bond GR: Vocational rehabilitation for persons with severe mental illness, in Handbook of Psychiatric Rehabilitation. Edited by Liberman RP. Elmsford, NY, Pergamon, 1991

Eckman TA, Liberman RP, Blair K, et al: Teaching medication management skills to schizophrenic patients. J Clin Psychopharmacol 10:33–38, 1990

Farkas MD, Anthony WA (eds): Psychiatric Rehabilitation Programs. Baltimore, MD, Johns Hopkins University Press, 1989

Jacobs HE: The Job Finding Module, 1991. [Available from Psychiatric Rehabilitation Consultants, Camarillo-UCLA Research Center, Box 6022, Camarillo, CA 93011]

Jacobs HE, Kardashian S, Kreinbring RK, et al: A skills-oriented model for facilitating employment among psychiatrically disabled persons. Rehabilitation Counseling Bulletin 28:87–96, 1984

Koegel P, Burnam MA: Alcoholism among homeless adults in the inner city of Los Angeles. Arch Gen Psychiatry 45:1011–1018, 1988

Koegel P, Burnam MA, Farr RK: The prevalence of specific psychiatric disorders among homeless individuals in the inner city of Los Angeles. Arch Gen Psychiatry 45:1085–1092, 1988

Liberman RP: Psychiatric Rehabilitation of the Chronically Mentally Ill. Washington, DC, American Psychiatric Press, 1988

Liberman RP (ed): Handbook of Psychiatric Rehabilitation. Elmsford, NY, Pergamon, 1991

Liberman RP, Eckman TA: Dissemination of skills training modules to psychiatric facilities. Br J Psychiatry 155(suppl):117–122, 1989

Liberman RP, DeRisi WJ, Mueser KT: Social Skills Training for Psychiatric Patients. Elmsford, NY, Pergamon, 1989

Schwitzgebel R: Street Corner Research. Cambridge, MA, Harvard University Press, 1966

Wirshing WC, Eckman T, Liberman RP, et al: Management of risk of relapse through skills training of chronic schizophrenics, in Current Research on Schizophrenia. Edited by Tamminga C, Schulz SC. New York, Raven, 1990

Appendix

Recommendations of the first American Psychiatric Association Task Force on the Homeless Mentally Ill

Major Recommendation

To address the problems of the homeless mentally ill in America, a comprehensive and integrated system of care for this vulnerable population of the mentally ill, with designated responsibility, with accountability, and with adequate fiscal resources, must be established.

Derivative Recommendations

1. *Any attempt to address the problems of the homeless mentally ill must begin with provisions for meeting their basic needs: food, shelter, and clothing.* The chronically mentally ill have a *right*, equal to that of other groups, to these needs being met.

2. *An adequate number and ample range of graded, stepwise, supervised community housing settings must be established.* While many of the homeless may benefit from temporary housing such as shelters, and some small portion of the severely and chronically mentally ill can graduate to independent living, for the vast majority neither shelters nor mainstream low-cost housing are appropriate. Most housing settings that require people to manage by themselves are beyond the capabilities of the chronically mentally ill. Instead, there must be settings offering different levels of supervision, both more and less intensive, including

Reprinted from Talbott JA, Lamb HR: Summary and recommendations, in The Homeless Mentally Ill: A Task Force Report of the American Psychiatric Association. Edited by Lamb HR. Washington, DC, American Psychiatric Association, 1984.

quarterway and halfway house, lodges and camps, board-and-care homes, satellite housing, foster or family care, and crisis or temporary hostels.

3. *Adequate, comprehensive, and accessible psychiatric and rehabilitative services must be available and must be assertively provided through outreach services when necessary.* First, there must be an adequate number of direct psychiatric services, both on the streets and in the shelters, when appropriate, that provide (a) outreach contact with the mentally ill in the community, (b) psychiatric assessment and evaluation, (c) crisis intervention, including hospitalization, (d) individualized treatment plans, (e) psychotropic medication and other somatic therapies, and (f) psychosocial treatment.

Second, there must be an adequate number of rehabilitative services, providing socialization experiences, training in the skills of everyday living, and social rehabilitation. Third, both treatment and rehabilitative services must be provided assertively—for instance, by going out to patients' living settings if they do not or cannot come to a centralized program. And fourth, the difficulty of working with some of these patients must not be underestimated.

4. *General medical assessment and care must be available.* Since we know that the chronically mentally ill have three times the morbidity and mortality of their counterparts of the same age in the general population, and the homeless even higher rates, the ready availability of general medical care is essential and critical.

5. *Crisis services must be available and accessible to both the chronically mentally ill homeless and the chronically mentally ill in general.* Too often, the homeless mentally ill who are in crisis are ignored because they are presumed, as part of the larger homeless population, to reject all conventional forms of help. Even more inappropriately, they may be put into inpatient hospital units when rapid, specific interventions such as medication or crisis housing would be more effective and less costly. Others, in need of acute hospitalization, are denied it because of restrictive admission criteria or commitment laws. In any case, it will be difficult to provide adequate crisis services to the homeless mentally ill until they are conceptualized and treated separately from the large numbers of other homeless persons.

6. *A system of responsibility for the chronically mentally ill living in the community must be established, with the goal of ensuring that ultimately each patient has one person responsible for his or her care.* Clearly the shift of psychiatric care from institutional to community settings does not in any way eliminate the need to continue the provision of comprehensive services to mentally ill persons. As a result, society must declare a public policy of responsibility for the mentally ill who are unable to meet

their own needs; governments must designate programs in each region or locale as core agencies responsible and accountable for the care of the chronically mentally ill living there; and the staff of these agencies must be assigned individual patients for whom they are responsible. The ultimate goal must be to ensure that each chronically mentally ill person in this country has one person—such as a case manager or resource manager—who is responsible for his or her treatment and care.

For the more than 50% of the chronically ill population living at home or for those with positive ongoing relationships with their families, programs and respite care must be provided to enhance the family's ability to provide a support system. Where the use of family systems is not feasible, the patient must be linked up with a formal community support system. In any case, the entire burden of deinstitutionalization must not be allowed to fall upon families.

7. *Basic changes must be made in legal and administrative procedures to ensure continuing community care for the chronically mentally ill.* In the 1960s and 1970s more stringent commitment laws and patients' rights advocacy remedied some egregious abuses in public hospital care, but at the same time these changes neglected patients' right to high-quality, comprehensive outpatient care as well as the rights of families and society. New laws and procedures must be developed to ensure provision of psychiatric care in the community—that is, to guarantee a right to treatment in the community.

It must become easier to obtain conservatorship status for outpatients who are so gravely disabled and/or have such impaired judgment that they cannot care for themselves in the community without legally sanctioned supervision. Involuntary commitment laws must be made more humane to permit prompt return to active inpatient treatment for patients when acute exacerbations of their illnesses make their lives in the community chaotic and unbearable. Involuntary treatment laws should be revised to allow the option of outpatient civil commitment; in states that already have provisions for such treatment, that mechanism should be more widely used. Finally, advocacy efforts should be focused on the availability of competent care in the community.

8. *A system of coordination among funding sources and implementation agencies must be established.* Because the problems of the mentally ill homeless must be addressed by multiple public and private authorities, coordination, so lacking in the deinstitutionalization process, must become a primary goal. The ultimate objective must be a true system of care rather than a loose network of services, and an ease of communication among different types of agencies (e.g., psychiatric, social, vocational, and housing) as well as up and down the governmental ladder,

from local through federal. One characteristic of a genuine system is the ability to flexibly alter roles, responsibilities, and programs as specific service needs change, and we must strive for this ultimate end.

9. *An adequate number of professionals and paraprofessionals must be trained for community care of the chronically ill.* Among the additional specially trained workers needed, four groups are particularly important for this population: (a) psychiatrists who are skilled in, and interested in, working with the chronically mentally ill; (b) outreach workers who can engage the homeless mentally ill on the streets; (c) case managers, preferably with sufficient training to provide therapeutic interventions themselves; and (d) conservators, to act for patients too disabled to make clinically and economically sound decisions.

10. *General social services must be provided.* Besides the need for specialized social services such as socialization experiences and training in the skills of everyday living (referred to in recommendation 3), there is also a pressing need for generic social services. Such services include escort services to agencies and potential residential placements, help with applications to entitlement programs, and assistance in mobilizing the resources of the family.

11. *Ongoing asylum and sanctuary should be available for that small proportion of the chronically mentally ill who do not respond to current methods of treatment and rehabilitation.* Some patients, even with high-quality treatment and rehabilitation efforts, remain dangerous or gravely disabled. For these patients, there is a pressing need for ongoing asylum in long-term settings, whether in hospitals or in facilities such as California's locked skilled-nursing facilities with special programs for the mentally ill.

12. *Research into the causes and treatment of both chronic mental illness and homelessness needs to be expanded.* While our knowledge has greatly advanced in recent years, it is still limited. Treatment of chronic mental illness remains largely palliative, and definitive treatment will occur only with an adequate understanding of etiologic processes. In addition, our understanding of differential therapeutics—that is, what treatment works for which patients in what settings—is in its infancy and requires increased resources and attention.

13. *More accurate epidemiological data need to be gathered and analyzed.* Currently the research findings of incidence of mental illness among homeless groups are highly variable, ranging up to 91%; these differences depend largely on such methodological issues as where the sample is taken, whether standardized scales or comparable criteria of illness are used, and theoretical biases. Better data, using recognized diagnostic criteria, need to be acquired.

14. *Finally, additional monies must be expended for longer-term solutions*

for the homeless mentally ill. Adequate new monies must be found to finance the system of care we envision, which incorporates supervised living arrangements, assertive case management, and an array of other services. In addition, financial support from existing entitlement programs such as Supplemental Security Income and Medicaid must be ensured.

In summary, the solutions to the problems of the mentally ill homeless are as manifold as the problems they seek to remedy. However, only with comprehensive short and long-term solutions will the plight of this most neglected population in America be addressed.

Index

Note: Page numbers in boldface type refer to figures and tables.